M000040562

THE TRANSMISSION OF DEPRESSION IN FAMILIES AND CHILDREN

THE TRANSMISSION OF DEPRESSION IN FAMILIES AND CHILDREN

ASSESSMENT AND INTERVENTION

Edited by
G. PIROOZ SHOLEVAR, M.D.
with
LINDA SCHWOERI, M.A., M.F.T.

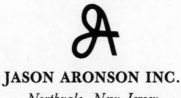

JASON ARONSON INC.
Northvale, New Jersey
London

Chapter 2 has been reprinted by permission of Gabor I. Keitner, M.D.

This book was set in 11 point Baskerville by Lind Graphics of Upper Saddle River, New Jersey, and printed and bound by Haddon Craftsmen of Scranton, Pennsylvania.

Library of Congress Cataloging-in-Publication Data

The transmission of depression in families and children : assessment and intervention / edited by G. Pirooz Sholevar.
    p. cm.
  Includes bibliographical references and index.
  ISBN 1-56821-088-4
   1. Depression in children. 2. Depression in adolescence.
3. Depressed persons—Family relationships. 4. Children of
depressed persons. 5. Family—Mental health. 6. Parent-Child
Relations. I. Sholevar, G. Pirooz.
  [DNLM: 1. Depression—diagnosis. 2. Depression—therapy.
3. Crisis Intervention. WM 171 D42317 1994]
RJ506.D4D464 1994
618.92'8527—dc20
DNLM/DLC
for Library of Congress   93-24688

Manufactured in the United States of America. Jason Aronson Inc. offers books and cassettes. For information and catalog write to Jason Aronson Inc., 230 Livingston Street, Northvale, New Jersey 07647.

CONTENTS

To
The Faculty and Medical Students
Robert Wood Johnson Medical School at Camden
University of Medicine and Dentistry of New Jersey

CONTRIBUTORS

WILLIAM BEARDSLEE, M.D.
Associate Professor of Psychiatry
Judge Baker Children's Center
Harvard Medical School
Department of Psychiatry
Cambridge, MA

JULES BEMPORAD, M.D.
Professor of Clinical Psychiatry
Cornell University
Director of Education
New York Hospital
Westchester, NY

ANTHONY J. COSTELLO, M.D.
Professor of Psychiatry
University of Massachusetts
Medical Director
Stoney Brook Counseling Center
Chelmsford, MA

JAMES COYNE, PH.D.
Professor of Psychology
Department of Psychiatry and Family Practice
University of Michigan Medical School
Ann Arbor, MI

GERALDINE DOWNEY, PH.D.
Assistant Professor of Psychology
Columbia University
New York, NY

RICHARD A. GARDNER, M.D.
Clinical Professor of Child Psychiatry
Columbia University
College of Physicians and Surgeons
New York, NY

GABOR I. KEITNER, M.D.
Professor of Psychiatry and Human Behavior
Brown University
Associate Medical Director for Inpatient Services
Butler Hospital
Providence, RI

IVAN W. MILLER, PH.D.
Associate Professor of Psychiatry and Human Behavior
Brown University
Director of Psychology and Research
Butler Hospital
Providence, RI

LINDA SCHWOERI, M.A., M.F.T.
Assistant Director, Division of Ambulatory Care and Faculty
Department of Psychiatry
Cooper Hospital/University Medical Center
Robert Wood Johnson Medical School
University of Medicine and Dentistry of NJ
Camden, NJ

G. PIROOZ SHOLEVAR, M.D.
Professor and Chairman
Department of Psychiatry
Cooper Hospital/University Medical Center
Robert Wood Johnson Medical School
University of Medicine and Dentistry of NJ
Camden, NJ

JOHN O. VIESSELMAN, M.D.
Medical Director
Pacific Shores Hospital
Oxnard, CA

ELIZABETH B. WELLER, M.D.
Professor of Psychiatry and Pediatrics
Director, Division of Child and Adolescent Psychiatry
The Ohio State University
Columbus, OH

RONALD A. WELLER, M.D.
Professor of Psychiatry
Director of Education and Training
Department of Psychiatry
The Ohio State University
Columbus, OH

SHAHNOUR YAYLAYAN, M.D.
Assistant Unit Director-Children's Unit
Kingwood Hospital
Michigan City, IN

JACQUELYN MILLER ZAVODNICK, M.D.
Faculty
Department of Psychiatry
Cooper Hospital/University Medical Center
Robert Wood Johnson Medical School
University of Medicine and Dentistry of NJ
Camden, NJ

OVERVIEW AND ETIOLOGY
Section I

1: INTRODUCTION

G. Pirooz Sholevar, M.D.

The publication of this volume is timely due to a number of factors. It has been established that depression is a prevalent condition, particularly among women of child-bearing age. The rate of depression and other types of childhood psychopathology is extremely high in the children of depressed parents, particularly depressed mothers. Once the depression is established in childhood or adulthood, the likelihood of its recurrence is very high, and it promises to be a periodic but lifelong disability. The present investigations suggest that an interactive process plays a fundamental role in the production of depression. The biological, psychological, and interpersonal processes are probably linked on many levels and are mutually provocative and complementary toward each other. The delineation of the vulnerabilities in the above areas is a highly desirable task for the present and the future. The collaboration of the investigator in the above three areas would be enhanced by adherence to a comprehensive model that can accommodate multiple sets of data.

The work of Patterson and his colleagues, described in Chapter 7, serves as an inspiring model for delineation of the underlying processes that produce apparently divergent behavioral pictures. The model proposed in this book is an expansion of well-accepted models in the field of mental health sciences, namely the biopsychosocial model of human behavior described initially by Adolf Meyer (1948–1952) and elaborated eloquently by George Engel (1977, 1980). An expansion of this model allows us to recognize infants and children genetically vulnerable to depression, the behavioral correlates of genetic vulnerability, and the role of stressful environmental events in precipitating a depressive disorder. The measurement of the level of stress sufficient for precipitating clinical depression in individuals with varying degrees of vulnerability is a challenging task. Delineation of the role of medication, psychological measures, and interpersonal interventions in reduction of environmental stress is a worthwhile and necessary goal. This paradigm underlines the importance of the diathesis-stress theory of Rosenthal (1970) and Zubin and Spring (1977), which has proved particularly helpful in the investigation of the role of high expressed emotion (EE) in the relapse of schizophrenic and depressed patients and the role of psychological and pharmacological measures in the reduction of this stress.

Section I provides an overview on depression in families and children as well as chapters on epidemiology, psychological factors, and the interrelatedness of aggression and depression in families. In Chapter 2, Keitner and Miller review the evidence supporting the concept that the family plays a major role in the development and course of major depression. The family pathology evident during an acute depressive episode continues after the patient's remission; the course of depressive illness, relapse rates, and suicidal behavior are all affected by family functioning; and children of depressed parents are at high risk for psychopathology. The authors conclude that there is evidence to support family and marital interventions, particularly in the treatment of depressed women.

In Chapter 3, Coyne, Schwoeri, and Downey examine the role of interpersonal and social stresses in the production of depression in a biologically vulnerable person. They specifically look at the marital and family relationships as risks as well as protective factors for depression. They describe the low affective involvement and poor problem solving in families of depressed patients as well as the high level of psychological disorders in the spouse and children of depressed patients.

In Chapter 4, Viesselman, Weller, and Weller describe the phenomenology of childhood depression, its diagnostic criteria according to *DSM-III-R*, the high level of psychopathology in the parents, and the natural course of the illness. The relationship between suicidal behavior and depression in youth is described.

In Chapter 5, Costello describes the epidemiology of depression in adulthood, childhood, and adolescence as well as the ratio of untreated or undertreated depressed patients to treated ones. The high prevalence of depression in child-rearing women and undetected and untreated depression contribute to the perpetuation and transmission of depression in families.

In Chapter 6, Schwoeri and Sholevar review the studies on transmission of depression from parents to children. They describe the alarmingly high rate of psychopathology including depression in children of depressed parents.

In Chapter 7, Schwoeri and Sholevar summarize the recent investigative findings of Patterson and Forgatch on the relationship of maternal depression and conduct disorders in children. They describe the impact of maternal depression and recent marital separation on parental management practices, resulting in unmanageable conduct problems in children.

In Chapter 8, Yaylayan, Weller, and Zavodnick summarize the neurochemical studies in childhood depression and the possible role of neurotransmitters such as norepinephrine and serotonin. Hormonal and polysomnographic studies and the role of the dexamethasone suppression test (DST) in the diagnosis of depression are also included in this chapter.

Section II describes multiple family, individual, and psychopharmacological therapeutic interventions with depression in children and families as well as preventive intervention with children of depressed parents. In Chapter 9, Coyne, Schwoeri, and Sholevar describe the general and specific strategies for therapeutic intervention with families, couples, and individuals in depressed families. The parenting of children is the special focus of the family-based interventions.

In Chapter 10, Gardner applies his gift for psychodynamic understanding of children and adolescents to provide for an understanding and management of depression and suicide in this group.

In Chapter 11, Bemporad, Sholevar, and Schwoeri look at different manifestations of depression in different developmental stages and provide a comprehensive guideline for recognition and treatment. The model is equally applicable to children, adolescents, and adults.

In Chapter 12, Viesselman, Weller, Weller, and Yaylayan review the latest clinical research and findings on the use of antidepressants with children and adolescents.

In Chapter 13, Beardslee and Schwoeri describe the rationale and methodology of a psychoeducationally based prevention program with children of depressed parents that has proven quite promising in its initial application.

In Chapter 14, Sholevar discusses the future course of the investigation of depression in families and endorses an adherence to a comprehensive model for investigation of the interaction between the interpersonal, psychological, and biological factors in depression.

It is hoped that this book is a facilitating step toward the creation of a refined model for assessment, diagnosis, and treatment of multiple aspects of depression.

REFERENCES

Engel, G. (1977). The need for a new medical model: a challenge for biomedicine science. *American Journal of Psychiatry* 196:129–136.

––––– (1980). The clinical application of the biopsychosocial model. *American Journal of Psychiatry* 137:535–544.

Meyer, A. (1948–1952). *Collected Papers of Adolf Meyer*. Vols. 1–4. Baltimore: Johns Hopkins University Press.

Rosenthal, D. (1970). *Genetic Theory and Abnormal Behavior*. New York: Brunner/Mazel.

Zubin, J., and Spring, B. J. (1977) Vulnerability: a new view of schizophrenia. *Journal of Abnormality* 486:103–126.

2: FAMILY FUNCTIONING AND MAJOR DEPRESSION

Gabor I. Keitner, M.D.
Ivan W. Miller, Ph.D.

INTRODUCTION

The importance of the role of the family in the development and course of major psychiatric illness has become increasingly recognized over the past 10 years. Patients with major psychiatric illnesses are spending more time with their families because of shorter hospital stays for acute episodes and deinstitutionalization policies that have forced these patients to rely more heavily on available family members. At the same time, despite the dramatic promises of pharmacotherapy, a substantial number of patients either fail to respond to pharmacotherapy or have residual symptoms requiring additional psychosocial care (Keller et al. 1982, 1984).

The earlier focus on the families of patients with schizophrenia has now shifted to include interest in what happens to the families of patients with major depression and how aspects of the family life of depressed patients may, in turn, affect the depressive illness itself. Sufficient empirical work has been done to warrant an overview of this new and increasingly important domain.

This chapter summarizes what is known about the impact of depression on families during an acute depressive episode, how family functioning changes as the depressive episode remits, and what factors in the family environment of depressed patients contribute to recovery, relapse, and suicidal behavior. We review the impact of major depression on parenting as well as the effect that major depression has on the children of depressed parents. We also review the evidence for the effectiveness of family treatments for patients with major depression. Finally, we identify several unresolved issues that may shed more light on the factors involved in these interactions and guide future directions in research. Our emphasis is on methodologically sound studies that have assessed patients with major depression.

FAMILY FUNCTIONING DURING AN ACUTE DEPRESSIVE EPISODE

One of the problems in studying the relationship between family processes and a relapsing and remitting illness is that both the family and the illness are changing over time. It is critical, therefore, to establish time frames when the relationship can be examined, both to obtain a clearer perspective on issues of causality and to allow for legitimate comparisons with other studies. The two most logical time frames for such studies are during an acute episode and at the time of remission of symptoms.

There are now many studies documenting the impact that depression has on the families of depressed patients during an acute depressive episode. Two studies reported more than 15 years ago (Hinchcliffe et al. 1975, Weissman and Paykel 1974) have paved the way. Weissman and Paykel (1974) studied the impact of the depression of forty moderately to severely depressed female out-patients on their families. They found that these depressed women were more reticent in their communications, were more submissive and dependent, were less affectionate toward their spouses, experi-enced more friction, and argued more frequently with their hus-bands than did nondepressed control subjects. These women also experienced more friction with their children and were reluctant to discuss personal feelings.

Hinchcliffe and colleagues (1975) used direct observational assessment techniques to assess twenty depressed psychiatric inpa-tients and their spouses during acute depressive episodes. Couples including the depressed patients had greater levels of negative hostile behavior, more self-preoccupation, more negative tension (tense, stuttering, and emotionally tinged speech), and more attempts at controlling other people than did couples including nondepressed surgical control subjects.

More recent studies using varied patient groups and assessment procedures have also found that families of depressed patients experience substantial problems during the most active phase of the illness. These disturbances are evident over a wide range of family functions. A unique study of twenty-seven depressed female outpatients observed in their homes while interacting with their families found that these women displayed less problem-solving behavior than their husbands and were less self-disclosing in their families than nondepressed women (Biglan et al. 1985). These depressed women and their families appeared to be locked into an interacting style that promoted high rates of aversive interchanges among family members (Hops et al. 1987).

Marital difficulties in depressed women were also identified in a study comparing family relationships in fifty depressed women and forty nondepressed women from working-class families (Birchnell 1988). The marriages of the depressed women were significantly worse than those of the control subjects, particularly because of the depressed wives' greater need for both intimacy and support.

Our research group (Keitner et al. 1986) found that forty-three depressed inpatients and their families reported significantly more dysfunction than did twenty-nine nonpsychiatric control families, particularly in the area of family communications and problem solving. Sixty-four percent of the families of depressed patients felt that their overall functioning was impaired (Keitner et al. 1987a).

It is not surprising that during the acute phase of an illness the patient's family is upset and feels more strain than normal or control families. However, a number of studies suggest that depressive illness is associated with more family distress and impairment than are other psychiatric illnesses and some medical conditions. In our studies, the families of patients with major depression consistently showed more impaired family functioning than families of patients with alcohol dependence, adjustment disorders, schizophrenia, or bipolar disorder (Miller et al. 1986). A similar finding was reported by Crowther (1985), who compared family functioning in twenty-seven inpatients with major depression with family functioning in patients with schizophrenia, bipolar disorder, anxiety disorder, and alcohol abuse. Crowther noted that depressed patients reported significantly more marital maladjustment and desired significantly more changes in their marriages than did the other psychiatric inpatients, with findings confirmed by the patients' therapists. A comparison with other chronically remitting and relapsing illnesses is also informative. Bouras, Vanger, and Bridges (1986) found that depression had a much greater impact on the marital life of depressed outpatients from the patients' and the spouses' points of view than did rheumatoid arthritis or cardiac illness.

The presence of a depressed family member has a major impact on other family members. Increased attention is being given to the difficulties experienced by family members who cope with a depressed relative on a daily basis. Coyne and colleagues (1987) noted that over 40 percent of adults living with a patient experiencing a depressive episode were distressed themselves to the point of meeting criteria for therapeutic intervention. Family members found the patient's lack of interest in social life, fatigue, feelings of hopelessness, and constant worrying to be the aspects most disturbing for them. The burden on family members was felt most substantially during the acute episode. Fadden and associates (1987) found that the negative effects rather than the florid symptoms of mental illness were the most problematic for family members, who resisted attributing the patients' worrying, social withdrawal, irritability, and nagging to the mental illness itself.

In summary, studies using various methodologies and fairly diverse groups of patients have consistently shown that during an acute episode the families of patients with major depression experience substantial difficulties in many areas of their family life. Communications in the family are particularly problematic, especially appropriate self-disclosure by the depressed patient. Depressed women tend to be aversive to others and exhibit impaired parenting; the families as a whole experience difficulties in their ability to solve problems. Overall, the families of depressed patients appear to experience more difficulties than do families of patients with rheumatoid arthritis or cardiac disease.

FAMILY FUNCTIONING AT REMISSION

The finding of family disturbances during acute depressive episodes leads to the following questions: Do the difficulties reported during an acute episode reflect the family's response to the patient's depression or do they represent a more chronic pattern of family dysfunction? More specifically, does family functioning change after recovery from the acute episode? If so, does family functioning return to a normal level after the acute episode has been resolved?

Studies of depressed outpatients (Dobson 1987, Goering et al. 1983) as well as inpatients (Hinchcliffe, Vaughn and Hooper 1977, Keitner et al. 1987a, Merikangas et al. 1985, Rounsaville et al. 1980) have shown that family functioning improves as depression remits, although the families still experience more dysfunction than nonclinical families. They still report significantly poorer functioning than control families, particularly in their ability to solve problems, to communicate with each other, and to feel generally satisfied with their overall functioning (Keitner et al. 1987a).

In general, there is striking consistency in the findings of studies that have examined changes in family functioning as a depressive illness remits. Even as depressive symptoms decrease and family functioning improves over time, these families continue to experience more problems than nonclinical families. It seems evident that continued work with and support for these families are warranted even after the depressive episode has subsided. It is still not clear, however, as to what extent the ongoing problems in these families are a function of the depressive illness itself rather than other factors.

FAMILY FUNCTIONING AND THE COURSE OF DEPRESSIVE ILLNESS

A further question concerns the relationship of family functioning to the course of depressive illness. Is family functioning associated with recovery rates? More specifically, are patients with poor family functioning during the acute phase of the illness more likely to have a slow rate of recovery? Does change in the quality of family life have any bearing on the course of depressive illness? Only four studies (Corney 1987, Keitner et al. 1987a, Rounsaville et al. 1979, Swindle et al. 1989) have addressed this issue.

Rounsaville, Weissman, and Prusoff (1979) reported that for depressed female outpatients a reduction in the number of marital disputes was associated with improved depressive symptoms and social functioning after 8 months of individual psychotherapy.

From a different perspective, Corney (1987) noted that women who had major marital problems were more likely to be depressed at follow-up than those with good relationships, and that women with no or minor marital problems improved more quickly than those with marital difficulties.

We found that among depressed inpatients who had recovered, those patients with families who improved in their general functioning had a significantly shorter time to recovery (4.1 months) than patients of families who did not improve (8.1 months) (Keitner et al. 1987a). Also, patients in families that improved in their communication, roles, and affective involvement showed nonsignificant trends toward having a shorter recovery time. Therefore, although family functioning during an acute episode was not associated with speed of recovery among recovered patients, positive changes in overall family functioning during the course of illness were associated with faster recovery times.

Swindle and colleagues (1989) assessed the effects of psychosocial factors on the course of unipolar depression in a large group of outpatients and inpatients ($N = 352$). Assessments were made during an acute episode and at 1-year and 4-year follow-ups. Swindle and colleagues concluded that a concurrent medical condition in the patient and family conflict at the index episode consistently predicted poorer long-term outcome for the depression.

Despite the very limited number of studies that have investigated the relationship between family functioning and recovery from depression, the available data suggest that problematic family functioning is associated with lower rates of recovery and slower recovery among patients who do recover. However, it is not possible to distinguish whether this association between family functioning and recovery occurs because impaired family functioning affects the patient's depression or because a chronic course of depression produces greater family impairment.

Relapse

Another critical question is whether the quality or type of family functioning is associated with relapse, that is, are patients in certain family environments more likely to have higher or lower rates of relapse? Two studies (Hooley et al. 1986, Vaughn and Leff 1976b) have investigated this issue.

Vaughn and Leff (1976a) reported that depressed patients whose family members had high levels of expressed emotion — critical, hostile, or emotionally overinvolved attitudes expressed by key relatives in reference to the depressed patient — were three times as likely to relapse within 9 months as were patients whose relatives had low levels of expressed emotion. Similar results were found in a replication study by Hooley and colleagues (1986). Over a 9-month follow-up period, Hooley and colleagues found that 59 percent of the patients whose spouses had high levels of expressed emotion relapsed, but that no patients living with spouses with low levels of expressed emotion did so. Furthermore, depressed patients tended to relapse at lower levels of criticism than did schizophrenic patients. Interestingly, of the nine patients in homes with high levels of expressed emotion who did not relapse, seven were men.

Expressed emotion is time-consuming to measure. In an attempt to find related but more easily assessed relationship variables that may predict relapse in depressed patients, Hooley and Teasdale (1989) examined the predictive utility of two other family measures — marital distress and perceived criticism — in the same group of patients used to study expressed emotion (Hooley et al. 1986). Marital satisfaction was measured by using the Dyadic Adjustment Scale (DAT; Spanier 1976). Perceived criticism was assessed on a 10-point Lykert-type scale in response to the question "How critical is your spouse of you?" Although all three family variables were significantly associated with 9-month relapse rates, the single best predictor of relapse was the patients' views of their spouses' criticalness. These results strongly suggest that a simple way to identify depressed patients at high risk for relapse is to ask them how critical they feel their relatives are toward them.

It is becoming increasingly apparent that a supportive, nonstressful social environment is important in sustaining remissions. Provoking factors like stressful life events are associated with a higher risk of relapse, especially in the presence of long-term vulnerability factors such as lack of supportive social networks (Brown and Prudo 1981) and even independent of frequency of depressive symptoms (Goering et al. 1983). Although conflict in the family is associated with relapse, an open, supportive discussion of feelings and problems in the family may predict lower rates of rehospitalization (Goldberg and Mudd 1968).

Again, despite the limited number of studies, the available data suggest that the family environment in which depression evolves does have a substantial relationship to the likelihood of recurrence of a depressive episode. A stressful, an unsupportive, or, particularly, a critical social environment has been found consistently to be associated with a higher rate of relapse. However, as with the relationship between family functioning and recovery, it is impossible to separate cause from effect in these studies.

SUICIDE AND FAMILY FUNCTIONING

Studies focusing on familial factors in suicidal behavior have tended to explore genetic associations, loss of family members, and nonspecific family stresses (Aldridge 1984, Richman 1978). Very few studies have attempted to assess the intrafamilial environment within which suicidal behavior emerges.

Our research group found that depressed inpatients who attempted suicide perceived their family functioning to be worse than did their families (Keitner et al. 1987b). Suicidal patients also viewed their families more negatively than did depressed nonsuicidal inpatients, who actually viewed their family functioning more positively than did their family members (Keitner et al. 1987b).

In a 2-year follow-up study (Keitner et al. 1990), we attempted to delineate which psychosocial factors were related to subsequent suicide attempts in depressed patients. We found that previous suicide attempts, interepisodic adjustment, changes in family constellation, and a negative perception of family functioning were characteristic of depressed patients with recurrent suicide attempts.

Although suicide attempts are certainly multidetermined acts, family functioning may be one of the important influences that helps to explain why a minority of depressed patients attempt suicide, whereas the majority do not.

CHILDREN AND PARENTING

The repeated findings of impaired family functioning in patients with major depression raise additional questions. What happens to the children of depressed parents? How is their upbringing affected by the patient's depression? Is the greater risk of psychopathology in these children a function of their parents' specific illness, or is it a nonspecific effect of distress in the family?

A number of review articles (Beardslee et al. 1983, Forehand et al. 1987, Orvaschel et al. 1980) have concluded that (1) depressed parents have impaired relationships with their children, (2) these impairments are greater in the families of depressed patients than they are in the families of nonclinical subjects, (3) there is a negative relationship between a parent's depressive mood and a child's functioning, and (4) the homes of depressed children are characterized by family discord and parental rejection.

An increasing number of controlled studies have looked at the issue of the impact of parental affective disorder on children. The results of these studies (Billings and Moos 1983, Gordon et al. 1989, Hammen et al. 1987, Lee and Gotlib 1989, Radke-Yarrow et al. 1985, Susman et al. 1985, Weissman et al. 1987) have been very consistent with previous findings of the negative impact of parental depression on children. Rates of major depression in the children of parents with affective disorder range from 23 percent to 38 percent, in contrast to ranges of 11–24 percent in control families; rates of any *DSM-III* diagnoses in children of depressed parents range from 65 percent to 73 percent, as opposed to 52–65 percent in control families (Keller et al. 1986, Merikangas et al. 1988). In addition, it has been noted (Weissman et al. 1987) that children of depressed parents have a younger age at onset of depression (12–13 years) than do children of normal parents (16–17 years).

It is not clear to what extent a child's psychopathology is a function of the parent's depressive illness or of the presence of any psychiatric or medical disorder (Hammen et al. 1987, Radke-Yarrow et al. 1985, Susman et al. 1985). Generally, psychiatric illness appears to create a greater burden than do nonpsychiatric illnesses (Lee and Gotlib 1989), but this may not be specific to depression. The severity and chronicity of the parent's illness also have substantial effects on the child's psychopathology and functioning (Hammen et al. 1987, Keller et al. 1986).

From a different perspective, depressed women complain of difficulties in coping with unruly and disobedient behavior in their children (Birchnell 1988). They also report high levels of inconsistency in discipline and control and tend to be highly protective of their children (Susman et al. 1985). It may be that a positive family environment (low levels of stress and high levels of support) is associated with lower rates of disturbance in children (Susman et al. 1985). However, even children in families where the parent's depression is remitted still function more poorly than do children in nonclinical control families (Billings and Moos 1985).

Overall, the findings of these studies are consistent in highlighting the substantial impact that major depression in a parent has on the functioning of children in these families. These children appear to be at much higher risk not only for affective illness but for psychopathology in general.

The cause of the higher rate of psychopathology in children of depressed parents is not clear. Both genetic and psychosocial factors have been hypothesized to be relevant (Blehar et al. 1988, Cadoret et al. 1985). Genetic vulnerability has been most clearly established for severe unipolar depression (McGuffin and Katz 1989). However, no studies have been conducted comparing the relative strength of genetic and psychosocial factors. Similarly, the direct contribution of family environment to child psychopathology has not been investigated. Despite this lack of direct evidence, it seems reasonable to hypothesize that there is an interactive effect among genetic vulnerability, deficient parenting skills, and overall family environment that contributes to the psychopathology in the children of depressed parents. Specific parental diagnosis, severity and chronicity of the affective illness, and the nonspecific stresses and strains brought about by having an ill parent appear to increase the risk.

TREATMENT

Because evidence for the substantial impact that depression has on the families of depressed patients and the role of the social environment on the course of depressive illness has only recently been established, it is not surprising that there are few controlled studies of family interventions with patients suffering from major depression. One of the earliest studies of marital treatment for patients with depression was undertaken by McLean and colleagues (1973). Their purpose was to determine whether a behavioral approach to the treatment of depressed patients and their spouses, with particular emphasis on modification of verbal interactional styles in addition to social learning training using behavioral contracts, would be more effective than standard community treatment. The experimental group receiving the behavioral marital treatment showed a more significant reduction of problematic behaviors, depressive symptoms, and negative actions and reactions than did the comparison group. In another study, using small numbers of patients, Beach and O'Leary (1986) noted that marital therapy showed promise in alleviating both depression and marital discord.

In the first well-controlled study comparing the effectiveness of an antidepressant drug (amitriptyline), marital therapy, and the combination of the two, Friedman (1975) found that the combination of the drug and marital therapy was more effective than either treatment administered separately. Drug therapy was faster and more effective in relieving symptoms and clinically improving the depression, and marital therapy was more effective in improving role task performance and perception of the marital relationship. Importantly, the patient group that received amitriptyline and marital therapy showed more improvement than any of the other three groups (drug plus minimal contact, placebo plus marital therapy, and placebo plus minimal contact).

A randomized clinical trial of family intervention for inpatients with schizophrenia or affective disorders was undertaken by the family research group at the Payne Whitney Clinic (Glick et al. 1985, Haas et al. 1988, Spencer et al. 1988). This study attempted to determine whether the inclusion of a family intervention package added any benefit to standard hospital treatment. The family intervention consisted of six psychoeducational family sessions over a 5-week hospital stay. These sessions were reality oriented and dealt with practical problems. The standard hospital treatment included a diagnostic workup, group therapy, milieu therapy, activity therapies, and pharmacotherapy. Patients were randomly assigned to hospitalization with or without the inpatient family intervention. The family intervention was provided by a social worker on the unit together with the psychology intern or psychiatry resident. Overall, the study found that at discharge from the hospital the inpatient family intervention had a positive effect on female patients with schizophrenia or affective disorders and their families. This positive effect was sustained at 7- and 18-month follow-ups. Surprisingly, not only was there no benefit but there actually was a slight worsening found with the family intervention for male patients.

Marital therapy may be selectively helpful for depressed patients who are involved in problematic relationships. In an unpublished 1987 paper, Jacobson and colleagues reported that patients with marital problems had lower relapse rates when given a treatment package including marital therapy, and that patients without marital problems did not require marital intervention.

Group therapy with the families of patients with major depression has become increasingly popular over the past 5 years. In an attempt to tease out the active ingredients in these large-group formats, Anderson and colleagues (1986) randomly assigned inpatients with affective disorders and their families to either a multiple-family group with a process orientation emphasizing support and self-help or a psychoeducational group emphasizing information about the illness. Both types of groups were found to be useful and desirable for the inpatients; very little difference was found between the two formats. The families of the patients receiving the psychoeducational program, however, were more satisfied with their experience.

In summary, preliminary evidence suggests that adding a family approach to the treatment of major depression may be helpful, especially for depressed female patients who are experiencing marital turmoil. Further research in this area is sorely needed, given the paucity of well-designed studies, the prevalence of the disorder, and the substantial family dysfunction associated with it.

UNRESOLVED ISSUES

It is evident from the literature reviewed that the families of patients with major depression have substantial impairments in family functioning during acute depressive episodes and also during remissions. Several issues remain unresolved and need further clarification, however. Particular issues requiring further study relate to the heterogeneity of depressive families, the congruence among perceptions of different family members, the instruments used to assess family functioning, sex differences in depressive illness, and the causal relationship between family functioning and major depression.

Heterogeneity

Although *DSM-III* has helped to define depressive illness more precisely, major depression most likely consists of a number of different disorders. In addition, the psychopathological problems of patients with major depression and of their families (Epstein et al. 1988) differ clinically. At present, there is little research support for the hypothesis that a particular family constellation or interactional style invariably leads toward or is associated with major depression. Factors such as the premorbid functioning of the family, the developmental stage of the family, the health of other family members (particularly the presence or absence of psychiatric illness), the family's social and financial situation, and the availability of external supports may all bear on the family's level of functioning and capacity to deal with crises, including an affective episode. The issue of assortative mating (Merikangas 1984) may also influence the burden felt by other family members and the support available to the depressed patient.

Nonfamily factors may also have a major impact on a family's response to depressive illness. There is marked heterogeneity in the patients themselves. Notable complicating factors are the finding of concurrent dysthymia and/or personality disorders of various types (Alnaes and Torgensen 1989, Keller and Shapiro 1982). What is the importance of the presence of such coexisting axis II diagnoses (Black et al. 1988, Charney et al. 1981)? Some depressive disorders coexist with a variety of other axis I and axis III disorders as well. This comorbidity has been found to have an additional deleterious effect on family functioning and on recovery rates (Keitner et al. 1989, Swindle et al. 1989). Most of the literature on comorbidity of depression and medical conditions explores the prevalence of depression and its impact on a variety of medical illnesses. Few have focused on the impact of medical illnesses on depression.

Current studies have paid little attention to these issues of heterogeneity. However, in the absence of studies investigating the relationship between family functioning and these other characteristics of depressed patients and their families, it is not clear whether family dysfunction is an independent prognostic factor or is an epiphenomenon strongly associated with other particular features or subgroups of depressed patients. This question has important implications regarding the most appropriate focus of treatment interventions. Studies investigating these issues are clearly needed.

Measurement of Family Functioning

One of the difficulties in reviewing studies of depressed families is that many different instruments are used to assess marital and family satisfaction, adjustment, and functioning. It is beyond the scope of this chapter to review all of these instruments. Some are well validated and psychometrically tested (Epstein et al. 1983, Locke and Wallace 1959, Moos and Moos 1981, Snyder et al. 1981, Vaughn and Leff 1976a). Others were not primarily designed or validated to assess family functioning, although some of their subscales have been used for that purpose (Weissman 1975). Still others were designed for a particular study and do not have much psychometric support (Targum et al. 1981, Waring et al. 1981). The instruments range from questions concerning general satisfaction (Locke and Wallace 1959, Spanier 1976) to schedules assessing multiple aspects of family life (Epstein et al. 1983, Moos and Moos 1981, Olson et al. 1982), Snyder et al. 1981). The relative validity of the results reported is very difficult to assess accurately.

It is unclear whether the same or similar family processes are being measured in these studies and to what extent the findings from the different studies can be merged. It is all the more striking, therefore, to note the remarkable uniformity of findings in different studies using widely disparate measures. Generally, almost all studies agree that families of depressed patients experience substantial disturbances through all of the stages of the illness.

A second problem in the assessment of families is that very few studies have actually attempted to evaluate family functioning using objective measures. Most studies have used the perceptions of family members as a reflection of family functioning. Only a few have attempted to observe and rate these families using trained interviewers (Hinchcliffe et al. 1975, Hooley et al. 1986); fewer still have attempted to observe depressed patients in their own home environments (Biglan et al. 1985, Hops et al. 1987). Without such studies, it is difficult to separate actual family dysfunction from potential negative biases on the part of depressed patients.

Congruence of Perceptions between Patients and Other Family Members

In describing and measuring family functioning, the issue of weighing the varying perspectives of family members creates a difficult methodological problem. Should one describe each family member's perception and give each equal weight? Should this be the same whether there are two family members or six? Should the same weight be given to the perceptions of children as to those of parents or grandparents? There are no easy answers to these questions.

Overall, studies have suggested that there is in fact good congruence between a depressed patient's description of his or her family functioning and that of other family members (Billings and Moos 1985, Merikangas et al. 1985).

For the sake of simplicity, our approach has been to use mean family scores in our preliminary analyses. Discrepancies between the patient's perceptions and those of other family members, however, can be an important indication of particular types of problems. We have found, for instance, that a discrepancy in perception of the family environment between the depressed patient and other family members is strongly associated with suicide attempts (Keitner et al. 1987b).

At this point, we do not know the best way to report family assessment measures. Further research is needed to determine not only how common agreement between family members is but what disagreement implies for the course of the illness, potential for relapse, and other clinical or theoretical issues.

Sex Differences

The suggestion of differences in the responses of male and female patients to depressive illness is of considerable interest. It is well known that the prevalence of depression in women is two to three times higher than it is in men (Boyd and Weissman 1981). Partly because of this disparity, most studies investigating depression and family functioning have focused on female patients. The few that have not have provided mixed results in terms of differential patterns between men and women in response to a depressive episode (Crowther 1985, Hinchcliffe et al. 1977, Hops et al. 1987, Keller et al. 1986, Radke-Yarrow et al. 1985, Spencer et al. 1988).

Overall, marriage appears to be less protective for women than for men (Gove 1972). Married men, for instance, have consistently lower rates of affective disorders than single men, but married women do not have lower rates than single women (Bebbington 1987). The women's role also appears to be more critical than does the man's in terms of the impact of depression on children. A father's depression has no effect on the attachment between his children and their mother (Radke-Yarrow et al. 1985) and has a negligible association with his children's adaptive functioning (Keller et al. 1986). Given the disproportionately important role of women and mothers in families, perhaps it is not surprising that children in families with depressed mothers direct more aversive behavior at the mothers than they do at the fathers (Hops et al. 1987).

Consistent with these findings, depressed men tend to rate their marriages as significantly better adjusted than do depressed women (Crowther 1985). As the depression resolves, depressed men tend to show a greater shift in reducing tension with their partners than do depressed women (Hinchcliffe et al. 1977).

It is interesting to note that family interventions not only may be more successful when the patient is a woman but may actually lead to some worsening with male patients (Spencer et al. 1988). It may be that female patients need greater support in order to maintain their multiple role functions within the family.

The question of sex differences in depression remains unresolved (Gotlib and Whiffen 1989) but certainly deserves further research. Attempts should be made to study more families with a male depressed patient to delineate more clearly what happens in these families and how they differ from those with a female depressed patient. In particular, the suggestion that differential treatment interventions may be indicated depending on the sex of the identified patient needs to be pursued.

Causality

It is not certain whether problematic family relationships predispose to or facilitate the emergence of depressive illness or whether the depressive illness and its attendant impact on patients' interpersonal styles create family difficulties in coping. There is evidence to support both points of view. In addition, the combination of a number of different stressors can obviously have an additive effect in leading to family dysfunction. Rounsaville and colleagues (1980), for instance, suggested that the marriages of depressed women tended to be either good or disturbed over time. They also found that when women who had had disputes with their husbands divorced and remarried, they had disputes with their new husbands as well. Because a number of depressed patients are able to sustain good marriages, the personality of the depressed person rather than the illness itself may be responsible for the marital strain.

The individual characteristics of depressed patients may create problems for family members, rather than the family environment being destructive to the patient (Hops et al. 1987). The patient's level of depression may be less involved in creating family and interpersonal disturbances than factors intrinsic to the situation and the personalities of the family members involved (Krantz and Moos 1987, Menaghan 1985). In fact, there is evidence to suggest that marital distress itself may affect the severity of depression (Birchnell and Kennard 1983). Up to 70 percent of depressed patients reported that their marriages were poor before the onset of depression (Roy 1985, 1987). A variety of factors that are antecedents or sequelae of depression may lead indirectly to depression through their effect on the quality of the marital relationship (Barnett and Gotlib 1988).

In fact, the question of causality may be the wrong question to ask. There is no reason to assume a single linear relationship between depression and family functioning. It seems more likely that a mutually reinforcing negative pattern of interaction between patient vulnerability and family competence may prove a more useful model (see Figure 2–1).

For a variety of reasons, certain patients are vulnerable to developing major depression. Their vulnerability may be genetically based and may be precipitated by a number of factors, such as illnesses, life events, personality variables, and early life experi-

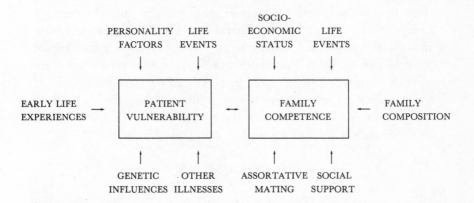

FIGURE 2–1. Depression Model: Interaction between Patient Vulnerability and Family Competence

ences. On the other hand, there is a range of competence within families that is influenced by a variety of factors, including socioeconomic status, family composition, availability of social support, presence or absence of other psychiatric and/or medical illnesses, and current life events. A patient's vulnerability may be readily influenced by family issues and forces at play at a given time. By the same token, a family's competence may be compromised greatly by the illness, particularly an affective illness, of one of its members.

According to this model, then, a patient who is vulnerable to major depression develops a depressive episode. The depressive episode may have been caused by a variety of factors, including family dysfunction. The family is now in the position of having to respond to the patient's illness. If the family is able to respond effectively, the depressive illness may last a relatively short time and may more readily remit. Conversely, if the family is unable to respond adequately to the patient's affective illness because of its own difficulties, there is evidence to suggest that the depressive episode will be prolonged and the patient will be more likely to relapse into subsequent episodes of depression. These subsequent episodes of depression may further impair the family's competence to cope, thereby setting up a vicious cycle. Patient vulnerability and family competence, therefore, can be seen as mutually reinforcing forces that may act either to further the depressive illness or to provide a way of lessening its impact and tendency to recur.

This model not only allows for but in fact calls for interventions that address both the patient's vulnerability and the family's competence. The patient's vulnerability can be diminished with the aid of individual psychotherapy and psychopharmacological agents. The family's competence can be reinforced through the use of family intervention techniques, including psychoeducational groups, family therapy, and self-help support programs. The critical point is that both aspects of the system need to be addressed to deal adequately with this mutually reinforcing pattern.

CONCLUSIONS

What do we know about the relationship between major depression and family functioning? The available evidence supports a number of conclusions. Substantial family dysfunction is a common accompaniment of an acute depressive episode. Even with remission of the depression, family strain often persists. Ongoing family problems, particularly if manifested by excessive criticism of the patient and an unsupportive family environment, are associated with a prolonged course of the depression, a greater tendency to relapse, and possibly a higher risk for suicide. Children of depressed parents are at high risk for both affective and nonaffective psychopathology.

It seems evident that the family system should be understood and worked with when treating a person with major depression. Unfortunately, it is not clear at this time what particular types of family approaches are most appropriate and for which patients. Studies assessing the usefulness of adding family therapy to the pharmacological and individual psychotherapeutic treatment of major depression are needed.

In the meantime, it seems reasonable to develop a heightened awareness of the social context in which affective illness emerges and evolves. There is a danger of losing sight of this broader psychosocial reality with our increasing focus on neurochemical, neurophysiological, and pharmacological issues in the understanding and treatment of depressive illnesses.

REFERENCES

Aldridge, D. (1984). Family interaction and suicidal behavior: a brief review. *Journal of Family Therapy* 6:309–322.

Alnaes, R, and Torgensen, S. (1989). Personality and personality disorders among patients with major depression in combination with dysthymia or cyclothymic disorders. *Acta Psychiatrica Scandinavica* 79:363–369.

Anderson, C. M, Griffin, S., Ross, A., et al. (1986). A comparative study of the impact of education vs process groups for families of patients with affective disorders. *Family Process* 25:185–205.

Barnett, P. A., and Gotlib, I. H. (1988). Psychosocial functioning and depression: distinguishing among antecedents, concomitants, and consequences. *Psychology Bulletin* 104:97–126.

Beach, S. R. H., and O'Leary, K. D. (1986). The treatment of depression occurring in the context of marital discord. *Behavior Therapy* 17:43–49.

Beardslee, W. R., Bemporad J., Keller, M. B., et al. (1983). Children of parents with major affective disorder: a review. *American Journal of Psychiatry* 140:825–832.

Bebbington, P. (1987). Marital status and depression: a study of English national admission statistics. *Acta Psychiatrica Scandinavica* 75:640–650.

Biglan, A., Hops, H., Sherman, L., et al. (1985). Problem-solving interactions of depressed women and their husbands. *Behavior Therapy* 16:431–451.

Billings, A. G., and Moos, R. H. (1983). Comparisons of children of depressed and nondepressed parents: a social-enviromental perspective. *Journal of Abnormal Child Psychology* 11:463–486.

———— (1985). Children of parents with unipolar depression: a controlled 1-year follow-up. *Journal of Abnormal Child Psychology* 14:149–166.

Birchnell, J. (1988). Depression and family relationships: a study of young, married women on a London housing estate. *British Journal of Psychiatry* 153:758–769.

Birchnell, J., and Kennard, J. (1983). Does marital maladjustment lead to mental illness? *Social Psychiatry* 18: 79–88.

Black, W. D., Bell, S., Hulbert, J., et al. (1988). The importance of axis II in patients with major depression: a controlled study. *Journal of Affective Disorders* 14:115–122.

Blehar, M. C., Weissman, M. M., Gershon, E. S., et al. (1988). Family and genetic studies of affective disorders. *Archives of General Psychiatry* 45:289–292.

Bouras, N., Vanger, P., and Bridges, P. K. (1986). Marital problems in chronically depressed and physically ill patients and their spouses. *Comprehensive Psychiatry* 27:127–130.

Boyd, J. H., and Weissman, M. M. (1981). Epidemiology of affective disorders: a reexamination and future directions. *Archives of General Psychiatry* 38:1039–1046.

Brown, G. W., and Prudo, R. (1981). Psychiatric disorder in a rural and an urban population, 2: sensitivity to loss. *Psychological Medicine* 11:601–616.

Cadoret, R. J., O'Gorman, W. T., Heywood, E., et al. (1985). Genetic and environmental factors in major depression. *Journal of Affective Disorders* 9:155–164.

Charney, D. S., Nelson, J. C., and Quinlan, D. M. (1981). Personality traits and disorder in depression. *American Journal of Psychiatry* 138:1601–1604.

Corney, R. H. (1987). Marital problems and treatment outcome in depressed women: a clinical trial of social work intervention. *British Journal of Psychiatry* 151:652–659.

Coyne, J. C., Kessler, R. C., Tal, M., et al. (1987). Living with a depressed person. *Journal of Consulting and Clinical Psychology* 55:347–352.

Crowther, J. H. (1985). The relationship between depression and marital maladjustment: a descriptive study. *Journal of Nervous Mental Disorders* 173:227–231.

Dobson, K. S. (1987). Marital and social adjustment in depressed and remarried women. *Journal of Clinical Psychology* 43:261-265.

Epstein, N. B., Baldwin, L. M., and Bishop, D. S., (1983). The McMaster family assessment device. *Journal of Marital and Family Therapy* 9:171-180.

Epstein, N. B., Keitner, G. I., Bishop, D. S., et al. (1988). Combined use of pharmacological and family therapy. In *Affective Disorders and the Family: Assessment and Treatment*, ed. J. F. Clarkin, G. Haas, and I. Glick. New York: Guilford.

Fadden, G., Bebbington, P., and Kuipers, L. (1987). Caring and its burdens: a study of the spouses of depressed patients. *British Journal of Psychiatry* 151:660-667.

Forehand, R., McCombs, A., and Brody, G. H. (1987). The relationship between parental depressive mood states and child functioning. *Advances in Behavior Research and Therapy* 9:1-20.

Friedman, A. S. (1975). Interaction of drug therapy with marital therapy in depressive patients. *Archives of General Psychiatry* 32:619-637.

Glick, I. D. Clarkin, J. F., Spencer, J. H. et al. (1985). A controlled evaluation of inpatient family intervention, I: preliminary results of the six-month follow-up. *Archives of General Psychiatry* 42:882-886.

Goering, P., Wasylenki, D., Lancee, W., et al. (1983). Social support and post hospital outcome for depressed women. *Canadian Journal of Psychiatry* 28:612-618.

Goldberg, M., and Mudd, E. (1968). The effects of suicidal behavior upon marriage and family. In *Suicidal Behaviors: Diagnosis and Management*, ed. H. L. P. Resnick. Boston: Little, Brown.

Gordon, D., Burge, D., Hammen, C., et al. (1989). Observations of interactions of depressed women with their children. *American Journal of Psychiatry* 146:50-55.

Gotlib, I. H., and Whiffen, V. E. (1989). Depression and marital functioning: an examination of specificity and gender differences. *Journal of Abnormal Psychology* 98:23-30.

Gove, W. R. (1972). Sex, marital status, and suicide. *Journal of Health and Social Behavior* 13:204-213.

Haas, G. L., Glick I. D., Clarkin, J. F., et al. (1988). Inpatient family intervention: a randomized clinical trial, II: results at hospital discharge. *Archives of General Psychiatry* 45:217-224.

Hammen, C., Gordon, D., Burge, D., et al. (1987). Maternal affective disorders, illness, and stress: risk for children's psychopathology. *American Journal of Psychiatry* 144:736-741.

Hinchcliffe, M., Hooper, D., Roberts, F. J., et al. (1975). A study of the interaction between depressed patients and their spouses. *British Journal of Psychiatry* 126:164-172.

Hinchcliffe, M., Vaughn, P. W., Hooper, D., et al. (1977). The melancholy marriage: an inquiry into the interaction of depression, II: expressiveness. *British Journal of Medical Psychology* 50:125–142.

Hooley, J. M., Orley, J. and Teasdale, J. D. (1986). Levels of expressed emotion and relapse in depressed patients. *British Journal of Psychiatry* 148:642–647.

Hooley, J. M., and Teasdale, J. D. (1989). Predictors of relapse in unipolar depressives: expressed emotion, marital distress and perceived criticism. *Journal of Abnormal Psychology* 98:229–235.

Hops, H., Biglan, A., Sherman, L., et al. (1987). Home observations of family interactions of depressed women. *Journal of Consulting Clinical Psychology* 55:341–346.

Keitner, G. I., Miller, I. W., Epstein, N. B., et al. (1986). The functioning of families of patients with major depression. *International Journal of Family Psychiatry* 7:11–16.

_____ (1987a). Family functioning and the course of major depression. *Comprehensive Psychiatry* 23:54–64.

Keitner, G. I. Miller, I. W., Furzzetti, A. E., et al. (1987b). Family functioning and suicidal behavior in psychiatric inpatients with major depression. *Psychiatry* 50:242–255.

Keitner, G. I., Ryan, C. E., Miller, I. W., et al. (1989). Compounded depression and family functioning during the acute episode and at 6-month follow-up. *Comprehensive Psychiatry* 30:512–521.

Keitner, G. I., Ryan, C. E., Miller, I. W., et al. (1990). Family functioning, social adjustment, and recurrence of suicidality. *Psychiatry* 53:17–30.

Keller, M. B., Beardslee, W. R., Dorer, D. J., et al. (1986). Impact of severity and chronicity of parental affective illness on adaptive functioning and psychopathology in children. *Archives of General Psychiatry* 43:930–937.

Keller, M. B., Klerman, G. L., Lavori, P. W., et al. (1984). Long term outcome of episodes of major depression: clinical and public health significance. *Journal of the American Medical Association* 252:788–792.

Keller, M. B., and Shapiro, R. W. (1982). "Double depression": superimposition of acute depressive episodes on chronic depressive disorders. *American Journal of Psychiatry* 139:438–442.

Keller, M. B., Shapiro, R. W., Lavori, P. W., et al. (1982). Recovery in major depressive disorder: analysis with the life table and regression models. *Archives of General Psychiatry* 39:905–910.

Krantz, S. E., and Moos, R. H. (1987). Functioning and life context among spouses of remitted and nonremitted depressed patients. *Journal of Consulting and Clinical Psychology* 55:353–360.

Lee, C. M., and Gotlib, I. H. (1989). Clinical status and emotional adjustment of children of depressed mothers. *American Journal of Psychiatry* 146:478–483.

Locke, H. J., and Wallace, K. M. (1959). Short marital adjustment and prediction tests: their reliability and validity. *Marriage and Family Living* 21:251-255.

McGuffin, P, and Katz, R. (1989). The genetics of depression and manic-depressive disorder. *British Journal of Psychiatry* 15:294-304.

McLean, P. D., Ogston, K., and Grauer, L. (1973). A behavioral approach to the treatment of depression. *Journal of Behavior Therapy and Experimental Psychiatry* 4:323-330.

Menaghan, E. G. (1985). Depressive affect and subsequent divorce. *Journal of Family Issues*, 6:295-306.

Merikangas, K. R. (1984). Divorce and assortative mating among depressed patients. *American Journal of Psychiatry* 141:74-76.

Merikangas, K. R., Prusoff, B. A., Kupfer, D. J., et al. (1985). Marital adjustment in major depression. *Journal of Affective Disorders* 9:5-11.

Merikangas, K. R., Prusoff, B. A., and Weissman, M. M. (1988). Parental concordance for affective disorders: psychopathology in offspring. *Journal of Affective Disorders* 15:279-290.

Miller, I. W., Kabacoff, R. I., Keitner, G. I., et al. (1986). Family functioning in the families of psychiatric patients. *Comprehensive Psychiatry* 27: 302-312.

Moos, R. J., and Moos, B. S. (1981). *Family Environment Scale Manual.* Palo Alto, CA: Consulting Psychologists.

Olson, D. H., Portner, J., and Bell, R (1982). *Faces-II: Family Adaptability and Cohesion Evaluation Scales.* St. Paul, MN: University of Minnesota, Family Social Science.

Orvaschel, H., Weissman, M. M., and Kidd, K. K. (1980). Children and depression—the children of depressed parents; the childhood of depressed parents; depression in children. *Journal of Affective Disorders* 2:1-16.

Radke-Yarrow, M., Cummings, E. M., Kuczinski, L., et al. (1985). Patterns of attachment in two- and three-year-olds in normal families and families with parental depression. *Child Development* 56:884-893.

Richman, J. (1978). Symbiosis, empathy, suicidal behavior, and the family. *Suicide and Life-Threatening Behavior* 8:139-149.

Rounsaville, B. J., Prusoff, B. A., and Weissman, M. M. (1980). The course of marital disputes in depressed women: a 48-month follow-up study. *Comprehensive Psychiatry* 21:111-118.

Rounsaville, B. J., Weissman, M. M., Prusoff, B. A., et al. (1979). Marital disputes and treatment outcome in depressed women. *Comprehensive Psychiatry* 20:483-490.

Roy, A. (1985). Depression and marriage. *Psychiatric Journal of the University of Ottawa* 10:101-103.

———— (1987). Five risk factors for depression. *British Journal of Psychiatry* 150:536-541.

Snyder, D. K., Wills, R. M., and Keiser, T. W. (1981). Empirical validation of the Marital Satisfaction Inventory: an actuarial approach. *Journal of Clinical Psychology* 49:262-268.

Spanier, G. B. (1976). Measuring dyadic adjustment: new scales for assessing the quality of marriage and other dyads. *Journal of Marital and Family Therapy* 38:15-28.

Spencer, J. H. Jr., Glick, I. D., Haas, G. I., et al. (1988). A randomized clinical trial of inpatient family intervention, III: effects at 6-month and 18-month follow-ups. *American Journal of Psychiatry* 145:1115-1121.

Susman, E. J., Trickett, P. K., Jannotti, R. J., et al. (1985). Child-rearing patterns in depressed, abusive, and normal mothers. *American Journal of Orthopsychiatry* 55:237-251.

Swindle, R. W. Jr., Cronkite, R. C., and Moos, R. H. (1989). Life stressors, social resources, coping, and the 4-year course of unipolar depression. *Journal of Abnormal Psychology* 98:468-477.

Targum, S. D., Dibble, E., Davenport, Y. B., et al. (1981). The Family Attitudes Questionnaire: patients' and spouses' views of bipolar illness. *Archives of General Psychiatry* 38:562-568.

Vaughn, C. E., and Leff, J. P. (1976a). The measurement of expressed emotion in the families of psychiatric patients. *British Journal of Social and Clinical Psychology* 15:157-165.

_____ (1976b). The influence of family and social factors on the course of psychiatric illness. *British Journal of Psychiatry* 129:125-137.

Waring, E. M., McElarth, D., Mitchell, P., et al. (1981). Intimacy and emotional illness in the general population. *Canadian Journal of Psychiatry* 26:167-172.

Weissman, M. M. (1975). The assessment of social adjustment: a review of techniques. *Archives of General Psychiatry* 32:357-365.

Weissman, M. M. Gammon, D. G., Karen, J., et al. (1987). Children of depressed parents. *Archives of General Psychiatry* 44:847-853.

Weissman, M., and Paykel, E. (1974). *The Depressed Woman: A Study of Her Relationships*. Chicago: University of Chicago Press.

3: DEPRESSION, THE MARITAL RELATIONSHIP, AND PARENTING: AN INTERPERSONAL VIEW

James Coyne, Ph.D.
Linda Schwoeri, M.A., M.F.T.
Geraldine Downey, Ph.D.

INTRODUCTION

A comprehensive perspective on depression should encompass its interpersonal context. In order to account for the depressed person's difficulties, consideration should be given to the social and familial as well as the biological factors that contribute to the onset and maintenance of depression. Research has shown that depression is concentrated in particular families (Coyne, Burchill, and Stiles 1991, Keitner and Miller 1990). Depression in a family member is a marker for more pervasive difficulties in the family. Other family members are vulnerable to psychiatric disturbance and adjustment problems. Families with a depressed family member are, as a whole, characterized by less affective involvement and poorer problem solving, communication, and general functioning.

This chapter looks at the role of interpersonal and social stresses in the onset of depression in a biologically vulnerable person. It looks specifically at the marital and family relationship as a risk as well as a protective factor for a person vulnerable to depression. There are likely to be marital problems associated with depression. Furthermore, we will see that depression in an adult can be associated with a considerable burden on family members. Their well-being may be at stake and, in turn, their response to depressed persons can affect patients' likelihood of relapse. Yet, more generally, spouses of depressed persons may bring their own vulnerabilities to the marriage or otherwise be implicated in depressed persons' problems. Children of depressed persons are at risk for a full range of psychological difficulties. Finally, depression in children is strongly suggestive of parental psychopathology, most notably depression.

As the range and concentration of family problems associated with depression become more clearly established, it is also apparent that no single set of factors will explain this patterning. For instance, although depression in a mother is associated with both her impairment as a parent and heightened risk for psychological disturbance in her children, it is possible that many of the children's difficulties may be more directly tied to marital conflict and the unavailability of the nondepressed parent. We should be conscious of drawing any premature conclusions from what are basically correlational data. Similarly, although this chapter reviews evidence that interpersonal factors contribute to the onset of most depressions, we will see that much of the importance of an interpersonal perspective on depression does not depend on any strong assumptions about etiology.

There has been a longstanding bias toward viewing depressed persons and their complaints in isolation from their interpersonal context. Recent decades have witnessed tremendous increases in our understanding of the biology of depression, and the efficacy of antidepressant medication has been well established. Yet these advances in no way contradict the need to better understand the interpersonal circumstances of depressed persons. Even when there is strong evidence that there is a biological component to a depressive episode, interpersonal factors are likely to play a key role as a precipitant. They may also be an important determinant of the response to treatment and how the episode is resolved. Interpersonal factors have an impact on the family as well as on the patient and may determine what residual problems remain. Moreover, such factors may not be influenced by biological treatments. By their persistence, interpersonal problems may remain a continued source of vulnerability for the recovering depressed person.

It is only recently that the study of interpersonal processes in depression has begun to achieve momentum. Our understanding of these processes remains limited and, for the most part, is based on provocative findings that particular phenomena co-occur, rather than a sense of precisely how they are linked. Thus, although there is evidence that spousal criticism at the time of hospitalization predicts subsequent relapse (Hooley et al. 1986, Vaughn and Leff 1976), we can only speculate about the mechanism that is involved. Being married is associated with slower recovery from a depressive episode (George et al. 1989) and poorer response to antidepressant medication (Keller et al. 1984). The explanation of this finding remains elusive. To the extent that findings from some of these studies can be replicated, there is the suggestion of complex links between interpersonal and biological processes that deserve considerably more attention than they have received.

Some well-established myths about the nature of depression pose barriers to a better understanding of interpersonal processes in depression. There is a tendency to interpret distinctions between endogenous and nonendogenous depression as if they represented a rigid division between those depressions for which we can afford to ignore the role of interpersonal factors and those for which there is some relevance of interpersonal factors. That is, a distinction between depression related to biological factors and one related to stress presents a misunderstanding of the nature of and correlates of endogenous depression. A set of symptoms such as sleep and appetite disturbance predicts a better response to antidepressant medication and electroconvulsive therapy. Endogenous depression and melancholia are now defined in part on this basis. Diagnosing a depression as endogenous does not depend on whether a precipitating stress can be identified. Reactivity to changes in the environment during a depressive episode, rather than the absence of precipitating stress, has been found to predict response to biologically oriented treatment (Fowles and Gersh 1979). This has now replaced the lack of antecedent stress as an additional criterion for endogenicity. There is evidence that endogenously depressed patients tend to have preexisting problems in their close relationships (Birchnell and Kennard 1983), and the overall association among depressed patients between endogenous features and the presence or absence of recent life events is weak at best (Dolan et al. 1985).

Thus, whether we consider depression in clinical populations, endogenous depression, or depression with an associated neuroendocrine abnormality, we are not precluding the importance of stressful life events in the onset of depression. The key question is not whether depression is to be explained in terms of the interactional context or biology, but how interaction and biological factors fit together. As yet, this question has not received the attention it deserves.

STRESS AND DEPRESSION

Exposure to severe life events and, to a lesser degree, chronic difficulties plays an important role in the onset of depression, even though these factors in themselves are insufficient to explain fully its occurrence. Paykel (1979) has calculated that, taking into account the occurrence of any of the major life events that he examined, the risk of depression is increased by a factor of 5.6 in the 6 months after the event. An event involving an exit from a significant role increases the risk of depression by a factor of 6.5.

Brown and Harris (1978) found that the relationship between severe life events and depression held across inpatient, outpatient, general practitioner, and community samples. For instance, as many as 80–90 percent of episodes of depression developing in the community sample were preceded by serious life events or ongoing major difficulties such as poor housing or an alcoholic husband.

> The distinctive feature of the great majority of the provoking events is the experience of loss or disappointment. This is defined broadly to include threat of or actual separation from a key figure, an unpleasant revelation about someone also, a life-threatening illness to a close relative, a major material loss or general disappointment or threat of them, and miscellaneous crises such as being made redundant after a long period of steady employment. [Brown and Harris, 1978, pp. 274–275]

Family and other close relationships are a major source of such events. In a subsequent review of seven studies of depressed patients using comparable measures of live events, Brown and Harris (1982) found that an average of 56 percent of the patients had an important life event before onset, compared with an average rate of 18 percent in a similar time period in the general population. In arriving at these estimates, Brown and Harris have taken great pains to not count any events that might conceivably be due to depressive symptoms. These figures are thus conservative, but they suggest that the onset of most episodes of depression in clinical populations is associated with major life events.

Most occurrences of major life events, however, are not associated with the onset of depression (Brown and Harris 1978), and so other factors are implicated, both individual and social. We next give attention to one such factor: involvement in an unsupportive or conflictful close relationship. Such a relationship can both generate major life events and be a source of vulnerability to depression in itself. Yet an interpersonal perspective sensitizes us to how being depressed can also negatively affect close relationships (Coyne 1976a, b) and even precipitate life events such as divorce (Briscoe and Smith 1973). A depressive episode can have a profound effect on family members. Over time, the behavior of depressed persons and family members can become interwoven or concatenated to the detriment of all who are involved. Understanding and renegotiating close relationships can therefore be a crucial part of the recovery process for a depressed person and can reduce the toll that depression takes on relatives, regardless of how the depression has come about.

DEPRESSION AND THE MARITAL RELATIONSHIP

Close Relationships as Risk and Protective Factors

Many life events associated with depression represent disturbances in close relationships, and the single most frequent event reported by depressed women is an increase in arguments with spouses (Paykel et al. 1969). As well as further establishing the importance of life events in the onset of depression, the Brown and Harris (1978) study appeared to demonstrate the protection against depression afforded by involvement in a confiding close relationship. Their data suggest that women who have such a relationship are only one-third as likely to become depressed in the face of life events as those who do not. Having a good, intimate relationship neutralizes the effects of other risk factors such as having three young children at home, being unemployed, and having lost one's mother before the age of 11 (Brown and Harris 1978).

An intimate relationship would seem to provide a secure source of meaning and self-esteem in the face of threatening events arising outside the relationship. It may also serve to preserve the sense of confidence that one's circumstances are predictable and things will work out as well as can reasonably be expected. The opportunities for self-disclosure, validation, and corrective emotional experiences provided by an intimate relationship may also serve to counter negative experiences that might otherwise result in depression. Finally, a spouse with whom there is a positive, intimate relationship may be more actively and collaboratively involved in the process of coping with a stressful life event in a way that reduces the burden or threat to the person at risk.

Yet it has not been demonstrated precisely how having a confiding relationship reduces the risk of depression, and it is unlikely to be via a single mechanism. It is possible to reinterpret the apparent beneficial effects of having a confiding relationship with a spouse as actually due to the absence of a close relationship that is conflictual, nonconfiding, or unsatisfactory. Roy (1978) found that women reporting an inability to confide in their husbands were but a subset of those reporting a bad marriage, and that it is having a bad marriage that leaves women at risk for depression, and not the lack of a confiding relationship per se.

The most provocative data relevant to this point come from the Yale Epidemiologic Catchment Area (ECA) Study (Weissman 1987). It found that being married and being able to talk to one's spouse provided a modest reduction in the risk for depression over that associated with being single, separated, or divorced. This is consistent with the usual interpretation of the effects of a confiding relationship. However, this effect was overshadowed by the negative effects of being married and indicating that one could not talk to one's spouse. The odds ratio for depression associated with being married and not being able to talk to one's spouse (i.e., the odds associated with not being able to talk to one's spouse versus the odds associated with all other conditions) was a striking 25.8 for men and 28.1 for women. Thus, it could be that most of the apparent protection from depression afforded by having a good relationship with one's spouse might better be seen as a reflection of the detrimental effects of being married but not getting along with one's spouse. These findings give added credibility to arguments that not having to deal with problematic features of bad relationships may be more powerful than the purported salutary effects of good relationships (Coyne and DeLongis 1986).

Coyne (1991a) found important differences in the marital

relationships of depressed inpatients depending on whether the patient was a man or woman. Although there was heightened marital distress in both instances, the marital distress and number of marital complaints endorsed by both patients and spouses were greater when the wife was the depressed inpatient. Furthermore, female patients and their spouses reported tactics for resolving conflict that were more destructive (yelling and name-calling) and less constructive (active listening and proposing compromises). These findings could be due to women being more crucial for the emotional functioning of the marriage or to their being more vulnerable to the effects of marital difficulties. Alternatively, men may simply be more intolerant of the dysphoria and dysfunction of a depressed spouse.

Kahn and colleagues (1985) found important similarities between depressed persons and their spouses in terms of overt hostility and lack of constructive problem solving. These authors suggested that depressed persons and their spouses may be involved in a cycle in which their unsuccessful efforts to resolve differences lead to withdrawal and avoidance and to negative affect, mistrust, and misgivings about each other. The accumulated effect of such interactions overwhelms the couple when they again attempt to settle specific differences, increasing their hopelessness about the possibility of improving their relationship.

The interactions between depressed persons and their spouses are considerably more negative than those between depressed persons and strangers (Hinchliffe et al. 1978), and differences in the marital interactions of couples with and without a depressed partner persist when marital dissatisfaction is controlled (Hautzinger et al. 1982). Observational studies suggest a particular patterning of the marital relationships of depressed persons. That is, depressed women's displays of distress tend to inhibit their husbands' aggressiveness temporarily, but aggressiveness by husbands also inhibits their wives' subsequent depressive behavior (Biglan et al. 1985). Other studies suggest that depressed women concede more in disagreements with their husbands (Merikangas et al. 1979), and that they are more likely than nondepressed women to be dominated by their husbands in decision making (Hoover and Fitzgerald 1981).

The dependency of depressed persons and their feelings of insecurity may be more congruent with the nature of their relationships with their spouses than has generally been supposed. Leff and

Vaughn (1985) found that the majority of depressed patients, particularly women, were fearful of loss and rejection and desirous of continual comfort and support. Yet as Leff and Vaughn (1985) also found, depression may be maintained in such fears and perceptions, namely, "few depressed patients described as chronically insecure or lacking in self-confidence were living with supportive or sympathetic spouses . . . " (p. 95). They found, in fact, that the majority of the spouses of depressed persons were critical of them. Although some of this criticism centered on the depressed partner's current symptomatic behavior, a considerable proportion of it was aimed at traits and behavior evident before the onset of the patient's depression. This hostile, critical environment can be the origin of the patient's self-complaints and hopelessness, a means of validating and expanding on existing self-criticism, and a buffer against change. Experimental studies suggest that intimates who agree with a person's negative self-view can effectively insulate that person from positive experiences that might otherwise challenge this view of him- or herself (Swann and Predmore 1985).

The Marital Relationships of Depressed Persons

In an early study, Weissman and Paykel (1974) found that although the difficulties of depressed women extended into all of their social roles, including worker and member of the community, they faced their greatest problems as wives and mothers. Structured interviews with these women indicated that their marriages were characterized by friction, hostility, poor communication, dependency, and diminished sexual satisfaction.

Subsequent studies have found that the marriages of depressed persons are beset by problems including general dissatisfaction and overt conflict. The majority of depressed persons have serious marital adjustment scales (Coyne 1990, Rounsaville et al. 1979). Whereas the complaints of the patients tend to center on the quality of the relationship, their spouses focus on the patients' depression (Coyne 1990).

In laboratory studies, the interactions of depressed persons and their spouses are uncomfortable, tense, and hostile. These interactions are characterized by disruptions and negative outbursts, discrepancies between verbal contention and tone of both spouses, avoidance and withdrawal, and little constructive problem solving

(Arkowitz et al. 1982, Hautzinger et al. 1982, Hinchliffe et al. 1978, Kahn et al. 1985, (McLean et al. 1973).

Rush and colleagues (1980) suggested that "the spouse of the depressed person cannot be considered neutral. He or she becomes frustrated, confused, overly solicitous or angry, or withdrawn emotionally" (p. 105). The picture emerging from recent research is even more complex. Spouses may have precipitated many of the difficulties of depressed persons, and they may be actively involved in their perpetuation. There is a definite burden associated with living with a depressed person. We need to develop an appreciation of how difficult the close relationships of depressed persons are for all involved, how they came to be this way, and how they can be effectively modified.

Spouses of Depressed Persons

There is evidence that the spouses of depressed persons have heightened psychological distress during their partners' episodes, and that they have personal and family histories of psychopathology themselves. Furthermore, some women who are particularly vulnerable to depression are more likely to marry men who contribute to their becoming depressed.

Spouses of patients currently in a depressive episode show considerable psychological distress themselves, much of which remits when the patients are not in an episode (Coyne et al. 1987). The spouse's distress is directly related to the burden imposed by the patient's symptoms. The chief spousal complaints are the patient's lack of energy, the possibility that the patient will become depressed again, the patient's sense of worthlessness, the patient's lack of interest in doing things, and the emotional strain the spouse feels.

On the other hand, there is evidence of assortative mating: spouses of depressed persons may bring their own liabilities and vulnerabilities to the marriage. Depressed women are more likely than other women to be married to a man with a history of depression or alcohol or substance abuse problems. Over half the depressed women drawn from clinical samples have husbands with a history of psychiatric disturbance, mostly affective disorders (Merikangas and Spiker 1982). In a community sample, a quarter of the husbands had a history of depressive disorder, and a fifth had a history of substance abuse (Peterson et al. 1991). These rates were substantially higher than for control women. Overall, assortative mating for psychopathology may more directly affect the social adjustment and quality of family life, rather than episodic disturbance of either spouse (Merikangas et al. 1988). Brown and colleagues (1986) found that over two-thirds of the women in their sample who lacked a quality relationship with their spouses were married to men whom raters considered grossly undependable as mates, parents, and providers.

Studies of the risk for depression due to adversity in early childhood may be largely indirect, such as through the selection of the spouse and the quality of the marital relationship (Parker and Hadzi-Pavlovic 1984, Quinton et al. 1984). These studies have shown that women with highly adverse childhood experiences such as being reared in an institution after death of the mother were quite prone to psychiatric disturbance and marital and parenting difficulties. Yet the minority of women who were largely free of disturbance or social difficulties had good, supportive relationships with their spouses. Whether they had such positive relationships with their spouses was tied in part to whether their spouses were currently having alcohol or drug problems or difficulties with the law. Furthermore, spouses' reports of their own problems in adolescence predicted whether these women had problems currently. Thus, taken together, these studies may be interpreted as suggesting that depression-prone women are more likely to be married to men with difficulties of their own and who may be less able to provide the secure, intimate relationship that would reduce the women's risk of depression.

Marital Quality and the Course and Outcome of Depression

The marital problems faced by many depressed persons are a negative prognostic indicator in treatment with antidepressant medication (Rounsaville et al. 1979). Those patients whose marriages improve show satisfactory response to medication, but the evidence is that medication has little direct effect on the quality of depressed persons' involvement in their marriages (Weissman et al. 1984.) Further, 4-year follow-up assessments of depressed persons with marital problems who have been treated with antidepressants suggest that they tend to continue to be vulnerable to depression and to have marital problems (Rounsaville et al. 1980). Courney (1984) found that depressed women with marital problems were less likely to improve in individual psychotherapy than those without problems. Taken together, findings that depression is associated with marital problems and that these problems have a negative impact on recovery may explain the overall tendency of married patients to respond less well to antidepressant medication (Keller et al. 1984) and to take longer to recover (George et al 1989).

A pair of studies suggested that the number of critical comments about a depressed patient that the spouse makes in an interview during the patient's hospitalization is predictive of post-hospital relapse, independent of the patient's level of symptomatology (Hooley et al. 1986, Vaughn and Leff 1976). In the Vaughn and Leff (1976) study, a cutoff of two critical comments by the spouse provided the best discrimination of those depressed patients who subsequently relapsed, whereas in the Hooley et al. (1986) study, the best discrimination was with three comments. In the latter study, none of the eight patients whose spouses were low in criticism relapsed, whereas twenty of the thirty-one patients whose spouses were high relapsed.

Taken together, these studies highlight the continued effects of interpersonal circumstances and specifically the marital situation beyond the instigation of a depressive episode. Findings that response to medication may be affected by marital problems point to the need to understand better the links between interpersonal circumstances and the biology of depression. Further, the finding that treatment with antidepressants may not resolve the marital problems associated with depression suggests the need to consider work with the close relationships of depressed persons either as a primary treatment or as an adjunct to medication. There is no incompatibility between medication and marital intervention, and for more severely depressed patients, a combination may be the approach of choice (Coyne 1988). However, the same difficulties that suggest the need for marital intervention may limit couples with a depressed partner from seeking or benefiting from conventional conjoint therapy. We discuss this problem and its solutions in the next chapter.

DEPRESSION AND PARENT–CHILD RELATIONSHIPS

Children of Depressed Parents

Characteristics of the Children

Children of depressed parents have behavior problems, more physical complaints, and difficulties at school and with their peers. They complain more about health problems, and they resemble other children who experience the stress and disruption that accompany serious parental psychiatric or medical illnesses. Available evidence suggests that child adjustment does not fluctuate as parents move in and out of episodes (Billings and Moos 1985, Richters and Pelligrini 1989). Perhaps the chronic impairment and family stress that often accompany parental depression have more serious implications for child development than the acute impairment associated with acute depressive episodes (Richters 1987).

Early uncontrolled studies of children with a depressed parent provide suggestive evidence that these children are at risk for a wide range of problems in psychological functioning (Beardslee et al. 1983). School-aged children of depressed parents generally showed higher levels of both externalizing and internalizing than normal children. This finding has emerged in reports by teachers, parents, and the children themselves. These children had more treatment for psychiatric disturbance and higher levels of functional impairment. A high proportion of the children score in the clinical range of symptom checklists. They have deficits in social and academic competence that are not due to intellectual limitation.

In addition to general adjustment difficulties and psychiatric conditions, children of depressed mothers show what have been interpreted as markers of risk for subsequent depression. Specifically, they are more self-critical than other children (Hammen et al. 1988), and they have difficulties with regulating emotion and social interaction (Zahn-Waxler, et al. 1990, Zahn-Waxler and Kochanska 1990, Zahn-Waxler et al. 1984). Because peers and adults react negatively to such inappropriate emotional and social behavior, children of depressed parents who show these problems will probably experience heightened levels of rejection and adversity in social interactions. This may further confirm their negative self-concepts and lead them to avoid social and emotional expression. Difficulties in socioemotional development may accrue over time because the children simply fail to keep pace with peers. Thus, we can see a potential interactional process linking these high-risk children and their social context in the accentuation of their difficulties.

Subsequent studies with diagnostic assessment of children of depressed parents found them at heightened risk for psychiatric disturbance, with as many as 40 percent having at least one diagnosis. It appears that depression, and especially major depression, is a more specific consequence of having a unipolar-depressed parent. Depression is the only diagnosable condition for which children of depressed parents consistently show significantly heightened risk across studies and comparison groups (see Downey and Coyne 1990 for a review). The rate of any affective disorder is three times higher in children of unipolar disorder parents than control children, and the rate of major depressive disorder is six times higher than in control children.

Children's Contribution to Depression in Parents and Parenting Difficulties

Evidence from multiple sources and across multiple situations shows that children of depressed parents pose a greater challenge to effective parenting than average children. The literature examining the impact of children's behavior on depressed parents is not a large one, but there are reasons to believe that child disturbance helps maintain parenting difficulties and parental depression. First, there is evidence that declines in maternal distress and improvements in the quality of parenting parallel the successful treatment of the children's behavior problems (Forehand et al. 1980, Lytton 1990, Patterson 1982). Second, there is evidence of reciprocal relations between maternal depression and child behavior problems (Hammen et al. 1990, Radke-Yarrow et al. 1988, Schwoeri and Sholevar, see Chapter 6). Depressed mothers report more hostile interactions with their children than with their spouses (Weissman and Paykel 1974). Observational studies substantiate that depressed mothers and their children engage in a reciprocal pattern of negativity and hostility. These patterns are evident even in infancy. Paralleling their depressed mothers' interactional pattern, children as young as 3 months direct their behavior toward their mothers less frequently, smile and express happiness less often, and are more irritable and fussy. This unrewarding interactional style generalizes to strangers, in whom it evokes a negative response (Field et al. 1988).

Whatever the origins of the problematic interactional style shown by infants and children of depressed parents, it is clear that the feedback available to depressed parents from interactions with their children may help maintain depression by validating feelings of ineptitude, worthlessness, and rejection. It is not simply a matter of depressed mothers being guilt-ridden and self-critical because they view their interactions with their children as unsatisfactory. Children are a major source of criticism directed at depressed mothers and, thus, undermine their mothers' self-esteem. With single depressed mothers, children may be the primary source of criticism (Brown et al. 1990, Patterson 1982).

Difficult child behavior also may indirectly contribute to the maintenance of depression by providing another source of marital conflict and opportunity for spouses to criticize and to undermine one another. Finally, child difficulties that extend to schools and that involve illegal activities (e.g., substance abuse, stealing) will foster depression through the additional stressors they impose on the family system. Thus, adequate models of depression in the family and of the links between parental depression and child adjustment should incorporate the reactive characteristics of children and the systemic nature of the family.

Family Context of Children's Depression

The literature on the family context of childhood depression is still woefully inadequate, but there are links that need to be considered. There are important similarities in families identified because of parental depression and families identified because of depression in a child. First, Puig-Antich and colleagues (1985a, b) report one-half to two-thirds of parents of depressed children are themselves depressed. Parental depression is probably the most prevalent etiological factor in childhood depression. The families of depressed children have been studied by a number of investigators in what are called bottom up studies. The studies include the ones by Strober (1984); Mitchell and colleagues (1989); Puig-Antich and colleagues (1989); and Weller (1990). The studies all compared depressed children and adolescents with control groups of normal children or children with other disorders. The studies have collectively supported the following conclusions:

1. There is a high rate of psychopathology in parents of children with major depressive disorder (MDD). Frequently, both parents of depressed children are affected by major depression and other psychopathologies.
2. Mothers of depressed children have high rates of MDD, bipolar illness, and anxiety disorder.
3. Fathers of MDD children have increased antisocial personality. These fathers also may have high rates of drug and alcohol abuse.

The association of other parental disorders with childhood depression may be spurious. It may reflect either comorbidity between depression and another disorder in the diagnosed parent or disorders in the nondepressed parent, a consequence of assortative mating for psychopathology. Thus, parental alcoholism may appear to be associated with childhood depression. However, this is true only if one of the parents is also depressed (Merikangas et al. 1985).

In summary, the apparent specificity of the association between depression in parents and depression in children, together with the high rates of depression in the parents of depressed children and in the children of depressed parents, suggests that these ostensively separate literatures are based on the same families.

Second, families of both depressed children and of depressed parents show similar parenting difficulties. Studies of clinically depressed children and of children with elevated depressive symptomatology characterize their families as emotionally distant, lacking in warmth, and poor in emotion regulation and conflict resolution, and their parents as inconsistent, controlling, and sometimes abusive (Amanat and Butler 1984, Asarnow et al. 1987, Cole and Rehm 1986, Kashani et al. 1987, Poznanski and Zrull 1970, Puig-Antich et al. 1985b). This description resembles the retrospective accounts of depressed adults about their childhood (Holmes and Robins 1988, Parker 1981, 1983, Perris et al. 1986).

Parenting is difficult when someone is depressed, and the parenting behavior of depressed persons has frequently been implicated in their children's problems. Weissman and Paykel (1974) observed that the helplessness and hostility associated with acute depression can interfere with the mother's ability to be effective and warm toward the children. This early study found that depressed mothers described themselves as being resentful and hostile toward their children, as well as being less affectionate, more emotionally distant, irritable, and preoccupied. Subsequent observational studies have verified these self-reports, for instance, showing that depressed mothers express considerable hostility toward their children (Hammen et al. 1987). Depressed parents show lower rates of behavior, particularly the expression of positive affect, and they respond slower and less contingently and consistently (Cohn et al. 1990, Field, et al. 1985). Surprisingly, the influence of sad affect has not received as much attention as hostility. However, Biglan and colleagues (1988) showed that depressed mothers' sad affect suppressed displays of hostility from their children. Results of other studies suggest that depressed mothers use less effortful strategies in dealing with their children than nondepressed mothers.

In controlled observations of mother–child interactions, it was noted that depressed mothers are less able to compromise in disagreements with their children and often confuse their children's normal attempts at independence as rule breaking. They also tend to back off when they encounter resistance from their children. They exhibit, instead, signs of helplessness and uncertainty in their interactions. Also, negative moods and emotions were found to occupy significantly more of the time during the observations of depressed mothers and their children than those of nondepressed mothers (Radke-Yarrow et al. 1990).

Radke-Yarrow et al. (1990) further discuss how mothers socialize their children's emotions. The mothers react variously by ignoring, explaining, denying, anxiously attending, punishing, consoling, and so forth. They respond differently according to the age and sex of the child. There is more tolerance for the younger than the older child (within a range of 2–3½ years). Anger in boys is likely to elicit concern and reward from the mother who gives in to what the child wants (Patterson 1990, p. 181).

The Interaction of Marital Conflict and Parenting Difficulties

Depression in a parent is only one source of the disadvantages and difficulties of the children of depressed parents, and depression is only one of the problems these parents have in dealing with their children. Families that include a depressed parent differ from other families in terms of high levels of marital conflict and adversity. Marital conflict has been implicated in the parenting problems of depressed persons and the difficulties of their children. It is fairly well established that adjustment problems in children, especially conduct disturbance, are influenced by marital conflict (Hetherington et al. 1989, Long et al. 1987). Marital conflict is a particularly credible alternative explanation for the general adjustment problems of children with a depressed parent. There are different hypotheses about the processes by which marital conflict, child adjustment problems, and parenting problems become associated. Some thoughts about this include (a) inconsistencies in child rearing, not only between the depressed parent and the spouse but also within the parents as they become embroiled in marital disputes; (b) lack of support for parenting; and (c) children witnessing and being unwilling participants in overt marital conflict. These factors may directly affect child well-being, interact with parental depression, or mediate its effects (Downey and Coyne 1990).

Depression interferes with being an effective parent and a responsive spouse as much as it interferes with all other social role performance. The demands of parenting add to the already existing interactional problems faced by depressed persons. Depression, because of its multiple levels of symptoms, reduces the person's focus — cognitive, behavioral, biological — to the self. Parenting, and marriage itself, requires attention to the needs of others. If marital conflict already exists in the family, the children are doubly at risk. They have to face the inevitable fallout from depression in terms of irritability, withdrawal, and loss of parental affect as well as experience their parents' marital conflict as it interferes with effective parenting. That is to say, the child with a depressed parent inevitably fails to receive effective parenting through the dysfunction brought on by the depression, and problems are intensified by the constant conflict in the marriage. This conflict is especially problematic if the nondepressed spouse absents himself from the parenting role. This aggravates the problems existing in the already conflictual parent–child dyad. It also exacerbates the mother's depressive mood state, further undermines her attempts at parenting, and undoubtedly perpetuates the marital conflict due to the lack of support she feels.

Dadds and his colleagues have provided some insight into the processes linking conflicted marriages, parental depression, parenting, and child difficulties (Dadds 1987). In these families, exchanges between parents are rarely supportive and often aversive, especially regarding issues posed by the children's behavior (Dadds et al. 1987). Dadds and colleagues argue that it is likely that the father withdraws from parenting and that the mother's exposure to coercive, emotionally taxing exchanges with the child increases. The increasing withdrawal of fathers as children become more difficult is consistent with the view that fathers' involvement in child care continues to be more discretionary than mothers', and that mothers' self-concept and well-being are more tied to the parenting role. The scenario outlined by Dadds and his colleagues may explain the link between marital conflict, maternal distress, parenting difficulties, and child-externalizing difficulties. However, it is unclear whether it explains the increased rates of depression in children with a depressed parent. In any case, we should be cautious about placing too much responsibility on depressed mothers or the mothers of depressed children for what are best seen as difficulties tied to the larger context and that may be contingent on the adjustment, behavior, or availability of the father as well. Clearly, clinical evidence of the father's reduced involvement in parenting in families with a depressed mother needs more scrutiny from researchers: Does reduced involvement precede and foster the difficulties between depressed mothers and their children? To what extent do the ensuing child difficulties and both parents' inability to cope with the difficulties serve to justify the nondepressed parent's further withdrawal?

Other Disruptions to Parenting

The major loss events that precipitate depression also disrupt parenting, as the research on divorce illustrates (Hetherington et al. 1989). Parents' attention is distracted from effective parenting as they deal emotionally and practically with a life crisis. The children's sense of the coherence of their world is challenged by the disruption in relations with their parents, in their living arrangements, and possibly in economic security. They react with limit testing to establish the parameters of their world. Their obnoxious behavior toward parents reflects both their sense of vulnerability and their anger about the disruption. These behaviors further tax custodial parents, usually mothers, who are already distressed by their loss, whose sense of self-worth is diminished, and whose sense of the future is disrupted. Adequate models of depression and child adjustment must take into account the likelihood of such reactive characteristics and reciprocal influences. The problems of the children may depend on the adjustment of the depressed person's spouse and whether there are marital problems or disruption. Thus, the risk of child disturbance increases when both parents are disturbed (Kuyler et al. 1980, Weissman et al. 1984).

Emery and colleagues (1982) concluded that in the absence of marital difficulties, the risk of problematic school behavior among the offspring of an affectively disturbed parent was no greater than among the offspring of normal control parents. Other studies have found that families in which there has been a divorce account for a considerable proportion of the psychological disturbance of children of depressed parents (Connors et al. 1979, Kuyler et al. 1980).

COMMENTS AND INTEGRATION

The research we have reviewed indicates that depression typically arises in the context of conflictful or attenuated relationships and severe life stress. Family members, both spouses and children, are vulnerable to disturbance themselves. However, limitations on the nature of available data restrict our ability to go beyond simple description to explanation of why depression proves to be such a marker for other problems in the family. The bulk of the research examines simple associations among pairs of phenomena such as lack of a confiding relationship and depression or depression and difficulties as a parent, with little effort to explicate more complex, systemic patterns. Yet, as noted elsewhere, the study of the interplay between depression and its social context is fraught with difficulties, and many more ambitious efforts fall prey to methodological difficulties that preclude confident generalization beyond the particular sample under study (Coyne 1992).

Depression is generally preceded by major losses or disappointments that become more potent when they occur in the context of a relationship with an undependable spouse. Such antecedents may directly explain some of the family problems that have been blamed on depression or the associated impairment of the depressed person. In other instances, these antecedent conditions may help explain why the family does not develop compensatory ways of coping with the problems posed by having depressed persons in the home. In general, the personal (Wells et al. 1989) and familial (Coyne et al.

1987) burden of life with depression has only begun to be appreciated. Furthermore, some of the limitations and maladaptive coping strategies of both the depressed person and the family members may continue to generate stress that taxes the family's ability to adapt, quite independent of the problems posed by depression.

The research that we have identified and summarized grants little acknowledgment to the heterogeneity of depressive disorders or the considerable diversity in the kinds of family circumstances and processes associated with them. However, we were able to dispense with one myth that has served to limit interest in the importance of psychological factors such as family functioning. Namely, we have shown that the identification of an episode of depression as endogenous or as being associated with an identifiable neuroendocrine abnormality does not preclude the importance of psychosocial factors in its onset or resolution. Although it is beyond the scope of this chapter, we should note that the best and most recent data concerning concordance for depression among twins suggest a relatively modest role for heredity in unipolar depression and perhaps a greater role for contemporary psychosocial factors, notably family life.

It has been suggested that families of depressed persons are characterized by emotional dysregulation (Coyne et al. in press). That is, they do not readily allow for negative interactions to be repaired or disagreements to be satisfactorily resolved. In these families, negative affect becomes contagious, and there is little chance for negative affect to be transformed into positive affect. Furthermore, how irritability, hostility, and anger are handled may be as crucial as the handling of sadness and depression. The depressed patient's condition may be seen as reflecting life in such a family but also as a contribution to the perpetuation of its dysregulation.

Clinically speaking, the range of problems that we have identified is somewhat daunting. There would seem to be little hope of finding solutions for all of them, and any effort to do so would run the risk of defusing the focus of treatment with the loss of whatever opportunity there might be to promote symptomatic improvement in the patient. Yet, even if practicing clinicians cannot hope to address all of these problems, neither can they afford to ignore them. The various studies that we have reviewed suggest that disharmony in close relationships may have an impact on the course of depression, and that continued problems may impede the recovery process, limit the response to treatment, and even be associated with higher rates of relapses. Furthermore, we noted that depressed persons are at continued risk for family problems beyond the acute episode, that such problems predict persistence or recurrence of depression, and that the difficulties of their children also persist beyond the acute episode.

FAMILY TREATMENT AND CONSIDERATIONS

We do not propose that family therapy is either the treatment of choice or even a workable alternative in all cases of depression. The findings that most underscore the importance of the family of depressed persons can also be construed as suggesting barriers to family-based treatment: family members may be too hostile, dysfunctional, or unmotivated to participate. We do, however, suggest the usefulness of a greater sensitivity to family factors and a heightened suspicion that family factors may be implicated when there is an unsatisfactory response to antidepressant medication or individual therapy. We should reiterate a caution about the dangers of overgeneralization, given the heterogeneity of both depressed persons and their family circumstances. Yet we still suggest that one particular focus may be more important than others to consider. Namely, depressed persons' involvement in a hostile, critical, or conflictual marital relationship may be a key to understanding many of their problems and the problems of the larger family system. Unfortunately, these relationship problems may be chronic and difficult to resolve.

REFERENCES

Amanat, E., and Butler, C. (1984). Oppressive behaviors in the families of depressed children. *Family Therapy* 11:67–77.

Arkowitz, H., Holliday, S., and Hutter, M. (1982). Depressed women and their husbands: a study of marital depression. Presentation at the Annual Meeting of the Association for the Advancement of Behavior Therapy, November.

Asarnow, J. R., Carlson, G. A., and Guthrie, D. (1987). Coping strategies, self-perceptions, hopelessness, and perceived family environments in depressed and suicidal children. *Journal of Consulting and Clinical Psychology* 55:361–366.

Beardslee, W. R., Bemporad, J., Keller, M. B., and Klerman, G. K. (1983). Children of parents with an affective disorder: a review. *American Journal of Psychiatry* 140:825–832.

Biglan, A., Hops, H., Sherman, L., et al. (1985). Problem-solving interactions of depressed women and their husbands. *Behavior Therapy* 16:431–451.

Biglan, A., Hops, H., and Sherman, L. (1988). Coercive family processes and maternal depression. In *Marriages and Families: Behavioral Treatments and Processes*, ed. R. J. McMahon and R. DeV. Peter. New York: Brunner/Mazel.

Billings, A. G., and Moos, R. H. (1985). Children of parents with unipolar depression: a controlled 1-year follow-up. *Journal of Abnormal Child Psychology* 14:149–166.

Birchnell, J., and Kennard, J. (1983). Does marital maladjustment lead to mental illness? *Social Psychiatry* 18:79–88.

Briscoe, C. W., and Smith, J. B., (1973). Depression and marital turmoil. *Archives of General Psychiatry* 29:811–817.

Brown, G. W., Bifulco, A., and Andrews, B. (1990). Self-esteem and depression: 3. Aetiological issues. *Social Psychiatry and Psychiatric Epidemiology* 25:235–243.

Brown, G. W., Bifulco, A., Harris, T., and Bridge, L. (1986). Life stress, chronic subclinical symptoms and vulnerability to clinical depression. *Journal of Affective Disorders* 11:1–19.

Brown, G. W., and Harris, T. (1978). *Social Origins of Depression: A Study of Psychiatric Disorder in Women*. New York: The Free Press.

_____ (1982). Disease, distress, and depression. *Journal of Affective Disorders* 4:1–8

Cohn, J. F., Campbell, S. B., Matias, R., and Hopkins, J. (1990). Face to face interactions of postpartum depressed and nondepressed mother–infant pairs at 2 months. *Developmental Psychology* 26:15–23.

Cole, D. A., and Rehm, L. P. (1986). Family interaction patterns and childhood depression. *Journal of Abnormal Child Psychology* 14:297–314.

Conners, C. K., Himmelhoch, J., Goyette, C. H., et al. (1979). Children of parents with affective illness. *Journal of the American Academy of Child Psychiatry* 18:600–607.

Courney, R. H. (1984). The effectiveness of social workers in the management of depressed female patients in general medicine. *Psychological Medicine* 14 (Monograph Supplement 6).

Coyne, J. C. (1976a). Toward an interactional description of depression. *Psychiatry* 39:28–40.

_____ (1976b). Depression and the response of others. *Journal of Abnormal Psychology* 2:186–193.

_____ (1988). Strategic therapy. In *Family Intervention in Affective Illness*, ed. G. Maas, I. Glick, and J. Clarkin. New York: Guilford.

_____ (1990). Depression and marital problems. Paper presented at the Annual Meeting of Association for the Advancement of Behavior Therapy, San Francisco, November.

———— (1991a). Depression and marital problems. Paper presented at the Annual meetings of the Association for the Advancement of Behavior Therapy, New York, November.

———— (1991b). The social context of depression: the spouses of depressed persons. Paper presented at the Annual Meeting of the Association for the Advancement of Behavior Therapy, New York, November.

———— (1992). Review of Beach, Sandeen, and O'Leary. Depression in marriage. *Journal of Marital and Family Therapy* 17:414–415.

Coyne, J. C., Burchill, S. A. L., and Stiles, W. B. (1991). An interactional perspective on depression. In *Handbook of Social and Clinical Psychology: The Health Perspective*, ed. C. R. Snyder and D. O. Forsyth. New York: Pergamon.

Coyne, J. C., and DeLongis, A. (1986). Going beyond social support: the role of social relationships in adaptation. *Journal of Consulting and Clinical Psychology* 54:454–460.

Coyne, J. C., Downey, G., and Boergers, J. (in press). Depression in families: a systems perspective. In *Developmental Approaches to the Affective Disorders: Rochester Symposium on Developmental Psychopathology*, vol. 4, ed. D. Cicchetti and S. L. Toth. Rochester: University of Rochester.

Coyne, J. C., Kessler, R. C., Tal, M., et al. (1987). Living with a depressed person: burden and psychological distress. *Journal of Consulting and Clinical Psychology* 55:347–352.

Dadds, M. R. (1987). Families and the origins of child behavior problems. *Family Process* 26:341–355.

Dadds, M. R., Sanders, M. R., Behrens, B. C., and James, J. E. (1987). Marital discord and child behavior problems. A description of family interactions during treatment. *Journal of Clinical Child Psychology* 16:192–203.

Dolan, R. J., Calloway, S. P. Fonagy, P., et al. (1985). Life events, depression and hypothalamic-pituitary-adrenal axis function. *British Journal of Psychiatry* 147:429–433.

Downey G., and Coyne, J. C. (1990). Children of depressed parents: an integrative review. *Psychological Bulletin* 108.

Emery, R., Weintraub, S., and Neale, J. (1982). Effects of marital discord on the school behavior of children of schizophrenic, affectively disordered, and normal parents. *Journal of Abnormal Child Psychology* 16:215–225.

Field, T., Healy, B., Goldstein, S., et al. (1988). Infants of depressed mothers show "depressed" behavior even with nondepressed adults. *Child Development* 60:1569–1579.

Field, T., Sandberg, D., Garcia, R., et al. (1985) Pregnancy problems, postpartum depression, and early mother–infant interactions. *Developmental Psychology* 21:1151–1156.

Forehand, R., Wells, K., and Griest, D. (1980). An examination of the social validity of a parent training program. *Behavior Therapy* 11:488-502.

Fowles, D. C., and Gersh, F. S. (1979). Neurotic depression: the endogenous-reactive distinction. In *The Psychology of Depressive Disorders*. New York: Academic Press.

George, L. K., Blazer, D. G., Hughes, D. C., and Fowler, N. (1989). Social outcome and the outcome of major depression. *British Journal of Psychology* 32:478-485.

Hammen, C., Adrian, C., and Hiroto, D. (1988). A longitudinal test of the attributional vulnerability model in children at risk for depression. *British Journal of Clinical Psychology* 27:37-46.

Hammen, C., Burge, D., and Stansbury, K. (1990). Relationship of mother and child variables to child outcomes in a high-risk sample. A causal modeling analysis. *Developmental Psychology* 26:24-30.

Hammen, C., Gordon, D., Burge, D., et al. (1987). Communication patterns of mothers with affective disorders and their relationship to children's status and social functioning. In *Understanding Major Mental Disorder: The Contribution of Family Interaction Research*, ed. K. Hahlweg and M. Goldstein. New York: Family Process Press.

Hautzinger, M., Linden, M., and Hoffman, N. (1982). Distressed couples with and without a depressed partner: an analysis of their verbal interaction. *Journal of Behavior Therapy and Experimental Psychiatry* 13:307-314.

Hetherington, E. M., Stanley-Hagen, M., and Anderson, E. R. (1989). Marital transitions. A child's perspective. *American Psychology* 44:302-312.

Hinchcliffe, M., Hopper, D., and Roberts, F. J. (1978). *The Melancholy Marriage*. New York: Wiley.

Holmes, S. J., and Robins, L. N. (1988). The role of parental disciplinary practices in the development of depression and alcoholism. *Psychiatry* 51:24-36.

Hooley, J. M., Orley, J., and Teasdale, J. D. (1986). Levels of expressed emotion and relapse in depressed patients. *British Journal of Psychiatry* 148: 642-647.

Hoover, C. F., and Fitzgerald, R. G. (1981). Dominance in the marriage of affective patients. *Journal of Nervous and Mental Disease* 169:624-628.

Kahn, J., Coyne, J. C., and Margolin, G. (1985). Depression and marital conflict: the social construction of despair. *Journal of Social and Personal Relationships* 2:447-462.

Kashani, J. H., Carlson, G. A., Beck, N. C., et al. (1987). Depression, depressive symptoms, and depressed mood among a community sample of adolescents. *American Journal of Psychiatry* 144:931-934.

Keitner, G., and Miller, I. (1990). Major depression and family function ing. *American Journal of Psychiatry* 147:1128-1137.

Keller, M. B., Klerman, G. L., Lavori, P. W., et al. (1984). Long-term outcome of episodes of major depression: clinical and public health significance. *Journal of the American Medical Association* 252:788-792.

Kuyler, P. L., Rosenthal, L., Igel, G., et al. (1980). Psychopathology among children of manic depressive patients. *Biological Psychiatry* 15:589-597.

Leff, J., and Vaughn, C. E. (1985). *Expressed Emotion in Families: Its Significance for Mental Illness.* New York: Guilford.

Long, N., Forehand, R., Fauber, R., et al. (1987). Self-perceived and independently observed competence of young adolescents as a function of parental marital conflict and recent divorce. *Journal of Abnormal Child Psychology* 15:15-27.

Lytton, H. (1990). Child and parent effects in boys' conduct disorder. A reinterpretation. *Developmental Psychology* 26:683-697.

McLean, P. D., Ogsten, K., and Grauer, L. (1973). A behavioral approach to the treatment of depression. *Journal of Behavior Research and Experimental Psychiatry* 4:323-330.

Merikangas, K. R., Prusoff, B. A., Kupfer, D. J., and Frank, E. (1985). Marital adjustment in major depression. *Journal of Affective Disorders* 9:5-11.

Merikangas, K. R., Prusoff, B., and Weissman, M. M. (1988). Parental concordance for affective disorders: psychopathology in offspring. *Journal of Affective Disorders* 15:279-290.

Merikangas, K. R., Ranelli, C. J., and Kupfer, D. J. (1979). Marital interactions in hospitalized depressed patients. *Journal of Nervous Mental Disease* 167:689-695.

Merikangas, K. R., and Spiker, D. G. (1982). Assortative mating among in-patients with primary affective disorder. *Psychological Medicine* 12:753-764.

Merikangas, K. R., Weissman, M., and Prusoff, B. (1988). Depressives with secondary alcoholism, psychiatric disorders in offspring. *Journal of Studies in Alcoholism* 46:199-204.

Mitchell, J., McCauley, E., Burke, P., et al. (1989). Psychopathology in parents of depressed children and adolescents. *Journal of the American Academy of Child and Adolescent Psychiatry* 28(3):352-357.

Parker, G. (1981). Parental reports of depressives, an investigation of several explanations. *Journal of Affective Disorders* 3:131-140.

――― (1983). Parental 'affectionless control' as an antecedent of adult depression. *Archives of General Psychiatry* 134:138-147.

Parker, G., and Hadzi-Pavlovic, D. (1984). Modification of levels of depression in mother-bereaved women by prenatal and marital relationships. *Psychological Medicine* 14:125-135.

Patterson, G. R. (1982). *Coercive Family Process.* Eugene, OR: Castilia.

_____ (1990). *Depression and Aggression in Family Interaction*. Hillsdale, NJ: Lawrence Erlbaum.

Paykel, E. S. (1979). Causal relationships between clinical depression and life events. In *Stress and Mental Disorder*, ed. J. E. Barrett. New York: Raven Press.

Paykel, E. S., Myers, J. K., Dienelt, M. N., et al. (1969). Life events and depression: a controlled study. *Archives of General Psychiatry* 21:753–757.

Perris, C., Arrindell, C., Perris, H., et al. (1986). Perceived depriving parental rearing and depression. *British Journal of Psychiatry* 148:170–175.

Peterson, P., Coyne, J. C., and Kessler, R. C. (1991). Assortative mating for psychopathology in a community sample. Unpublished manuscript, University of Michigan.

Poznanski, E., and Zrull, J. P. (1970). Childhood depression. *Archives of General Psychiatry* 23:8–15.

Puig-Antich, J., Goetz, D., Davies, M., et al. (1989). A controlled family history study of prepubertal major depressive disorder. *Archives of General Psychiatry* 46:406–418.

Puig-Antich, J., Lukens, E., Davies, M., et al.(1985a). Psychosocial functioning in prepubertal major depressive disorders. *Archives of General Psychiatry* 42:500–507.

Puig-Antich, J., Lukens, E., Davies, M., et al. (1985b). Controlled studies of psychosocial functioning in prepubertal major depressive disorders, II. Interpersonal relationships after sustained recovery from the affective episode. *Archives of General Psychiatry* 42:511–517.

Quinton, D., Rutter, M., and Liddle, C. (1984). Institutional rearing, parenting difficulties and marital support. *Psychological Medicine* 14:107–124.

Radke-Yarrow, M., Richters, J., and Wilson, W. E. (1988). Child development in a network of relationships. In *Individual in a Network of Relationships*, ed. R. Hinde and J. Stevenson-Hinde. Cambridge, England: Cambridge University Press.

Radke-Yarrow, M., Belmont, B., Nottelman, E., and Bottomly, B. (1990). Young children's self-conceptions. Origins in the natural discourse of depressed and normal mothers and their children. In *The Self in Transition*, ed. D. Cicchetti and M. Beeghley. Chicago, IL: University of Chicago Press.

Richters, J. (1987). Chronic versus episodic stress and the adjustment of high-risk offspring. In *Understanding Major Mental Disorder: The Contribution of Family Interaction Research*, ed. K. Hahlweg and M. J. Goldstein, (pp. 74–90). New York: Family Process.

Richters, J., and Pelligrini, D. (1989). Depressed mothers' judgements about their children: an examination of the depression-distortion hypothesis. *Child Development* 60:1068-1075.

Rounsaville, B. J., Prusoff, B. A., and Weissman, M. M. (1980). The course of marital disputes in depressed women: a 48-month follow-up study. *Comprehensive Psychiatry* 21:111-118.

Rounsaville, B. J., Weissman, M. M., Prusoff, G. A., and Herceg-Baron, R. L. (1979). Marital disputes and treatment outcome in depressed women. *Comprehensive Psychiatry* 20:483-490.

Roy, A. (1978). Risk factors and depression in Canadian women. *Journal of Affective Disorders* 3:69-70.

Rush, A. J., Shaw, B., and Khatami, M. (1980). Cognitive therapy of depression: utilizing the couples system. *Cognitive Therapy and Research* 4:103-113.

Strober, M., (1984). Familial aspects of depressive disorders in early adolescence. In *Current Perspectives on Major Depressive Disorder in Children*, ed. E. B. Weller and R. A. Weller, pp. 37-48. Washington, DC: American Psychiatric Press.

Swann, W. B., Jr., and Predmore, S. C. (1985). Intimates as agents of social support: sources of consolation or despair? *Journal of Personality and Social Psychology* 49:1609-1617.

Vaughn, C. E., and Leff, J. (1976). The influence of family and social factors on the course of psychiatric illness. *British Journal of Psychiatry* 129:125-137.

Weissman, M. M. (1987). Advances in psychiatric epidemiology: rates and risks for depression. *American Journal of Public Health* 77:445-451.

Weissman, M. M., and Paykel, E. S. (1974). *The Depressed Woman.* Chicago: University of Chicago Press.

Weissman, M. M., Prusoff, B. A., Gammon, G. D., et al. (1984). Psychopathology in children (ages 6-18) of depressed and normal parents. *Journal of the American Academy of Child Psychiatry* 23:78-84.

Weller, R. (1990). Parents of depressed children and adolescents. Presentation: Institute VI. Childhood Depression and Its Family Context: Explorations and Interventions. Chicago, IL, October.

Wells, K. B., Stewart, A., Hays, R. D., et al. (1989). The functioning and well-being of depressed patients. Results from the Medical Outcomes Study. *Journal of the American Medical Association* 262:914-919.

Zahn-Waxler, C., Iannotti, R. J., Cummings, E. M., and Denham, S. (1990). Antecedents of problem behaviors in children of depressed mothers. *Development and Psychopathology* 2:271-291.

Zahn-Waxler, C., and Kochanska, G. (1990). The origins of guilt. In *Thirty-Sixth Annual Nebraska Symposium on Motivation*, ed. R. Thompson, pp. 183-258.

Zahn-Waxler, C., McKnew, D. H., Cummings, E. M., et al. (1984). Problem behaviors in peer interaction of young children with a manic-depressive parent. *American Journal of Psychiatry* 141:236-240.

4: DEPRESSION IN CHILDREN AND ADOLESCENTS

John O. Viesselman, M.D.
Elizabeth B. Weller, M.D.
Ronald A. Weller, M.D.

INTRODUCTION

Until the past decade, the presence of depression in children as a diagnostic entity was doubted. Rie (1966) stated that "the familiar manifestations of adult, nonpsychotic depression are virtually non-existent in childhood. There is remarkable consensus about this finding" (p. 654). He goes on to give examples of children who demonstrate the features of adult depression and then dismisses these findings on theoretical grounds. Much of his argument against the existence of depression in childhood assumes that because the dynamics of depression do not seem to be the same as in adult depression, then depression in children does not exist. This implies that depression springs from a common dynamic. The doubt about the existence of childhood depression was due mainly to these assumptions about etiology and not to the presence of the observable signs and symptoms of depression. The signs and symptoms were clearly stated in the examples he used in his discussion.

Since the advent of the *Diagnostic and Statistical Manual of Mental Disorders* (*DSM-III-R* [3rd ed.–rev.] American Psychiatric Association 1987), psychiatrists are more familiar with diagnosing conditions according to an operationally defined set of criteria. In

Rie's (1966) paper the children he uses as examples from the literature meet criteria for one of the affective disorders; however, the underlying assumptions about etiology prevented him from seeing this. From our current perspective, we view these cases as examples of depression in children. It is hoped that our current scientific process will yield results based on scientific findings rather than a priori theories about etiology, pathogenesis, and outcome. As Puig-Antich (1987) states, "the main research question being asked a decade ago, namely, 'Do affective disorders exist in children and adolescents?' [is] obsolete" (p. 843). This is due to the large body of knowledge that has accumulated about affective disorders in children and the current focus of research on delineating the features, course, and outcome of childhood depression, including their relationship to adult affective disorders.

HISTORY

One form of childhood depression described historically is *anaclitic depression* (Spitz and Wolfe 1946). Anaclitic depression is a condition occurring in infancy upon separation from the mother for longer than a 3-month period of time during the second 6-month period of the first year of life. For anaclitic depression to occur, adequate attachment and bonding to the mother must have occurred. The clinical picture of anaclitic depression is one of withdrawal and regression. Bowlby (1969) describes the infant's response to separation as being protest, despair, and detachment. In anaclitic depression, the infant regresses over the 3-month period from being clingy, demanding, weepy, and wailing to being withdrawn, being apathetic, and having motor retardation. Insomnia and anorexia as well as weight loss are present. Conditions similar to these have also been described as nonorganic failure to thrive (Chatoor and Egan 1983, English 1978), environmental failure to thrive (Barbero and Shaheen 1967), psychosocial deprivation (Caldwell 1971), maternal deprivation (Patton and Gandner 1962), and deprivation dwarfism (Silver and Finkelstein 1967). Some of these may represent other disorders; however, the depressive features of the disorders appear to stem from the breaking of the attachment bond between infant and mother over a long period of time (Blumberg 1977). These disorders can also occur when maternal deprivation comes about due to changes in job schedules and caretaking arrangements

(Agarwal et al. 1985). The difference between Spitz and Wolfe's anaclitic depression and Bowlby's characterization of the response of the infant to separation is the duration of the separation. Bowlby (1969) means immediate and short-term separation responses, and Spitz and Wolfe (1946) mean responses to separation of 3 months or greater.

Kashani and colleagues (1981b) review some of the dynamics of depression in childhood. One dynamic is the loss of a desired object or goal. The desired object might be a love object, such as a mother or father, and the desired goal might be the desire to be loved and nurtured by a parent. In this formulation, depression is an ego-state that is brought about when an infant is aware of what it desires and wishes to obtain and is unable to do so. The infant needs to be aware that "I want . . . " and be unable to get it for depression to occur. This ego-state is "independent of the aggressive drive." One major theoretical objection to depression in children was that the ego in children, by definition, is just beginning to develop. In addition, the superego in children is also primitive and incompletely developed. Because of this lack of fully developed egos and superegos, it was theoretically believed that depression as seen in adults could not occur in children (Rie 1966).

Kashani and colleagues (1981b) trace the development of depression from being a reaction to loss or separation to its current status as a diagnosable disorder. As awareness of the presence of depressive symptoms in children increased, there began to be attempts to characterize and classify childhood depression. In 1966, Kurt Glaser stated that "In the child and adolescent, depression is often not recognized as such because it may be hidden by symptoms not readily identified with this condition" (p. 565), which gave rise to the concept of *masked depression*. In his paper he stated that "symptoms which in adults are usually considered diagnostic for depression — such as suicidal attempts or suicide — do not necessarily point toward the same diagnosis in children but may be impulsive acts, indicating acute anger or rebellion, rather than chronic depression" (p. 565). The concept of masked depression was often related to the underlying feelings of unhappiness and low self-esteem often elicited from delinquent children in psychotherapy. These were children whom we might currently consider dysthymic. In developing the concept of masked depression in children, Glaser (1967) also discounted the obvious possibility that children who attempt or commit suicide may be depressed. He also stated that "behavioral problems and delinquent behaviors, such as temper tantrums, disobedience, truancy, and running away from home, may indicate depressive feelings but may not be manifested as such" (p. 567). Thus, masked depression requires the belief that what seems to be depression is not, and what appears not to be depression is.

Carlson and Cantwell (1980a) examined 102 children systematically, using a semistructured interview to elicit symptoms to diagnose children according to *DSM-III* criteria. They used research diagnostic criteria (RDC) (Spitzer et al. 1979) to assess the occurrence of depressive symptoms. They demonstrated that affective disorders in children could be diagnosed according to adult criteria. In their study, children who met criteria for affective disorders could have behavior disorders, and children with behavior disorders could have affective disorders. Half of the children with affective disorders had behavior disorders or other *DSM-III* disorders. They concluded that the lack of systematic inquiry into symptoms of depression in children and adolescents was a more likely explanation for the appearance of masked depression than the true existence of a separate hidden syndrome. Many of the children had behavior problems, but depression was also quite apparent when systematically assessed.

If conduct and affective disorders were merely different manifestations of the same disorder, then one would expect that over time a number of children with just conduct disorders would eventually appear as having affective disorders, and a number of children with just affective disorders would eventually appear as having conduct disorders. Cantwell and Baker's (1989) 3-to 5-year follow-up study shows a general low stability of the affective and conduct diagnoses over time, mostly due to recovery. The authors mention that the children with affective disorders seem less likely to develop conduct disorders than children with other emotional disorders. Conversely, it appears from their data that children with conduct disorders are less likely to develop affective disorders than children with other behavioral disorders. If children with affective disorders tend not to develop conduct disorders and vice versa, this suggests that these disorders are distinct and that one of the disorders is not simply a masked version of the other.

The question of masked depression in children and adolescents raised the issue about the presence of conduct symptoms in children with depression. Carlson and Cantwell (1980b) looked at children who had the onset of depression symptoms before their behavior symptoms (primary affective disorder) and compared them with children who had the onset of behavior problems before the depression symptoms (secondary affective disorder). The authors noted that 71 percent of children who had a diagnosis of primary affective disorder had behavior problems such as fighting, arguing, and being disobedient. However, these problems were *not* seen by the parents as being the child's major problem. In contrast, in the children with secondary affective disorder, 75 percent of the children had major behavior problems such as reckless hyperactivity, truancy, and antisocial acts, which were seen by the parents as the major problem causing them to seek treatment.

Children with affective disorders do have conduct and behavioral symptoms. If the behavioral symptoms are chronic and antedate the affective symptoms, then they are much more likely to be severe and the chief reason for seeking help. If the affective symptoms antedate the behavioral symptoms, then the behavioral problems are likely to be seen by the parents as mild and incidental. In summary, conduct symptoms certainly do occur, but their temporal relationship to the onset of the depression seems to be the crucial factor in determining their severity and persistence.

Somatic symptoms were mentioned as well in a number of early studies (Brumbach et al. 1977, Frommer 1968, Ling et al. 1970, Mendelson et al. 1971, Ossofskey 1974, Poznanski and Zrull 1970). The somatic symptoms include headaches, stomachaches, muscle aches, nausea, vomiting, colic, allergies, anorexia, enuresis, and encopresis. Some of these symptoms, particularly headaches, were thought to be depressive equivalents. However, Ling and colleagues (1970) studied children who presented with a chief complaint of headache at a neurology clinic. When these children were asked about depressive symptoms, ten out of twenty-five met full criteria for depression. These criteria were essentially the same as current *DSM-III* criteria for a depressive episode. Headache and somatic symptoms appear from these early studies to be additional symptoms that were associated with depression and not necessarily depressive equivalents concealing an underlying depression. The symptoms of depression were not concealed when asked about.

Much of the confusion in the early studies seems to have come about due to difficulty in deciding which symptoms to include in the definition of depression. Which symptoms were necessary and sufficient for a diagnosis of depression? Should headaches be included? Should aggressive symptoms be included? Was the presence of depressive symptoms simply due to a phase of development or a child's immature way of expressing rebellion and anger? Was depression in children a disorder as in adulthood? Were conduct and behavioral symptoms really a manifestation of underlying depression?

In an attempt to clarify some of the confusion about these issues, Cantwell (1983) discussed and pointed out the differences between depression as a symptom, a syndrome, and a disorder. He believed that the symptom of dysphoric mood could be multidetermined. It may not be part of a depressive disorder but could be due to disappointment, loss, or another psychiatric disorder or merely as part of a naturally occurring variability of mood. He emphasized the need to distinguish among these possibilities. The depressive syndrome is dysphoric mood, plus a cluster of other symptoms that can present as a primary problem or be associated with a variety of other medical and psychiatric disorders. *Depressive disorder* implies a depressive syndrome plus some degree of functional impairment and a specific clinical picture, natural history, and response to treatment.

Because disorder implies impairment, what are the kinds of impairment that occur in children who are depressed? The major work that children do is school work, therefore, declining grades may be a type of impairment. Also, the child is involved in relationships with peers, family, and teachers, so impairment may show up in those areas. Puig-Antich and colleagues (1985a) looked at impairment in psychosocial functioning in prepubertal children with a major depressive disorder. They diagnosed the children using RDC, compared them with a neurotic group and a normal control group; measured the children's relationships with mother, father, and peers; and collected information on school functioning. The results showed that the children who met criteria for a depressive disorder had more impairment in school behavior, academic achievement, relationships with teachers, reading, spelling, and arithmetic than did the nondepressed neurotic children or the normal controls. They also had more impaired relationships with mother, father, and peers. The areas that were affected included amount and depth of communication, warmth, hostility, tension, group activities, punishment, and maintenance of friendships, the depressed children being impaired in all of these. The parents of depressed children had more conflict about child rearing. The children with endogenous depression were sexually more impaired than those with nonendogenous depression. In a follow-up study of a treated subsample of these children, Puig-Antich and colleagues (1985b) found that school impairments improved; however, the children still showed residual impairments in relationships. This study demonstrates the importance of considering impairment when distinguishing between disorder and syndrome.

PHENOMENOLOGY

A number of attempts were made to describe the signs and symptoms of depression in children and to characterize the phenomenology of the disorder. Because different investigators were using different criteria to diagnose depression in children and adolescents (Frommer 1968, Malmquist 1971a,b, Poznanski and Zrull 1970, Weinberg et al. 1973), the National Institute of Mental Health (NIMH) convened a conference in 1975 to attempt to coordinate this effort. As a result of this conference, a series of recommendations were made. First, the committee reached an agreement to consider depression in childhood as a syndrome that manifests observable impairment in functioning. Second, they recommended approaching this problem by using four strategies: (1) assume that the syndrome of depression exists in children as it does in adults and attempt, via research, to validate this; (2) survey professionals who have worked with children to attempt to elicit core and auxiliary symptoms of depression; (3) (the strategy favored by the committee) define the problem as the systematic description of the grief reaction (such as due to loss of a parent or loved one) at various ages and define depression as the statistically deviant response to loss; and (4) study at risk children whose parents have an affective disorder and could be considered high risk. Since the conference, a number of investigators have concluded that childhood and adolescent depression can be diagnosed according to adult criteria (Weller and Weller 1990b). Several authors then studied the application of adult criteria to depressive disorders in children and adolescents. Puig-Antich and Chambers (1978) demonstrated that children could be diagnosed according to adult criteria. He used unmodified RDC for major depressive disorder in thirteen prepubertal children and found the children met criteria for major depressive disorder including endogenous and psychotic subtypes (with hallucinations). All of the children showed separation anxiety, and five of the older boys had conduct symptoms as well.

In addition, Carlson and Cantwell (1979) surveyed a population of children according to RDC and *DSM-III* criteria to assess the utility of using adult criteria for affective disorders. They found 27 percent of their children met criteria for an affective disorder. Although affective symptoms were present in the children with other *DSM-III* disorders, they were much more prevalent in the children with affective diagnoses. Strober and colleagues (1981) used the Schedule for Affective Disorders and Schizophrenia (SADS) and categorized the affective disorder diagnoses into their respective subtypes for forty adolescents who met *DSM-III* criteria for major depression. These adolescents demonstrated high interrater reliability for individual symptoms. Strober and colleagues noted that the core symptoms of *DSM-III* depression were present in 65–95 percent of their sample. Other symptoms were present with less frequency. They noted the presence of somatic concerns (30 percent, delusions (13 percent), and affective hallucinations (10 percent). The distribution of affective subtypes (e.g., psychotic, endogenous, etc.) did not differ from the distribution seen in adults, with one exception. Endogenous and incapacitating affective disorders occurred less frequently in the adolescents.

Strober and colleagues (1981) also looked at the incidence of depressive equivalent symptoms in adolescents with affective disorders and in adolescent psychiatric controls with nonaffective diagnoses. They noted a 23 percent incidence of school avoidance, a 20 percent incidence of somatic complaints, and a 10–18 percent incidence of acting-out and conduct problems (aggression, running away, disobedience, etc.) in the adolescents with affective disorders. Except for somatic complaints, the incidence of these symptoms was higher in the psychiatric controls than in the adolescents with affective disorders. The nonaffective psychiatric controls had diagnoses of conduct, personality, somatoform, dissociative, adjustment, oppositional, and substance abuse disorders. Furthermore, the depressive equivalents that were present in the adolescents with affective disorders usually developed concurrently or after the onset of the affective symptoms.

Chambers and colleagues (1982) looked for the presence of psychopathologically meaningful psychotic symptoms in prepubertal children using a semistructured diagnostic interview. They found meaningful hallucinations present in 38 percent of their entire sample of children who met RDC for major depressive disorder (MDD). Forty-eight percent of the endogenously depressed and 28 percent of the nonendogenously depressed had psychopathologically significant hallucinations. Only four of fifty-eight prepubertal children reported significant delusions.

Livingston and colleagues (1988) looked at the frequency of somatic symptoms by *DSM-III-R* diagnosis in ninety-five hospitalized children. They showed that the only somatic symptom that was characteristically more common in depression was abdominal pain. Often this was seen more frequently in separation anxiety disorder and psychosis as well.

Carlson and Cantwell (1982) evaluated two sets of criteria for affective disorders in children. They compared children who met *DSM-III* criteria with children who met Weinberg criteria (Weinberg et al. 1973) and with children who met both. The different criteria did not identify the same group of children although there was considerable overlap. The *DSM-III* criteria were more restrictive. The children in the *DSM-III* groups rated themselves as more depressed on the Children's Depression Inventory (CDI) than did the children in the Weinberg-only group. The family histories, according to family history research diagnostic criteria (FHRDC) (Andreasen 1977), showed that children who met Weinberg criteria had less family history of pure depression. They were unable to say which set of criteria was more useful because there was no criterion by which to judge. They concluded that biological, treatment, and follow-up studies would be necessary to determine this.

Poznanski and colleagues (1985) compared four different sets of diagnostic criteria for depression (RDC, *DSM-III*, Weinberg, and Poznanski) in a sample of sixty-five prepubertal outpatients. They were different in the following ways: RDC and *DSM-III* criteria do *not* include looking sad, poor self-esteem, social withdrawal, somatic complaints, and change in attitude toward school.

Poznanski's criteria do not include pervasive anhedonia, loss of self-esteem, agitation, appetite change, somatic complaints, and change in attitude toward school. Weinberg's criteria do not include pervasive anhedonia, psychomotor retardation, anhedonia, and pathological guilt. All children who met *DSM-III* criteria for depression met RDC and vice versa. *DSM-III*, RDC, Poznanski, and Weinberg criteria agreed on the presence or absence of depression in 86 percent of the sample. The criteria sets disagreed on only nine children. There were seven children diagnosed depressed by both Weinberg's and Poznanski's criteria, and not depressed according to *DSM-III* and RDC. Six of these children were diagnosed because Weinberg's and Poznanski's criteria allow nonverbal dysphoria to qualify as one of the essential necessary symptoms of depression, whereas *DSM-III* and RDC do not. Nonverbal dysphoria is dysphoria inferred from the child's sad and depressed appearance (which is allowed by *DSM-III* if the child is under 6). If *DSM-III* and RDC had allowed nonverbal dysphoria to substitute for child or parent verbal reports of dysphoria in these 6- to 12-year-old children, then the four sets for of criteria would have agreed on forty-four out of forty-five of the diagnoses of depression and eighteen out of twenty of the children diagnosed as not depressed. This would be an overall agreement rate among the four sets of criteria of sixty-two out of sixty-five cases (95 percent). The authors looked at the *sensitivity* (the symptom's ability to identify true cases) and *specificity* (the symptom's ability to exclude false cases). Pervasive anhedonia was not a very sensitive symptom of depression because it did not occur often; however, it occurred exclusively in children who met criteria for depression (very specific). Nonverbal dysphoria was both sensitive and specific, showing good ability to both pick true cases and exclude false cases.

In summary, children and adolescents show similarities to and differences from adults in their manifestations of depression. Depressed prepubertal children differ from depressed adolescents. The specific criteria selected to diagnose depression in children and adolescents can also influence the number that will be diagnosed as depressed or as having some other psychiatric diagnosis. Finally, it has been demonstrated that, despite the differences from adults, depression in children and adolescents can be diagnosed by adult criteria.

CRITERIA

Which criteria should be used? Most of the criteria sets are similar, and depression in children can be diagnosed accurately according to *DSM-III-R* criteria (Weller and Weller 1990a). These criteria need to be modified somewhat to take into account the child's developmental level. Information is obtained from both parent and child. Additional information can be obtained from teachers and previous clinicians.

Reich and Earls (1987) proposed a strategy for making psychiatric diagnoses when there are multiple sources of information. They discuss how to resolve differences between the parent and child reports. They conclude that usually, the child's report alone is sufficient for diagnosis and is the most important source of information. The diagnoses of depression (in older children), separation overanxious disorder, conduct disorder, and alcohol and substance abuse can be made from the child interview alone in most cases. Parental and school information is adjunctive and helps confirm or deny diagnoses. Teacher information is particularly helpful in behavioral diagnoses. The reliability of children in the 6- to 9-year-old range is the lowest and needs to be taken into consideration for that age range.

DSM-III-R Diagnoses

Several diagnostic conditions are represented in *DSM-III-R*. These are major depressive disorder, depression with seasonal pattern, dysthymia, major depressive disorder superimposed on dysthymia (double depression), bipolar disorder-depressed, depressive disorder not otherwise specified, cyclothymia, major depression with psychotic features, organic mood disorder-depressed, adjustment disorder with depressed mood, uncomplicated bereavement, and melancholia.

A diagnosis of *major depressive disorder* requires that a depressive episode be present for at least 2 weeks. A depressive episode is defined as five or more of the following signs and symptoms: depressed (dysphoric) mood, loss of interest or pleasure, significant weight loss or weight gain, psychomotor agitation or retardation, loss of energy or fatigue, feelings of worthlessness or excessive inappropriate guilt, diminished concentration, recurrent thoughts of death, suicidal ideation, suicide attempt, or specific plan for committing suicide.

Major depression with seasonal pattern is diagnosed when the onset of a recurrent major depression occurs during a specific 60-day period from the beginning of October to the end of November, and the depression remits during a specific 60-day period that occurs from mid-February to mid-April. Seasonal affective disorder has clearly been defined in children (Rosenthal et al. 1986, Sonis et al. 1987, Sulik and Sonis 1987). Children show the same impairment at school as adults do at work. They also show irritability and impaired concentration. Most seem to have hypersomnia, and about 40 percent of those with hypersomnia have increased appetite and carbohydrate craving. They also respond to light therapy similarly to adults (Rosenthal et al. 1986, Sonis et al. 1987).

Dysthymia is defined as a depressed or irritable mood for at least one year and the presence of two or more of the following: poor appetite or overeating, insomnia or hypersomnia, low energy or fatigue, low self-esteem, poor concentration, and feelings of hopelessness.

Major depression superimposed on dysthymia (or double depression) is a major depressive episode occurring in the presence of a preexisting dysthymic disorder.

Bipolar disorder-depressed is a disorder in which a child or adolescent presents with a major depressive episode and has a history of one or more past manic episodes.

Cyclothymia is a disorder in which there is a history of numerous hypomanic episodes alternating with periods of depressed mood and loss of interest or pleasure of at least one year's duration.

Major depression with psychotic features is the presence of a depressive episode with mood congruent or mood incongruent psychotic features. As previously mentioned, significant hallucinations occur in about 38 percent of depressed children and adolescents and delusions in about 8 percent (Puig-Antich 1982).

Organic mood disorder — depressed is a depressive episode with prominent and persistent depressed mood and the evidence from history, physical examination, or laboratory tests of a specific organic factors(s) judged to be etiologically linked to the mood disturbance.

Adjustment disorder with depressed mood is defined as a reaction to an identifiable psychosocial stressor that occurs within 3 months of the onset of the stressor. The maladaptive reaction is either impaired occupational or school functioning or symptoms such as depressed mood, fearfulness, and feelings of hopelessness that are in excess of a normal reaction to the stressor.

Uncomplicated bereavement is a normal reaction to the death of a loved one. Weller and Weller (1990b) have demonstrated that a full depressive syndrome is the most frequent response of children to parental death. The reaction includes feelings of depression, poor appetite, weight loss, and insomnia.

Melancholia is a subtype of major depression. It consists of depressed mood and five of the following signs and symptoms: lack of interest or pleasure in all or almost all activities, lack of reactivity to usually pleasurable stimuli, depression being worse in the morning, psychomotor agitation or retardation, significant anorexia or weight loss, no significant personality disturbance before the first major depressive episode followed by complete or nearly complete recovery, and previous good response to specific and adequate somatic antidepressant therapy.

Differential Diagnosis and Co-morbidity

Although childhood and adolescent depressions can be diagnosed according to *DSM-III-R* criteria, certain differential diagnostic problems exist. For example, the criteria for melancholia for children are too strict. Children usually have not had previous depressive episodes, and a presenting episode of depression in children is usually the first episode. Children have not usually been previously treated with somatic antidepressant therapy and do not usually have personality diagnoses. Therefore, in order to meet criteria for melancholia, a child or adolescent would have to meet five out of six of the remaining criteria. This makes it harder to fulfill criteria for melancholia in children than in adults.

Also, major depression with seasonal pattern needs to be distinguished from an adjustment disorder with depressed mood that might occur at the beginning of the school year. Because the beginning of the school year and the onset of seasonal affective disorder coincide, this distinction is often difficult to make. The stresses and strains of new schools, new classes, new friends, or new academic pressures may precipitate an episode of dysphoria that may appear as seasonal affective disorder. A key feature that may help to distinguish between these disorders may be a seasonal pattern occurring over several years that does not seem to change with yearly circumstances.

Because a substantial number of children have conduct and somatic symptoms, determining the chronology and chronicity of the behavioral and conduct symptoms can help differentiate between conduct symptoms that are related to the affective disorder and affective symptoms that are part of the conduct disorder.

The differential between affective and anxiety disorders also needs to be considered. Mitchell and colleagues (1988) evaluated 125 children who presented with depression, school refusal, or suicidal ideation with the Kiddie Schedule for Affective Disorders and Schizophrenia (K-SADS). The symptom profile for the prepubertal children and the adolescents who met RDC for major depression basically did not differ except for hypersomnia, which was reported more frequently by the adolescents. Anxiety disorders coexisted in almost half of the total sample with no real difference between children and adolescents. The symptoms of depression were rated as much more severe in children who had both depression and anxiety disorder than in those with depression alone.

The rate of anxiety disorders coexisting with depression varies depending on the study. Asarnow and Ben-Meir (1988), using the K-SADS-E (epidemiological version), diagnosed coexisting anxiety disorders in 19 percent of the patients with major depression and 11 percent of the patients with dysthymic disorder. Hughes and colleagues (1989), using the Diagnostic Interview for Children and Adolescents (DICA) (Herjanic and Reich 1982) to diagnose children between 6 and 12 years of age, found only a 4.4 percent incidence of anxiety disorders.

The rate of associated conduct disorder varies from a low of 15–20 percent (Asarnow and Ben-Meir 1988, Mitchell et al. 1988) to a high of 49 percent (Hughes et al. 1989). The differences may be related to the different types of interviews used and the outpatient/inpatient mix of patients.

Hershberg and colleagues (1982) interviewed 102 children and adolescents according to *DSM-III* criteria. Of the 102 children, 28 met criteria for depressive disorders and 14 for anxiety disorders. They compared the frequency of occurrence of depressive and anxiety symptoms in these 42 children. The frequency of depressive symptoms in the anxiety disorder group was lower than in the depressive disorder group. Conversely, the frequency of anxiety symptoms in the depressive disorder group was lower than in the anxiety disorder group. These observations support the proposition that the two disorders are discrete. The anxiety disorder group had similar frequencies for poor school performance, appetite changes or weight gain, fatigue, sleep disturbance, hopelessness, and somatic complaints. The depressed group had dysphoric mood, poor self-esteem, anhedonia, and suicidal ideation more frequently. The anxiety group had a higher rate of situation-specific anxiety than the depressed group.

A number of studies have looked at the incidence of depressive disorders in patients with anxiety disorders (Anderson et al. 1987, Bernstein 1991, Kovacs et al. 1989, McGee 1990, Mitchell et al. 1988, Ryan et al. 1987a). The frequency of depressive disorders in children with anxiety disorders varies from 12 percent to 47 percent in different studies. The severity of the anxiety or depressive disorder is greater in those children who have both depressive and anxiety symptoms.

Geller and colleagues (1985) specifically assessed fifty-nine children with major depression for anxiety and conduct symptoms. They found that the onset of anxiety symptoms occurred after major depression 81 percent of the time, whereas the onset of antisocial behavior occurred after major depression 100 percent of the time. This data confirms the importance of determining the chronology of affective, anxiety, and conduct symptoms. The chronology of onset of symptoms is one of the best ways of differentiating between affective disorder, anxiety disorder, and conduct disorder.

AFFECTIVE DISORDERS AND SUICIDE

Shaffer (1974) studied suicide in children. Suicide was noted to be rare in children under the age of 12. In fact, Shaffer found no suicides before the age of 12. Seven years later, he stated that this low rate had been stable worldwide since 1955. The increase in the suicide rate occurs in adolescents 14 years and older. Carlson (1983) mentioned the rate in adolescents was 10 times the rate in 10- to 14-year-olds, and about 600 times the rate in children 9 and under (because of the virtual absence of suicides in that age range). Although the rate fluctuates, the rate for young adults from 15 to 24 is about 47.5/100, 000. This rate is close to the rate for adults. Since in adults suicide is a serious consequence of depression, is this the same for children and adolescents?

Brent and colleagues (1988) looked at a sample of children who were assessed for depression according to the Diagnostic Interview Schedule for Children (DISC). They classified suicidal ideation along a continuum from none to specific attempts. They demonstrated a correlation of the severity of the suicidal thought with the severity of the depression. Suicidal thought seemed to occur in a wide range of child and adolescent pathology. The frequency and severity of the symptoms of depression, however, accounted for the most statistically significant correlations.

Some investigators believe that suicide is a continuous phenomenon that ranges from death thoughts and preoccupation on one end to suicide on the other (Pfeffer 1991a). Others believe that the diagnostic characteristics of suicide attempters are different from those of suicide completers (Carlson and Cantwell 1982). This latter view is mostly based on data from adult studies and not on data from studies of children and adolescents who commit or attempt suicide. Brent and colleagues (1988) noted that adolescents who actually commit suicide are more severely ill than those who attempt it. They have more severe disorders (e.g., bipolar disorder, affective disorder with co-morbidity) and also have higher suicide intent. The current evidence is that those children who commit suicide are more severely ill than those who do not.

Hoberman and Garfinkel (1988) looked at the characteristics of 229 children and adolescents who had committed suicide. They generally used violent means to kill themselves. The most common methods were the use of firearms, hanging, carbon monoxide poisoning, drug ingestion, jumping from heights, and suffocation. Boys used firearms more frequently than girls, and girls overdosed more frequently than boys. Seventy percent of the suicides had precipitants associated with them, usually occurring in the 24-hour period preceding the suicide. The two most common precipitants were arguments with girlfriend, boyfriend, or parents and school problems, and they were the precipitants in one-third of the cases of completed suicide. At least 50 percent of the sample could retrospectively be diagnosed as having a psychiatric disorder. The most frequent diagnoses were depression, alcohol abuse, and drug abuse.

Although it is clear that suicide victims have high incidences of antisocial behavior, previous suicide attempts, and prior psychiatric treatment (Shafii et al. 1985), it is not clear how well these factors predict suicide. Borderline personality in females is associated with a higher frequency of suicide attempts (Friedman et al. 1983); however, because the percentage of actual suicides is so low, the significance of this finding can be applied only to suicide attempters and not generalized to suicide completers. Kupferman and colleagues (1988) followed up on 1, 331 child psychiatry inpatients and found only 11 suicides. The diagnoses of the suicidal patients based on chart review were schizophrenia (4), organic mental disorder (2), conduct disorder (1), personality disorder (1), neurotic disorder (1), mental retardation (1), and undiagnosed psychiatric disorder (1). However, these patients were all older than 17 at the time they committed suicide, so they really do not represent the population of child and adolescent suicide victims.

In summary, suicides in children less than age 13 are rare, and in children 13 and older more frequent. The rate of suicide in adolescents approaches adult levels in late adolescence. The characteristics of completed suicides resemble those seen in adults. The combination of affective disorders with drug and alcohol abuse is common. The same lethal means are used by those children and adolescents who complete suicide as are used by adults. Suicide among children who have had psychiatric treatment is 0.5–1 percent (Kupferman et al. 1988) and is infrequent even in follow-ups of suicide attempters (Pfeffer et al. 1991). It is not clear if the diagnostic characteristics of children who attempt suicide are the same as those of children who complete suicide.

EPIDEMIOLOGY

Fleming and Offord (1990) have stated that an understanding of the epidemiology of depression is important for three reasons: (1) to help in planning services, (2) to generate and test hypotheses about etiology, and (3) to eventually launch effective preventive efforts. The distinction between depression as a symptom, syndrome, or disorder has been mentioned. The epidemiology of depression differs depending on how depression is defined.

The epidemiology of depression as a symptom in children in the general population was addressed by Kashani and Sherman (1988). Of 109 children enrolled in nursery school, only 9 had depressive symptoms (8 percent), and only one child had a major depression. This illustrates that the prevalence of the individual symptoms of a disorder in a population is higher than the prevalence of the disorder (which by definition is more restrictive). A number of studies have examined the prevalence of depression in children and adolescents in the general population.

Fleming and Offord (1990) reviewed fourteen recent epidemiological studies to assess the prevalence of major depression, dysthymic disorders, and other depression in children and adolescents in the general population. The limitations of the studies are cited. The authors emphasized the need for proper sampling techniques, consistency in diagnostic criteria, and accurate measurement and methods of assessment. The prevalence of major depression in prepubertal children varied from 0.4 percent to 2.5 percent in seven studies. When parents were used as informants, the prevalence was lower than when child or teacher reports were used. The prevalence rates for major depression in adolescents varied from 0.4 percent to 6.4 percent in eight studies cited. One study gave a lifetime prevalence rate of 8.3 percent for major depression. Again, when the parent rather than the child was used as the informant, the prevalence rates differed by as much as a factor of five. This suggests that parents underreport depression in their children. The combined prevalence rate for all children and adolescents for major depression was 5.9 percent. The prevalence of dysthymic disorder ranged from 0.6 percent to 1.7 percent in children and 1.6 percent to 8.0 percent in adolescents. Rates of child-reported and adolescent-reported depression were consistently higher than parent-reported depression.

Fleming and Offord (1990) also looked at the issue of comorbidity. The most frequent disorders co-occurring with depression are anxiety disorders (in 32–75 percent of the sample) and conduct disorders (in 17–50 percent of the sample). Attention deficit hyperactivity disorder (ADHD) was seen in about 50 percent of the children and in 8–31 percent of the adolescents. Only two studies looked at drug and alcohol abuse and found that 23–25 percent of the depressed adolescents had these comorbid disorders.

The prevalence of depression also varies depending on the setting. Kashani and Carlson (1987) diagnosed depression in 0.9 percent of 1, 000 preschoolers who had been referred to a child development unit. In a pediatric hospital setting, depression was diagnosed in 7 percent of the patients. The rates of depression are higher in psychiatric samples. When depression is diagnosed by different clinicians in different populations of general psychiatric inpatients, differing prevalence rates are found. For example, Robbins and colleagues (1982) found depression in 27 percent of adolescent psychiatric inpatients, Petti (1978) in 59 percent of general psychiatric inpatients, Kashani and colleagues (1982) in 13 percent of children admitted to a community mental health center, and Carlson and Cantwell (1980a) in 28 percent of the patients in a child psychiatry clinic.

The rates in differing settings vary, but as Fleming and Offord (1990) point out, the rates in the general population also vary. The sources of variability appear to be due to factors such as sampling, the definition of a case (Beardslee et al. 1985), differing diagnostic instruments (e.g., DICA, DISC, K-SADS, CDI, CAS, etc.), and differing screening procedures. Also, in half of the studies reviewed by Fleming and Offord (1990), less than 75 percent of the target sample were actually evaluated. This response rate variability also was cited as a factor explaining differing prevalence rates.

Brandenburg and colleagues (1990) reviewed eight studies and suggested that the multimethod and multistage approach to ascertaining cases holds the most promise for more definitive epidemiological studies. Because of the large amount of variability present in current epidemiological studies, a large scale multicenter epidemiological study of the prevalence of psychiatric disorders in children needs to be undertaken. The scientific methodology and approach to conducting such a study have been amply described in the NIMH epidemiologic catchment area (ECA) program (Eaton and Kessler 1985).

FACTORS RELATED TO DEPRESSION

A number of factors can be related to depression (Birleson 1986): family relationships (Goodyer 1990), psychopathology in the parents (Klein et al. 1988, Mitchell et al. 1989, Rutter and Quinton 1984; Weissman et al. 1987), stressful life events (Goodyer et al. 1988,) Kashani et al. 1986), lack of support for parents (Goodyer et al. 1988), parenting styles and family interaction patterns (Cole and Rehm 1986), abuse and neglect (Livingston 1987), alcohol and drug abuse in parents (Strober 1984), and parental self-esteem (Cooper-smith 1967).

Rutter and Quinton (1984) did a 4-year prospective study of the families of 137 adult psychiatric patients who had children under the age of 15 living at home. The children of psychiatric patients were compared with a comparison group of school-age children. Their families were compared with a family comparison group. The children of the psychiatric patients were more frequently exposed to hostile and anxious/depressive behavior by the parents and were exposed to more extreme parental behaviors more frequently than the comparison group. They were also more physically involved in the extreme parental behaviors than the children in the comparison group. The extreme parental behaviors were related to the presence of marital discord, parental personality disorder, and affective disorders in the parent. Personality disorder was associated with persisting marital discord and an increased frequency of affective disorders in the spouses. Persistence of marital discord was associated with persistence of behavioral and emotional problems in the children, as assessed both by teacher questionnaire and by interview. The rate of depression in children with a psychiatric diagnosis whose parents did not have affective or personality disorder was 18 percent, whereas the rate of depression in children who had a psychiatric diagnosis whose parents had an affective disorder was 57 percent. This suggests a link between affective disorders in parents and their children.

Klein and colleagues (1988) compared the rate of affective disorders in the offspring of patients with primary unipolar major depressive disorder with the rate in the offspring of patients hospitalized with chronic orthopedic and rheumatologic conditions and normal controls. The offspring were diagnosed using the SADS-L (lifetime version). Thirty-two percent of the children of the parents with affective disorders had a *DSM-III* affective disorder diagnosis compared with 6 percent of the medical controls and none of the normal controls. Seventeen percent of the children of the depressed parents had a diagnosis of *DSM-III* dysthymia compared with none of the controls. The mean age of onset was 15.1 years of age, and the mean duration was 3.1 years.

Klein and colleagues (1988) also looked for the presence of subaffective dysthymia using the criteria of Akiskal and colleagues (1985). These criteria require that five of the following seven traits be present since the onset of adolescence: (1) quiet, nonassertive, preferring others to take the lead; (2) gloomy, pessimistic, serious, not having a great deal of fun; (3) self-critical, self-reproaching, self-derogatory; (4) skeptical, critical of others, hard to please; (5) conscientious, responsible, self-disciplined; (6) brooding, tending to worry a lot; and (7) preoccupied with negative events, feelings of inadequacy, and personal shortcomings. Twenty-one percent met these criteria in the unipolar offspring group compared with 6 percent and 3 percent in the medical and normal offspring group, respectively. In addition, having multiple relatives with affective disorders, persistence of parental depression, early onset of parental depression, and an increased number of hospitalizations for depression were associated with an increased risk for dysthymia in the offspring.

Weissman and colleagues (1987) demonstrated an increased risk for major depression, substance abuse, and multiple *DSM-III* diagnoses in the offspring of parents who met RDC for major depression compared with nonpsychiatrically ill controls. They showed that the age of onset of depression is lower in these children (12.7 years of age) than in the control children (16.8 years of age). More of the depressed children of depressed parents reported anhedonia than the depressed children of normal parents. Similar results were suggested in a study of the offspring of bipolar parents. Zahn-Waxler and colleagues (1988) followed the offspring of a small sample of bipolar parents. More of the children of the bipolar parents had two or more psychiatric diagnoses than did the controls. There was a tendency for the children of bipolar parents to have more depression, conduct problems, and anxiety problems than the control children. Internalizing problems, as identified from the Child Behavior Checklist (CBCL), were significantly more frequent in the offspring of bipolar parents. These are emotional and affective problems and support the suggestion that the children of bipolar parents are more likely to show disorders in the regulation of affect than control children. From these studies, it appears that having a parent with a psychiatric or personality disorder predisposes children to have affective disorders. Specifically, having a parent with a unipolar or bipolar affective disorder predisposes the child to have an affective disorder.

In addition to specific factors related to the occurrence of depression in children and adolescents, there are general risk factors to consider. Rutter and Quinton (1984) measured family adversity in a study of the children of psychiatrically disturbed parents. The measures of adversity that were associated with an increased risk of psychiatric or behavioral problems are the following: (1) psychiatric disorder/criminality in the mother or father, (2) marked marital discord, (3) children in foster care or admitted to a hospital, (4) four or more children at home, (5) overcrowding with 1.1 or greater persons per room, and (6) the head of the household in a semi- or unskilled job. In their study, the rates of emotional and behavioral problems in the children rose directly in proportion to the number of factors present.

Goodyer (1990) reviewed the family factors associated with increased psychopathology. He summarized research that demonstrated that depressed mothers hit and criticized their children more often than nondepressed mothers. The depressed mothers were distracted, preoccupied, and not as emotionally available to their infants. They did not smile or hug their children and often did not respond to their infant's cues. These findings were related to the presence of personality disorder in the mother. The mothers who had both personality disorder and depression were emotionally unavailable and did not interact with their children. The mothers who had just depression and no personality disorder showed sensitivity to their infants and interacted more positively with their children. Thus, as in the Rutter and Quinton (1984) study, personality disorder seems to be the mediating factor associated with dysfunctional parental patterns of interacting with children. These dysfunctional patterns may lead to later child pathology and increased childhood depression. It is clear that personality disorder in the parents is a risk factor for increased child behavior and emotional problems.

Goodyer and colleagues (1988) identified maternal factors that were related to increased frequency of anxiety and depression in children. Emotional disorders in the children consisted of anxiety and depressive disorders and were diagnosed by interview and questionnaire. They examined the role that lack of emotional support in the mother's life played in the rates of pathology in their children. They identified three factors: recent stressful life events in the mother's life, the degree to which the mother was distressed (maternal distress), and the quality of the mother's supportive confiding relationships. Maternal confiding relationships were defined as consisting of partners or close personal friends to whom the mothers could talk about their worries and spend time with and who would listen with interest and understanding. Recent stressful life events were determined by interview and were limited to undesirable recent stressful life events. Maternal distress was assessed by a valid and reliable questionnaire. The risk of emotional disorder in the child was multiplied by the presence of these adverse factors. The odds of emotional disorder in a child with recent stressful life events were 5:1, with maternal distress 5.5:1, and with poor maternal confiding relationships 3.5:1. If all three of these factors were present, the odds were 96.25:1 (5.5 × 5 × 3.5). In other words, the effects were independent and multiplicative rather than merely additive.

Divorce also produces a number of psychiatric conditions in children going through the breakup of their family. Depression occurs in about 30 percent of these children (Wallerstein 1985). It is difficult to disentangle the consequences of the predivorce marital discord from the divorce and dissolution itself. Because marital discord is associated with increased child and adolescent psychopathology, both the divorce process and the marital discord may be related to the child's problems. Persistence of marital discord has been mentioned as a factor and may persist as long as 11 years (Block et al. 1988). Younger children show more regression. Affective symptoms appear more frequently in children and adolescents. Tearfulness, fearfulness, confusion, anger, irritability, declining school performance, withdrawal, and acting-out behavior in previously well-cared-for children are not uncommon (Goodyer 1990). The incidence of depression of 30 percent is at least five to six times higher than the prevalence of depression in children and adolescents in the general population. It is also estimated that 38 percent of all children born in the mid-eighties will experience divorce (Wallerstein and Corbin 1991). According to these figures, 11.4 percent of children born in the mid-eighties will experience a depression related to divorce. This could account for a large number of cases of depression seen in clinical practice.

In summary, parenting styles and parental dysfunction have a significant association with child psychopathology. The specific effects, however, that may produce depression may be due to a combination of genetic and familial effects. Parental psychiatric disorder produces patterns of neglect, conflict, exposure to hostility, abuse, deviant value systems, and family discord. Chronic psychiatric disorders, criminality, and personality disorder are also associated with the persistence of the above-mentioned parenting behaviors. Persistence of these problems increases the frequency of psychopathology in the children. Family factors play a major role in the genesis and maintenance of child and adolescent depression. The main family factors associated with affective disorders in children are the presence of an affectively ill parent, negative and neglectful interactions with the children, bereavement, and divorce.

Developmental Factors

The manifestations of depression may not be the same over all ages. Many biological and behavioral functions vary over the course of development. Lapouse and Monk (1964) showed developmental differences in the types of fears and phobias children experience. Kovacs and Paulauskas (1984) were unable to demonstrate any developmental trends based on a Piagetian cognitive model of development in a sample of 8-to 13-year-old children. Ryan and colleagues (1987a) examined the symptom frequency and severity in both prepubertal and adolescent depressed children who met RDC for depression. They studied the symptom profiles to see if the symptom pattern varied based on age. Prepubertal children look depressed and have somatic complaints, psychomotor agitation, separation anxiety, phobias, and hallucinations more often than adolescents. Adolescents exhibit anhedonia, hopelessness, hypersomnia, change in weight, drug or alcohol abuse, and severe suicide attempts more often than prepubertal children.

Carlson and Kashani (1988) analyzed three studies done with different-aged children to assess developmental changes in symptom expression. The three studies were done with preschool children (Kashani and Carlson 1987), prepubertal children (Ryan et al. 1987a), and adults (Baker et al. 1971). The researchers were able to obtain relatively consistent symptom descriptions and frequencies for preschoolers, school-age children, adolescents, and adults. They concluded that anhedonia, diurnal variation of mood, psychomotor retardation, and delusions increase in frequency with age, whereas depressed appearance, somatic complaints, and hallucinations decreased with age.

In a later study, Kashani and colleagues (1989) directly

examined the frequency of symptoms in a sample of 8-, 12-, and 17-year-olds and had much the same findings as the earlier studies. Psychomotor agitation seems to occur more frequently in children and adults and drops to a low in adolescence. In summary, prepubertal depressed children tend to look sad and to be more somatic, anxious, and agitated, and adolescents tend to be more anhedonic and hopeless.

Temperamental Factors

Rutter and Quinton (1984) discussed the temperamentally difficult child and the difficult child's attributes of negative mood, low regularity, low malleability, and low fastidiousness. If a child had two or more of these temperamental characteristics, he was said to be of high temperamental risk. All of the children (100 percent) who had these characteristics had disturbance based on interview, as compared with 41 percent who did not have these characteristics.

Chess and colleagues (1983) reported on the development of depression in six of the cases in their New York longitudinal study. Although the number is small, this is the only prospective study that examined temperament, parenting, and the subsequent development of depression in children and adolescents. Their cases did not show a tendency to have temperamentally negative mood; however, four of the six cases did show extremes of one form of temperamental characteristic or another. Two of the cases had the temperamental pattern of the difficult child, one showed extreme persistence, and one showed extreme distractibility and short attention span. Chess and colleagues concluded that the interaction of these extreme temperamental characteristics with excessive parental or environmental demands appeared to have played a major historical role in the genesis of the depressions.

THEORIES OF DEPRESSION

A number of theories exist about the etiology of depression in children. These can be subsumed under the biopsychosocial rubric. The main theories are genetic, parent–child interactive, neuroendocrine, cognitive, psychoanalytic, behavioral, learned helplessness, and decreased self-esteem. All of these factors can play a role in depression; however, the relative contribution of each is currently unknown.

Genetic Factors

Genetic theories state that the etiology of depression is a predisposition that is transmitted genetically from parent to child. If twin studies show a higher rate of concordance for depression in children who are monozygotic twins than in children who are dizygotic twins, then this would be evidence supporting genetic factors. Also, if the frequency of depression is higher in the relatives of children who had depression than in the relatives of children who did not, this would further support genetic factors. If genetic factors were involved, one would expect that the frequency of depression would be higher in children whose parents had depression than in those who did not.

Concordance rates for depression are 76 percent for monozygotic twins who are raised together and 67 percent when they are raised apart. Concordance rates for dizygotic twins are 19 percent Akiskal and Weller 1989), which supports a strong genetic loading for affective disorders. Puig-Antich and colleagues (1989) showed an increased rate of depression, alcoholism, and anxiety disorders in the first-degree relatives of prepubertal children with affective disorders. Strober (1984) also found higher than expected rates of affective disorders in the relatives of depressed adolescents than would be expected from the adult epidemiological data. Finally, Weissman and colleagues (1987) found increased affective disorders in the children of parents with affective disorders. These studies are preliminary but provide support for a genetic component to affective disorders in children. In addition, these studies also suggest a possible parent–child relational component. Depression is seen in abused and neglected children. Depressed parents can be distracted and inattentive to their children and may be less involved. Depressed parents may model for their children anxious, pessimistic, and depressive ways of viewing the world and perhaps teach them cognitively distorted views of the world and the future. Chronically depressed parents may be irritable and subject their children to harsh and excessive criticism. These parent–child factors may also be operable in the genesis of the higher observed rates.

Neuroendocrine Factors

Neuroendocrine and neurophysiological theories predict that the genesis of depression will be found to be related to underlying neurochemical, hormonal, or electrophysiological abnormalities. Biological markers are classified into *state* or *trait* markers. *State* markers are those that are present during episodes of illness and absent during health or remission. *Trait* markers are those that can be measured even in the absence of active illness. Trait markers would be extremely helpful in identifying biologically vulnerable children who have not yet manifested depression. There are no known trait markers at present.

The dexamethasone suppression test (DST) is a state marker. Although it is associated with episodes of depression in some children, it is not present in all children with a diagnosis of depression. When it is present, however, it can be clinically helpful. It is positive in approximately 54 percent of depressed children and adolescents during episodes of depression (Weller and Weller 1988). Response to treatment and recovery are both correlated with DST results (Weller et al. 1986). When depression remits with treatment, the DST often returns to normal. The DST abnormalities in children and adolescents with depression imply a dysfunction of the hypothalamic-pituitary-adrenal axis.

As with many biochemical tests in children, the response to the test may be influenced by the stage of the child's development. This seems to be the case for the DST. In fact, the DST is more sensitive in children than in adolescents, either because prepubertal depression is more severe than depression occurring in adolescence, or because of some other unrecognized developmental reason. The DST, however, is as useful an empirical test in depressed children as it has been in depressed adults.

Other biological markers that have been studied in adult affective disorders include sleep parameters, growth hormone levels, and thyroid-stimulating hormone (TSH). A few studies have looked at these variables in children. The results of sleep studies in children are equivocal. The studies in adults show a decrease in stage 3 and stage 4 sleep, shortened rapid eye movement (REM) latency, and increased REM density (Kupfer et al. 1985). Three studies (Goetz et al. 1987, Puig-Antich et al. 1982, Young et al. 1982) were unable to find any differences in sleep architecture between depressed children and adolescents and controls. Two other studies found shorter REM latencies and increased REM density (Emslie et al. 1987, Lahmeyer et al 1983). The findings at the current time are equivocal, therefore further well-controlled research will be needed to answer these questions.

The findings with regard to growth hormone secretion are more positive. The secretion of growth hormone has been shown to be decreased in depressed children and adolescents in response to insulin-induced hypoglycemia (Meyer et al. 1985, Puig-Antich et al. 1984a), clonidine (Jensen and Garfinkel 1990, Meyer et al. 1985), apomorphine (Meyer et al. 1985), and desmethylimipramine (Ryan et al. 1987b). Growth hormone secretion in depressed children and adolescents was found to be elevated during sleep compared to controls (Kutcher et al. 1988, Puig-Antich et al. 1984b). Puig-Antich and colleagues (1984c,) found that children who had recovered from endogenous depression continued to show a blunted growth hormone secretory response to insulin and increased secretion during sleep. This occurred even after the children had 3–4 months of recovery and were off medication for at least 1 month. This suggests that growth hormone may be a trait marker; however, follow-up is still too short for a definitive conclusion. These findings in children are similar to those in depressed adults. They are preliminary and still represent only a small population of children actually studied.

The studies of thyroid-releasing hormone (TRH) stimulation completed to date have been negative (Chabrol et al. 1983, Greenberg et al. 1985). In depressed adults, the usual pattern is a blunted response of TSH to intravenous TRH injection. This response is seen in about 24 percent of depressed adults (Loosen and Prange 1982). From the studies cited, there is no evidence that this response occurs in children or adolescents who meet criteria for depression.

Cognitive Theories

Cognitive theories of depression in adults emphasize the kinds of cognitive distortions that occur in depression (Beck et al. 1979). These include magnification, minimization, selective abstraction, overgeneralization, dichotomous thinking, superstitious thinking, and personalization and self-reference. These distortions are cognitively employed to support the cognitive triad that maintains the depressive state. The cognitive triad refers to a negative and pessimistic view of the self, the world, and the future. These distortions are seen in the depressive state and less in the recovered state. In children, this theory has been tested in controlled studies only in group treatment (Reynolds and Coats 1986). In these studies, the children with depression seemed to respond to simple relaxation training as well as to the more complex cognitive approach. Further controlled studies are needed to assess if this theory applies in children the same as in adults, and if treatment based on this theory works as effectively as other treatment approaches.

Learned Helplessness

According to the theory of learned helplessness (Seligman 1975), learned helplessness occurs when people learn that they are helpless to control the outcome of seemingly uncontrollable events. This produces the expectation that nothing the person does will alter the outcome so there is no further motivation to try assertive or problem-solving behavior. This pattern of behavior deficits becomes global and, once established, persists. These deficits persist even when assertive problem-solving behavior has a high probability of being effective and successful. These deficits lead to sadness, lowered self-esteem, and a sense of personal ineffectiveness. These deficits are collectively known as learned helplessness deficits.

Abramson and colleagues (1978) have emphasized the effect of attributional style in maintaining learned helplessness deficits. Attributional style means that the person with learned helplessness deficits will attribute the causes of misfortune to be internal, unchangeable over time, and global. In effect, the person believes that the causes of problems are due to defects within him- or herself that will not change and shows more depression than the person who believes the causes of problems are due to external, specific, and temporary circumstances. Nolen-Hoeksema and colleagues (1986) looked at these deficits in children and found that these attributional styles were stable over a 1-year period, and that they were correlated with depression and underachievement in the predicted direction. Some of these findings are reminiscent of the cognitive distortions seen in cognitive theories of depression.

OUTCOME OF CHILDHOOD DEPRESSION

Kovacs and colleagues (1984a, b) demonstrated that major depression, adjustment disorder with depression, dysthymia, and major depression with dysthymia (double depression) have somewhat different outcomes. The length of time to recovery for the disorders varied. Children with adjustment disorders with depressed mood recovered on the average in about 5 months and remained well on 5-year follow-up without recurrences of depression. Children with major depression took 7 months to recover, and those with dysthymia took 45 months. There was also considerable variability in recovery times because these were given as median times to recovery. The likelihood of a recurrence in a child with a *DSM-III* diagnosis of major depression or dysthymia was about 69–72 percent. None of the children studied with a diagnosis of adjustment disorder had a recurrence.

The factors related to the likelihood of a recurrence were due to the presence or absence of comorbid disorders, specifically the diagnosis of dysthymia. In the absence of a comorbid diagnosis of dysthymia, the likelihood of a subsequent major depression over a 5-year period for the children with only major depression as an initial diagnosis was 32 percent. Patients with the presence of an initial primary diagnosis of dysthymia had a cumulative probability of having an episode of major depression of 59 percent over the same 5-year period. This implies that dysthymia is a poor prognostic sign. Kovacs and colleagues (1984b) also looked at the likelihood of recurrence of depression in cases who had been classified as recovered. When recovery was defined as 2 months free of symptoms of depression, the probability of having a subsequent depression during the next 4 years was 40 percent.

Kovacs and colleagues (1988) reported that on follow up, 36 percent of depressed children developed conduct disorders. Anxiety symptoms and disorders are also likely to occur (Kovacs et al. 1989). Conduct symptoms may be a consequence of affective disorders in children and may be preventable with proper treatment. Puig-Antich (1982) noted that among children whose conduct symptoms followed the onset of their affective disorder, successful treatment of the affective episode was associated with remission of the conduct symptoms. Although conduct symptoms remitted, children with a sustained recovery often continued to show difficulty in relationships with their mothers and fathers (Puig-Antich et al. 1985a, b). The presence or absence of anxiety disorders or symptoms did not influence the likelihood of having a recurrence or a later episode of major depression. If depression is associated with conduct symptoms, one of the outcomes may be conduct disorder unless the depression is adequately treated.

Adult outcomes for childhood and adolescent depression are still the subject of ongoing research. Harrington and colleagues (1990) blindly assessed the adult outcome of children who had been depressed and matched nondepressed psychiatric controls. The average follow-up period was 18 years after the initial contact. As adults, the formerly depressed children were at significantly greater risk for any depression and for major depression than the controls. More of them had also received psychotropic medication, other treatment for a psychiatric disorder, and psychiatric hospitalization and had impairment of their usual social role due to psychiatric disorder. In light of current findings, childhood depression does not bode well for the future. It is associated with increased risk for adult depression, adult psychiatric care, adult social role impairment, adult conduct and anxiety symptoms, and possibly chronicity.

SUMMARY AND CONCLUSIONS

A growing literature points to the existence of depression in childhood and adolescence. Depression appears to be composed of a number of diagnostic categories similar to those seen in adults. Current *DSM-III-R* criteria can be used to diagnose these disorders by adjusting the wording to accommodate the developmental level of the child. The best model for childhood depression may be bereavement or the grief response to the recent loss of a significant other. The symptoms and signs in child and adolescent depression are the same as those in adults; however, there are developmental differences. Children generally appear sadder than adolescents and do not necessarily vocalize their dysphoria. They somatize more than adolescents. Adolescents develop separation anxiety and conduct symptoms frequently after the onset of affective symptoms. The anxiety symptoms and conduct problems often remit upon recovery.

Epidemiological studies indicate that depression is a substantial problem, and suicide in adolescents is a risk as in adults. Depression is also associated with parental affective disorder, abuse, neglect, and dysfunctional families. It is associated to a high degree with divorce and family dissolution. Psychological theories of depression in adults have their counterparts and some supporting evidence in children. Psychotherapies based on some of these findings have had some success.

Depression in children and adolescents runs in families and may have a genetic component. A number of the neuroendocrine and neurophysiological findings are similar to the findings in adults, but there are differences as well. Evidence from objective controlled studies at the current time is limited in this regard.

Follow-up studies suggest that depression in children may more easily become chronic than in adults. They also suggest that the dysthymic disorders of adulthood may have their genesis in childhood. Depression in childhood places children and adolescents at risk for adult depression, anxiety, conduct problems, and job impairment.

Although specific treatment has not been addressed as part of this overview, the seriousness of depression in childhood and its later consequences imply the potentially positive benefit of effective treatment. Long-term suffering and impairment could be ameliorated. Much further epidemiological, treatment, and outcome research needs to be done to address these issues.

REFERENCES

Abramson, L. Y. Seligman, M. E. P. and Teasdale, J. D. (1978). Learned helplessness in humans: critique and reformulation. *Journal of Abnormal Psychology* 87:49–74,

Agarwal, R. K. Moudgil, A., Visivas, D., et al. (1985). Anaclitic depression—an attachment disorder of infancy. *Indian Journal of Pediatrics* 52:197–199,

Akiskal, H. S., Downs, J. S., Jordan, P., et al. (1985). Affective disorders in referred children and younger siblings of manic-depressives: mode of onset and prospective course. *Archives of General Psychiatry* 42:996–1003.

Akiskal, H. S., and Weller, E. B. (1989) Mood disorders and suicide in children and adolescents. In *Comprehensive Textbook of Psychiatry*, vol. 2, ed. H. I. Kaplan and B. J. Sadock, 5th ed. Baltimore: Williams & Wilkins.

American Psychiatric Association (1987). *Diagnostic and Statistical Manual of*

Mental Disorders. 3rd ed.-rev. Washington, DC: American Psychiatric Association.

Andersen, J. C., Williams, S. McGee, R., et al. (1987). *DSM-III* disorders in preadolescent children: prevalence in a large sample from the general population. *Archives of General Psychiatry* 44:69-76.

Andreasen, N. C., Endicott, J., Spitzer, R. L., et al. (1977). The family history method using diagnostic criteria: reliability and validity. *Archives of General Psychiatry* 34:1229-1235.

Asarnow, J. R., and Ben-Meir, S. (1988). Children with schizophrenia spectrum and depressive disorders: a comparative study of premorbid adjustment, onset pattern and severity of impairment. *Journal of Child Psychology and Psychiatry* 29:477-488.

Baker, M., Dorzab, J., Winokur, G., et al. (1971). Depressive disease. Classification and clinical characteristics. *Comprehensive Psychiatry* 12:354-365.

Barbero, G. J. and Shaheen, E. (1967). Environmental failure to thrive: a clinical review. *Journal of Pediatrics* 71:639-644.

Beardslee, W. R., Klerman, G. L., Keller, M. B., et al. (1985). But are they cases? Validity of *DSM-III* major depression in children identified in a family study. *American Journal of Psychiatry* 142:687-691.

Beck, A. T., Rush, A. J., Shaw, B. J., and Emery, G. (1979). *Cognitive Therapy of Depression*. New York: Guilford.

Bernstein, G. A. (1991). Co-morbidity and severity of anxiety and depressive disorders in a clinic sample. *Journal of the American Academy of Child and Adolescent Psychiatry* 30:43-50.

Birleson, P. (1986). Annotation - depression in childhood. *Australian Paediatric Journal* 22:7-10.

Block, J., Block, J. H., and Gjerde, P. (1988). Parental functioning and home environment in families of divorce: prospective and concurrent analyses. *Journal of the American Academy of Child and Adolescent Psychiatry* 27:207-213.

Blumberg, M. L. (1977). Depression in children on a general pediatric service. *American Journal of Psychotherapy* 38:20-32.

Bowlby, J. (1969). *Attachment and Loss. Vol. I. Attachment*. New York: Basic Books.

Brandenburg, N. A., Friedman, R. M., and Silver, S. E. (1990). The epidemiology of childhood psychiatric disorders: prevalence findings from recent studies. *Journal of the American Academy of Child and Adolescent Psychiatry* 29:76-83.

Brent, D. A., Perper, J. A., Goldstein, C. E., et al. (1988). Risk factor for adolescent suicide: a comparison of adolescent suicide victims with suicidal inpatients. *Archives of General Psychiatry* 45:581-588.

Brumbach, R. A., Dietz-Schmidt, S. G., and Weinberg, W. A. (1977).

Depression in children referred to an educational diagnostic center: diagnosis and treatment and analysis of criteria and literature review. *Diseases of the Nervous System* 529–534.

Caldwell, B. M. (1971). The effects of psychosocial deprivation on human development in infancy. In *Annual Progress in Child Psychiatry and Human Development* pp. 3–22. New York: Brunner/Mazel

Cantwell, D. P. (1983). Depression in childhood: clinical picture and diagnostic criteria. In *Affective Disorders in Childhood and Adolescence — An Update*, ed. D. P. Cantwell and G. A. Carlson, pp. 3–38. New York: Spectrum.

_____ (1985). Depressive disorders in children. Validation of clinical syndromes. *Psychiatric Clinics of North America* 8:779–792.

Cantwell, D. P., and Baker, L. (1988). Issues in the classification of child and adolescent psychopathology. *Journal of the American Academy of Child and Adolescent Psychiatry* 27:521–533.

_____ (1989). Stability and natural history of *DSM-III* childhood diagnoses. *Journal of the American Academy of Child and Adolescent Psychiatry* 28:691–700.

Cantwell, D. P., and Carlson G. (1979). Problems and prospects in the study of childhood depression. *Journal of Nervous and Mental Disorders* 167:522–529.

Carlson, G. A. (1983). Depression and suicidal behavior in children and adolescents. In *Affective Disorders in Childhood and Adolescents. An Update*, ed. D. P. Cantwell and G. A. Carlson. New York: Spectrum.

Carlson, G. A., and Cantwell D. P. (1979). A survey of depressive symptoms in a child and adolescent psychiatric population. Interview data. *Journal of the American Academy of Child Psychiatry* 18:587–599.

_____ (1980a). A survey of depressive symptoms, syndrome, and disorder in a child psychiatric population. *Journal of Child Psychology and Psychiatry*, 21:19–25.

_____ (1980b). Unmasking depression in children and adolescents. *American Journal of Psychiatry* 137:445–449.

_____ (1982). Diagnosis of childhood depression: a comparison of the Weinberg and *DSM-III* criteria. *Journal of the American Academy of Child Psychiatry* 21:247–250.

Carlson, G. A., and Kashani, J. H. (1988). Phenomenology of major depression from childhood through adulthood: analysis of three studies. *American Journal of Psychiatry* 145:1222–1225.

Chabrol, H., Chaverie, J., and Moron, P. (1983). DST, TRH test and adolescent suicide attempts. *American Journal of Psychiatry* 140:265.

Chambers, W. J., Puig-Antich, J., Tabrizi, M. A., et al. (1982). Psychotic symptoms in prepubertal major depressive disorder. *Archives of General Psychiatry* 39:921–927.

Chatoor, I., and Egan, J. (1983). Nonorganic failure to thrive and dwarfism due to food refusal: a separation disorder. *Journal of the American Academy of Child Psychiatry* 22:294–301.

Chess, S., Thomas A., and Hassibi, M. (1983). Depression in childhood and adolescence. A prospective study of six cases. *Journal of Nervous and Mental Disorders* 171:411–420.

Cole, D. A., and Rehm, L. P. (1986). Family interaction patterns and childhood depression. *Journal of Abnormal Child Psychology* 14:297–314.

Coopersmith, S. (1967). *The Antecedents of Self-Esteem*. San Francisco, CA: W. H. Freeman and Co.

Eaton, W. W., and Kessler, L. G., eds. (1985). *Epidemiologic Field Methods in Psychiatry*. Orlando, FL: Academic.

Emslie, G. H., Roffwarg, H. P., Rush, J., et al. (1987). Sleep EEG findings in depressed children and adolescents. *American Journal of Psychiatry* 144:668–670.

English, P. C. (1978). Failure to thrive without organic reason. *Pediatric Annals* 7:774–781.

Epidemiologic Field Methods in Psychiatry (1985). *The NIMH Epidemiologic Catchment Area Program*, ed. W. W. Eaton and L. G. Kessler. Orlando, FL: Academic.

Fleming, J. E., and Offord, D. R. (1990). Epidemiology of childhood depressive disorders: a critical review. *Journal of the American Academy of Child and Adolescent Psychiatry* 29:571–580.

Friedman R. C., Aronoff, M. S., Clarkin, J. F., et al. (1983). History of suicidal behavior in depressed borderline inpatients. *American Journal of Psychiatry* 140:1023–1026.

Fristad, M. A., Weller, E. B., Weller, R. A., et al., (1988). Self-report vs biological markers in assessment of childhood depression. *Journal of Affective Disorders* 15:339–345.

Frommer, E. A. (1968). Depressive illness in childhood. In *Recent Developments in Affective Disorders*, ed. A. Coppen, and A. Walk, pp. 117–136. (*British Journal of Psychiatry Special Publication*) London: RMPA.

Geller, B., Chestnut, E. C., Miller, D., et al. (1985). Preliminary data on *DSM-III* associated features of major depressive disorder in children and adolescents. *American Journal of Psychiatry* 142:643–644.

Glaser, K. (1967). Masked depression in children and adolescents. *American Psychotherapy* 21:565–574.

Goetz, R. R., Puig-Antich, J., Ryan, N., et al. (1987). Electroencephalographic sleep of adolescents with major depression and normal controls. *Archives of General Psychiatry* 44:61–68.

Goodyer, I. M. (1990). Family relationships, life events and childhood psychopathology. *Journal of Child Psychology and Psychiatry* 31:161–192.

Goodyer, I. M., Wright, C., and Altham, P. M. E. (1988). Maternal adversity and recent stressful life events in anxious and depressed children. *Journal of Child Psychology and Psychiatry* 29:651–667.

Greenberg, R., Rosenberg, G., Weisberg, L., et al. (1985). The dexamethasone suppression test and the thyrotropin-releasing hormone test in adolescent major depressive disorder (abs). *Proceedings of the 32nd Annual Meeting of the American Academy of Child and Adolescent Psychiatry*, San Antonio, Texas. Washington, DC, American Academy of Child and Adolescent Psychiatry 42.

Haley, G. M. T., Fine, S., Marriage, K., et al. (1985). Cognitive bias and depression in psychiatrically disturbed children and adolescents. *Journal of Counseling and Clinical Psychology* 53:535–537.

Harrington, R., Fudge, H., Rutter, M., et al. (1990). Adult outcomes of childhood and adolescent depression. I. Psychiatric status. *Archives of General Psychiatry* 47:465–473.

Herjanic, B., and Reich, W. (1982). Development of a structured psychiatric interview for children: agreement between parent and child on individual symptoms. *Child Psychiatry* 10:307–324.

Hoberman, H. M., and Garfinkel, B. D. (1988). Completed suicide in children and adolescents. *Journal of the American Academy of Child and Adolescent Psychiatry* 27:689–695.

Hughes, C. W., Preskorn, S. H., Weller, E. B., et al. (1989). A descriptive profile of the depressed child. *Psychopharmacology Bulletin* 25:232–237.

Jensen, J. B., and Garfinkel, B. D. (1990). Growth hormone dysregulation in children with major depressive disorder. *Journal of the American Academy of Child and Adolescent Psychiatry* 29:295–301.

Kashani, J. H., Barbero, G. J., and Bolander, F. D. (1981b). Depression in hospitalized pediatric patients. *Journal of the American Academy of Child Psychiatry* 20:123–134.

Kashani, J. H., Cantwell, D. P., Shekim, W. O., et al. (1982). Major depressive disorder in children admitted to an inpatient community mental health center. *American Journal of Psychiatry* 139:671–672.

Kashani, J. H., and Carlson, G. A. (1987). Seriously depressed preschoolers. *American Journal of Psychiatry* 144:348–350.

Kashani, J. H., Holcomb, W. R., and Orvaschel, H. (1986). Depression and depressive symptoms in preschool children from the general population. *American Journal of Psychiatry* 143:1138–1143.

Kashani, J. H., Husain, A., Shekim, W. O., et al. (1981b). Current perspectives on childhood depression: an overview. *American Journal of Psychiatry* 138:143–153.

Kashani, J. H., McGee, R. O., and Clarkson, S. E. (1983). Depression in a sample of 9-year-old children. Prevalence and associated characteristics. *Archives of General Psychiatry* 40:1217–1223.

Kashani, J. H., Rosenberg, T. K., and Reid, J. C. (1989). Developmental perspectives in child and adolescent depressive symptoms in a community sample. *American Journal of Psychiatry* 146:871–875.

Kashani, J. H., and Sherman, D. (1988). Childhood depression, epidemiology, etiological models, and treatment implications. *Integrative Psychiatry* 6:1–21.

Klein, D. N., Clark, D. C., Dansky, L., et al. (1988). Dysthymia in the offspring of parents with primary unipolar affective disorder. *Journal of Abnormal Psychology* 97:265–274.

Kovacs, M., Feinberg, T. L., Crouse-Novak, M. A., et al. (1984a). Depressive disorders in childhood: I. A longitudinal prospective study of characteristics and recovery. *Archives of General Psychiatry* 41:229–237.

———— (1984b). Depressive disorders in childhood: II. A longitudinal study of the risk for a subsequent major depression. *Archives of General Psychiatry* 41:643–649.

Kovacs, M., Gatsonis, C., Paulauskas, S. L., et al. (1989). Depressive disorders in childhood: IV. A longitudinal study of co-morbidity with and risk for anxiety disorders. *Archives of General Psychiatry* 46:776–782.

Kovacs, M., and Paulauskas, S. (1984). Developmental stage and the expression of depressive disorders in children: an empirical analysis. In *Childhood Depression*, ed. D. Cicchetti and K. Schneider-Rosen. (New Directions for Child Development, No. 26.) San Francisco: Jossey-Bass.

Kovacs, M., Paulauskas, S., Gatsonis, C., et al. (1988). Depressive disorders in childhood: II. A longitudinal study of comorbidity with and risk for conduct disorders. *Journal of Affective Disorders* 15:205–217.

Kupfer, D. F. Ulrich, R. F. Coble, P. A., et al. (1985). Electroencephalographic sleep of young depressives. *Archives of General Psychiatry* 42:806–810.

Kupferman, S., Black, D. W., and Burns, T. L. (1988). Excess suicide among formerly hospitalized child psychiatry patients. *Journal of Clinical Psychiatry* 49:88–93.

Kutcher, S. P., Williamson, P., Silverberg, J., et al. (1988). Nocturnal growth hormone secretion in depressed older adolescents. *Journal of the American Academy of Child and Adolescent Psychiatry* 27:751–754.

Lahmeyer, H. W., Poznanski, E. O., and Bellur, S. N. (1983). EEG sleep in depressed adolescents. *American Journal of Psychiatry* 140:1150–1153.

Lapouse, R., and Monk, M. A. (1964). Fears and worries in a representative sample of children. *American Journal of Orthopsychiatry* 29:803–818.

Ling, W., Oftedal, G., and Weinberg, W. (1970). Depressive illness in childhood presenting as severe headache. *American Journal of Disabled Children* 120:122–124.

Livingston, R. (1987). Sexually and physically abused children. *Journal of the American Academy of Child and Adolescent Psychiatry* 26:413–415.

Livingston, R., Taylor, J. L., and Crawford, S. L. (1988). A study of somatic complaints and psychiatric diagnosis in children. *Journal of the American Academy of Child and Adolescent Psychiatry* 27:185–187.

Loosen, P. T., and Prange, A. J. (1982). The serum thyrotropin (TSH) response to thyrotropin-releasing hormone (TRH) in depression: a review. *American Journal of Psychiatry* 139:405–416.

Malmquist, C. P. (1971a). Depression in childhood and adolescence. (First of two parts). *New England Journal of Medicine* 284:887–893.

_____ (1971b). Depression in childhood and adolescence. (Second of two parts). *New England Journal of Medicine* 284:955–961.

McGee, R., Feehan, M., Williams, S., et al. (1990). *DSM-III* disorders in a large sample of adolescents. *Journal of the American Academy of Child and Adolescent Psychiatry* 26:611–619.

Mendelson, W. B., Reid, M. A., and Frommer, E. A. (1971). Some characteristic features accompanying depression, anxiety and aggressive behavior in disturbed children under five. In *Depressive States in Childhood and Adolescence* ed. A. L. Annell, pp. 151–158. (Proc. 4th UEP Congress.) Stockholm: European Congress of Pedopsychiatry.

Meyer, W. J., Richards, G. E., and Cavallo, A., et al. (1985). Growth hormone and cortisol secretion dynamics in children with major depressive disorder. Presentation at the American Academy of Child Psychiatry Annual Meeting, San Antonio, Texas, 1985.

Mitchell, J., McCauley, E., Burke, P. M., et al. (1988). Phenomenology of depression in children and adolescents. *Journal of the American Academy of Child and Adolescent Psychiatry* 27:12–20.

Mitchell, J., McCauley, E., Burke, P., et al., (1989). Psychopathology in parents of depressed children and adolescents. *Journal of the American Academy of Child and Adolescent Psychiatry* 28:352–357.

Myers, K. M., Burke, P., and McCauley, E. (1985). Suicidal behavior by hospitalized preadolescent children on a psychiatric unit. *Journal of the American Academy of Child and Adolescent Psychiatry* 24:474–480.

Nolen-Hoeksema, S., Girgus, J. S., and Seligman, M. E. P. (1986). Learned helplessness in children: a longitudinal study of depression, achievement, and explanatory style. *Journal of Personality and Social Psychology* 51:435–442.

Ossofskey, H. J. (1974). Endogenous depression in infancy and childhood. *Comprehensive Psychiatry* 15:19–25.

Patton, R. G., and Gandner, L. I. (1962). Influence of family environment on growth: the syndrome of "maternal deprivation." *Pediatrics* 30:957–962.

Pearce, J. B. (1978). The recognition of depressive disorder in children. *Journal of the Royal Society of Medicine* 71:494–500.

Petti, T. A. (1978). Depression in hospitalized child psychiatry patients: approaches to measuring depression. *Journal of the American Academy of Child Psychiatry* 17:49–59.

Pfeffer, C. R. (1991a). Attempted suicide in children and adolescents: causes and management. In *Child and Adolescent Psychiatry. A Comprehensive Textbook*, ed. M. Lewis, pp. 664–672. Baltimore: Williams & Wilkins.

———— (1991b). The child and the vicissitudes of divorce. In *Child and Adolescent Psychiatry. A Comprehensive Textbook*, ed. M. Lewis, pp. 1108–1118. Baltimore: Williams & Wilkins.

Pfeffer, C. R., Klerman, G. L., Hunt, S. W., et al. (1991). Suicidal children grown up: demographic and clinical risk factors for adolescent suicide attempts. *Journal of the American Academy of Child and Adolescent Psychiatry* 30:609–616.

Poznanski, E., Mokros, H. B., and Grossman, J. (1985). Diagnostic criteria in childhood depression. *American Journal of Psychiatry* 142:1168–1173.

Poznanski, E., and Zrull, J. P. (1970). Childhood depression. Clinical characteristics of overtly depressed children. *Archives of General Psychiatry* 23:8–15.

Puig-Antich, J. (1982) Major depression and conduct disorder in prepuberty. *Journal of the American Academy of Child Psychiatry* 21:118–128.

———— (1987). Affective disorders in children and adolescents: diagnostic validity and psychobiology. In *Psychopharm: The Third Generation of Progress*, ed. H. Y. Metzer, pp. 843–859. New York: Raven.

Puig-Antich, J., and Chambers, W. (1978). Schedule for Affective Disorders and Schizophrenia for School Aged Children, Epidemiologic Version. K-SADS-E, 3rd version.

Puig-Antich, J., Goetz, R., Davies, M., et al. (1984a). Growth hormone secretion in prepubertal children with major depression: II. Sleep-related plasma concentrations during a depressive episode. *Archives of General Psychiatry* 41:463–466.

Puig-Antich, J., Goetz, R., Davies, M., et al. (1984b). Growth hormone secretion in prepubertal children with major depression: IV. Sleep related plasma concentrations in a drug-free fully recovered clinical state. *Archives of General Psychiatry* 41:479–483.

Puig-Antich, J., Goetz, D. M., Davies, M., et al. (1989). A controlled family history study of prepubertal major depressive disorder. *Archives of General Psychiatry* 46:406–418.

Puig-Antich, J., Goetz, R., Hanlon, C., et al. (1982). Sleep architecture and REM sleep measures in prepubertal children with depression. A controlled study. *Archives of General Psychiatry* 39:932–939.

Puig-Antich, J., Lukens, E., Davies, M. et al. (1985a). Psychosocial functioning in prepubertal major depressive disorders: I. Interpersonal relationships during the depressive episode. *Archives of General Psychiatry* 42:500–507.

—— (1985b). Psychosocial functioning in prepubertal major depressive disorders: II. Interpersonal relationships after sustained recovery from affective episode. *Archives of General Psychiatry* 42: 511–517.

Puig-Antich, J., Novacenko, H., Davies, M., et al. Growth hormone secretion in prepubertal children with major depression: I. Final report on response to insulin-induced hypoglycemia during a depressive episode. *Archives of General Psychiatry* 41:455–460.

Reich, W., and Earls, F. (1987). Rules for making psychiatric diagnoses in children on the basis of multiple sources of information: preliminary strategies. *Journal of Abnormal Child Psychology* 15:601–616.

Reynolds, W. M., and Coats, K. I. (1986). A comparison of cognitive-behavioral therapy and relaxation training for the treatment of depression in adolescents. *Journal of Counseling and Clinical Psychology* 54:653–660.

Rie, H. E. (1966). Depression in childhood: a survey of some pertinent contributors. *Journal of the American Academy of Child Psychiatry* 5:653–685.

Robbins, D. R., Alessi, N. E., Cook, S. S., et al. (1982). The use of the research diagnostic criteria (RDC) for depression in adolescent psychiatric inpatients. *Journal of the American Academy of Child Psychiatry* 21:251–255.

Rogeness, G. A., Maas, J. W., Javors, M. A., et al. (1988). Diagnoses, catecholamine metabolism, and plasm dopamine-B-hydroxylase. *Journal of the American Academy of Child and Adolescent Psychiatry* 27:121–125.

Rosenthal, J. E., Carpenter, C. J., James, S. P., et al. (1986). Seasonal affective disorder in children and adolescents. *American Journal of Psychiatry* 143:356–358.

Rutter, M., and Quinton, D. (1984). Parental psychiatric disorder: effects on children. *Psychological Medicine* 114:853–880.

Ryan, N. D., Puig-Antich, J., Ambrosini, P., et al. (1987a). The clinical picture of major depression in children and adolescents. *Archives of General Psychiatry* 44:854–861.

Ryan, N. D., Puig-Antich, J., and Meyer, V. (1987b). Growth hormone secretion during sleep in depressed adolescents. Presentation at the Consortium on Affective, Disorders in Children, Boston.

Seligman, M. E. P. (1975). *Helplessness: On Depression, Development and Death*. San Francisco: Freeman.

Shaffer, D. (1974). Suicide in childhood and early adolescence. *Journal of Child Psychology and Psychiatry and Allied Disciplines* 15:275–291.

Shaffer, D., and Fisher, P. (1981). The epidemiology of suicide in children and young adolescents. *Journal of the American Academy of Child Psychiatry* 20:545–565.

Shafii, M. Camigan, S., Whittinghill, J. R., et al. (1985). Psychological autopsy of completed suicides in children and adolescents. *American Journal of Psychiatry* 142:1061–1064.

Silver, H., and Finkelstein, M. (1967). Deprivation dwarfism. *Journal of Pediatrics* 70:317–324.

Sonis, W. A., Yellin, A. M., Garfinkel, B. D., et al. (1987). The antidepressant effect of light in seasonal affective disorder of childhood and adolescence. *Psychopharmacology Bulletin* 23:360–363.

Spitz, R. A., and Wolfe, K. M. (1946). Anaclitic depression. An inquiry into the genesis of psychiatric conditions in early childhood. *Psychoanalytic Study of the Child* 2:313–342. New York: International Universities Press.

Spitzer, R. L., Endicott, J., and Robins, E. (1979). Research diagnostic criteria: rationale and reliability. *Archives of General Psychiatry* 36:47–56.

Strober, M. (1984). Familial aspects of depressive disorder in early adolescence. In *An Update of Childhood Depression*, ed. E. B. Weller and R. A. Weller. Washington, DC: American Psychiatric Association Press.

Strober, M., Green, J., and Carlson, G. (1981). Phenomenology and subtypes of major depressive disorder in adolescence. *Journal of Affective Disorders* 3:281–290.

Sulik, L. R., and Sonis, W. A. (1987). Winter depression: the characteristics of children and adolescents with seasonal affective disorder. Presented at the First Annual National Conference on Undergraduate Research, University of North Carolina, Asheville, NC, April.

Velez, C. N., Johnson, J., and Cohen, P. (1989). A longitudinal analysis of selected risk factors for child psychopathology. *Journal of the American Academy of Child and Adolescent Psychiatry* 28:861–864.

Wallerstein, J. S. (1985). Children of divorce: preliminary report of a ten-year follow-up of older children and adolescents. *Journal of the American Academy of Child and Adolescent Psychiatry* 24:545–554.

Wallerstein, J. S., and Corbin, S. B. (1991). The child and the vicissitudes of divorce. In *Child and Adolescent Psychiatry*, ed. M. Lewis, pp. 1108–1118. Baltimore, MD: Williams & Wilkins.

Weinberg, W. A., Rutman, J., Sullivan, L., et al. (1973). Depression in children referred to an educational diagnostic center. Diagnosis and treatment. *Journal of Pediatrics* 83: 1065–1072.

Weissman, M. M., Gammon, G. D., John, K., et al. (1987). Children of depressed parents. Increased psychopathology and early onset of major depression. *Archives of General Psychiatry* 44:847–853.

Weller, E. B., and Weller, R. A. (1988). Neuroendocrine changes in affectively ill children and adolescents. *Psychiatric Clinics of North America* 6:41–54.

_____ (1990a). Depressive disorder in children and adolescents. In *Psychiatric Disorders in Children and Adolescents*, ed. B. D., Garfinkel, G. A. Carlson, and E. B. Weller. Philadelphia, PA: W. B. Saunders.

_____ (1990b). Grief in children and adolescents. In *Psychiatric Disorders in Children and Adolescents*, ed. B. D. Garfinkel, G. A. Carlson, and E. B. Weller. Philadelphia, PA: W. B. Saunders.

Weller, E. B., Weller, R. A., and Fristad, M. (1986). Dexamethasone suppression test and clinical outcome in prepubertal depressed children. *American Journal of Psychiatry* 143:1469–1470.

Weller, E. B., Weller, R. A., Fristad, M. A., et al. (1984). The dexamethasone suppression test in hospitalized prepubertal depressed children. *American Journal Psychiatry* 141:290–291.

Young, W., Knowles, J. B., MacLean, K. W., et al. (1982). The sleep of childhood depressives. Comparison with age matched controls. *Biological Psychiatry* 17:1163–1168.

Zahn-Waxler, C., Mayfield, A., Radke-Yamow, M., et al. (1988). A follow-up investigation of offspring of parents with bipolar disorder. *American Journal of Psychiatry* 145:506–509.

5: THE EPIDEMIOLOGY OF DEPRESSION

Anthony J. Costello, M.D.

INTRODUCTION

Epidemiology is the study of health and illness in human populations. In order to study a disease or disorder, it is obviously necessary to be able to identify it with confidence and distinguish it from other similar conditions. Unfortunately, our knowledge of the affective disorders before adulthood is still so incomplete that we cannot even make so basic a claim. Epidemiological data have to be treated as only some of the many pieces of information that are needed to establish the validity of the concept of childhood depression.

EPIDEMIOLOGY OF ADULT DEPRESSION

Our current knowledge of the epidemiology of affective disorders in adults is based on a long history of development and refining of both the concepts of the disorder and the methods of epidemiological study. The best available data come from the National Institute of Mental Health Epidemiological Catchment Area (ECA) program, in which over 18, 000 individuals were interviewed at five different sites in the United States (Regier et al. 1988). The weighted 1-month prevalence of any psychiatric disorder was on average 15.4 percent, varying between sites from 12.9 to 19.3 percent, and for all affective disorders 5.1 percent (range 3.5–5.8 percent). Dysthymia was more common (mean 1-month prevalence 3.3 percent, range 2.1–4.2

percent) than a major depressive episode (mean 2.2 percent, range 1.5–2.6 percent). Affective disorders were more common in women (6.6 percent) than in men (3.5 percent). This difference between the sexes was particularly marked for a major depressive episode, in which the rate for women was 2.6 percent, compared with 1.6 percent for men. For major depressive episodes, the rate peaks during the child-bearing and child-rearing years. The rate for 18- to 24-year-old women was approximately 3 percent, increasing to 4 percent for 25- to 44-year-olds, and then falling again to 3 percent for the 45- to 65-year-old group. For dysthymia, a similar picture emerged, with the rate of 5 percent for women aged 25 to 64 about twice that for all the remaining age/sex groups.

The vast majority of individuals in the community who meet criteria for a current psychiatric disorder never receive any treatment. In the New Haven ECA study, for example, only 14 percent of the individuals meeting *DSM-III* criteria in the 6 months before the interview said that they had seen a mental health specialist, compared with only 7 percent of those who had a past but not recent disorder. A further 6.3 percent contacted a general medical physician for mental or emotional problems (Leaf et al. 1988). Married individuals are less likely to make use of mental health specialists, but the age group in the sample most likely to have children, 25- to 44-year-olds, were more likely to consult a mental health specialist. So there appears to be no particular tendency for parents of children or adolescents to seek specialist help, though this question was not specifically analyzed. Blacks are known to be less likely to seek help for depression than whites (Sussman et al. 1987). Data on the proportion who were depressed, sought specialist mental health services, and were correctly diagnosed are not available, but in any case the number must be only a very small minority. Similarly, though the overall results of treatment in the community are not known, the proportion receiving treatment is so small that the question of whether treatment was adequate or effective is almost irrelevant.

The age of onset of major depression was found to be on average about 27 (Weissman et al. 1988). If lifetime prevalence is estimated, the prevalence rate for major depression climbs to 4.0 percent for women aged 18 to 44 and 4.8 percent for women aged 45 to 64. Though different diagnostic criteria and sampling strategies may give somewhat different estimates, there is surprising consistency between these and other epidemiological studies of adult depression (Weissman et al. 1988). It should be noted that the prevalence of depressive symptoms, and perhaps of depressive syndromes other than those defined by *DSM-III*, has generally been found to be even higher (Blazer et al. 1988), which may explain such startling claims as Richman's (1974) than 41 percent of mothers with young children in her sample were depressed. Such findings are of course very relevant when one is considering the family environment in which children grow up.

In examining prevalence rates, a number of caveats must be made. Prevalence measures the number of cases that can be found during a particular time. During this time, new cases will occur, and some will recover. If the time window is extended, then the number of cases identified will increase. However, the course of depression is so chronic that the incidence rate (i.e., the rate at which new cases develop) is very low. Longitudinal data on a population are needed to estimate incidence, and few such studies are as yet completed, but from such studies (Hagnell et al. 1982, Murphy et al. 1988) it appears that for women under 40, the annual incidence is approximately 1–2 per 1,000.

The ECA studies suggest that there are marked cohort effects. Individuals born between 1935 and 1945 were particularly vulnerable to depression, but this seems to have stabilized for women born after 1945. However, for those women born more recently, the age at which depression begins seems to be falling (Wickramaratne et al. 1989). Separation or divorce or unhappiness in marriage increases the risk of depression more than 25-fold, both for women and men (Weissman 1987). However, poverty, occupational status, and minority status have relatively little effect on the rate of major depression, though the lower rates tend to be found in rural areas. Though education is generally believed to have little impact on the rate of depression, in a middle-aged cohort of women, college education seemed to protect against depressive symptomatology (Costello 1991). Similarly, if depressed mood is analyzed, which is only one component of major depression, low socioeconomic status, social isolation, and poor education are all found to be factors associated with this affective state (Golding and Lipton 1990, Kaplan et al. 1987). Family history is an important but less powerful risk factor. The lifetime rate for depression of first-degree adult relatives of probands with major depression is about three times that found in controls, particularly if the age of onset is young. Thus, all the adult data suggests that depression in children and adolescents may be very common, and that the age of onset of much adult depression may be very early, particularly in the families of depressed adults.

Until the 1970s, depression in children was usually recognized only as a dysphoric mood state and not as a consistent syndrome. It was generally believed that the affective disorders of adults were rarely if ever seen until late adolescence. The awareness of familial risk factors for depression, possibly based on genetic transmission, and the recognition that psychiatric illness in a parent predisposed to behavioral problems in the child, made it reasonable to search for evidence of a depressive syndrome in childhood. The search was confused by the suggestion that a depressive condition in children might be manifest by symptoms other than the overt depressive symptoms found in adults, so that, for example, somatic complaints or conduct disorder might indicate that a child was suffering from a depressive disorder, even though there was slight or no evidence of depressed mood. This concept of masked depression proved unhelpful, if only because it was difficult to either refute or support the claim.

By the mid-1970s, the consensus was that the most usetul empirical strategy was to adopt the criteria used to diagnose adult depression with only minor modifications (Schulterbrandt and Raskin 1977), and this was the approach adopted in *DSM-III* and *DSM-III-R* (American Psychiatric Association 1980, 1987). Though this strategy is a reasonable first approach, by now it is evident that adult criteria have not defined a condition identical with depression in adults. The response to treatment with antidepressants is very unpredictable in prepubertal children (Puig-Antich et al. 1987, Weller et al. 1982), and in adolescents it is arguable that there may be no response at all (Ryan et al. 1986, 1988). Though our concepts of the longitudinal course in adults are changing, in children it seems that a diagnosis of depressive disorder using *DSM-III* criteria has a very poor prognosis, with a very high risk of recurrence. Only studies of children at risk because of parental depression show results consistent with the belief that the phenomenology of depression in adults and children is similar.

There are other strong reasons for supposing that the criteria for diagnosing depressive disorder in children should be more age specific. Symptoms associated with a child's depressed mood or unhappiness, such as crying, guilt, and carelessness about personal safety, are more prominent at one age than another (Kashani et al. 1989, Ryan et al. 1987). Some, such as tearfulness, diminish with age, whereas mood swings, irritability, and suicidal ideation become more prominent in adolescence.

Epidemiological studies of child and adolescent depression should therefore be considered only first approximations, which will probably be subject to much adjustment as our understanding of the affective disorders in children is refined.

PROBLEMS IN OBTAINING DIAGNOSTIC INFORMATION

It is by now a truism that a very large proportion of depression in children and adolescents remains undetected. Studies of samples representative of the whole population have invariably revealed more cases than are referred for help of any sort, and as in adults, only a minority of those who receive help are seen by mental health professionals. Moreover, the severity of symptomatology or the degree of disability distinguishes only a few of the most severely affected identified individuals from those in the community who are not identified, and the overlap of severity between the clinical and the community groups is large. There is some suggestion that this overlap may be most marked for children and adolescents whose symptomatology is mainly depressive. Teachers and parents appear to have more difficulty in recognizing depression in children than in recognizing more overt disorders such as conduct disorder or attention deficit hyperactivity disorder. There is also a substantial body of evidence to show that parents are less aware of unhappiness and anxiety that their children report than of other symptoms (e.g., see Edelbrock et al. 1986, Leon et al. 1982, Orvaschel et al. 1982, Weissman et al. 1987).

Though this data might suggest that the child's report is the most useful source of diagnostic information, unfortunately it also seems to be the case that children are the least reliable reporters of symptoms. When children are asked about their symptoms a second time a few days after the first interview, they often report fewer symptoms, and frequently the reduction is enough so that the child no longer meets criteria for a diagnosis. This is particularly true of depressive symptoms and is most marked in younger children (Edelbrock et al. 1985). The same phenomenon has been observed in adults (Robins 1985) but usually is smaller. The conclusion most investigators have reached is that a diagnosis of depression should be made if any informant reports that the child has sufficient symptoms, but this may inflate rates substantially. For clinical research, where it is usually more important to be sure that a case is a true case than to be confident that no possible cases have been missed, the usual practice has been to include only those cases for study for whom all informants consistently report the relevant symptoms on more than one occasion. This rigorous standard has not yet been applied in epidemiological studies, and it may be misleading to infer that cases diagnosed in the community are strictly comparable with those studied in clinical research.

In comparing rates of depression for different age groups, one has to consider not only the reliability of the child's self-report over time but also that there may be true developmental effects on the content of the report. Angold and colleagues (1991) for example, found that 16- to 18-year-old adolescent girls retrospectively reporting described an earlier onset and more symptomatology for the worst episode than younger girls, even after statistical correction was made for the longer risk exposure. By ingeniously sampling current mood states with an electronic pager, Larson and colleagues (1990) were able to show that even those prepubertal children with high depression scores on the Child Depression Inventory (CDI) (Kovacs 1985) were less likely to report negative affect than similarly identified older children. Similar studies of adolescents might help to explain the apparently heightened awareness of depressed mood that develops later, particularly in girls.

CHARACTERISTICS OF REFERRED CASES

The act of referring a child for mental health services is influenced by many considerations besides the extent and nature of symptoms and the resultant handicap. It has been known for some time that the psychological discomfort of a parent may prompt referral. Availability of services also plays an obvious part in determining referral rates, and because many referrals are initiated by general practitioners or teachers, these professionals' knowledge and awareness of depression in children may play an important part in deciding whether or not a child is referred (Costello et al. 1988). This means that the utilization of services is not very helpful in estimating the rate of disorder in the population at large, and indeed that even the patterns of symptomatology found in referred cases may not be typical of the whole population of depressed children and adolescents. Further, because the *DSM-III* classification describes "pure" syndromes, in most cases depending more on traditional clinical concepts of disorder than empirically established patterns of symptomatology, diagnoses recorded by clinicians may be even more misleading if there is reluctance to make all of the axis I diagnoses that the symptoms elicited permit (Costello et al. 1984, Weinstein et al. 1989).

CO-MORBIDITY

Co-morbidity is said to occur when two or more disorders are found together in individuals more often than would be expected by chance alone, given the base rates for each condition. Various explanations are offered for this phenomenon. The most mundane explanation is that if two conditions are very common it will be difficult to distinguish co-morbidity from a chance finding. Another is that a wider spread of symptoms may increase the chances of detection or referral. In passing, it should be noted that for detection of a case most first-stage screening instruments (in studies in which a two-stage design is adopted for reasons of economy) depend more heavily on a large number of symptoms than on weightings of the severity of symptoms. However, given the uncertainty that surrounds the concept of depression in young people, it is also possible that co-morbidity is in fact a phenomenon reflecting patterns of psychopathology other than those usually recognized in clinical classifications. Even though the concept of masked depression has been unhelpful, it has to be recognized that in childhood and adolescence depressed mood, in both clinical and epidemiological samples, is often found in association with symptoms of anxiety (Fleming et al. 1989), conduct problems (Cole and Carpentieri 1990), attention deficit hyperactivity disorder, and learning problems (Cole 1990). Between 79 percent and 100 percent of children and adolescents identified as depressed in community samples have other *DSM-III* diagnoses (Anderson et al. 1987, Fleming et al. 1989, Kashani et al. 1987). Not surprisingly, empirical analyses of the association of symptoms, whether reported by parents, teachers, or the child, do not support the syndromic constellation of symptoms that we believe characterizes depressive disorder (Achenbach 1991, Achenbach and Edelbrock 1983). The suspicion that the definition of depression according to *DSM-III* or *DSM-III-R*, or similar systems, may not represent a true syndrome is supported by data from studies of adults suggesting, for example, that the combination of anxiety and depression has different implications for prognosis and family history (Clayton et al. 1991).

CASE IDENTIFICATION IN THE COMMUNITY

Given this background, a reasonable first approach to improving our understanding of the phenomenology and psychopathology of depression in childhood is to conduct community surveys. The rate of depression found in clinically referred populations is often of the order of 25 to 30 percent, but it is usually accepted that only 10 to 15 percent of the population in need of psychiatric help actually see a mental health professional in most North American settings. Estimates of all psychiatric disorders in the child and adolescent population vary widely but are in the range of 10 to 20 percent. Thus, it seems reasonable to suppose that the point prevalence of childhood depression lies in the range between 25 per 1, 000 and 60 per 1, 000. Prevalence rates of this order demand large samples for an estimate with a reasonable confidence interval, a problem aggravated by the poor precision of case identification. To make a diagnosis consistent with *DSM-III* or *DSM-III-R* criteria, it is necessary to conduct an interview, because the extent of detail required goes beyond what can reasonably be achieved by question- naires. The daunting cost of interviewing every individual in large population samples has not, up to now, seemed warranted given the dubious usefulness of the additional information that might be obtained by this strategy, and nearly all research so far has instead either used a two-stage design or resorted to instruments that can be administered at less expense but that do not so accurately reflect current *DSM-III* criteria for the diagnosis of depression. A few studies have used a longitudinal approach, in which the trade-off is obtaining better data on the course of symptoms at the expense of more reliable estimates of prevalence. Longitudinal studies are, of course, essential if an estimate of incidence is to be made, but because most clinical follow-up research suggests that the course of much childhood depression is lengthy, the incidence is likely to be low, and even larger samples would be needed to make a good estimate of the incidence of new cases.

Two-stage designs have generally depended on a general checklist of psychopathology, such as the Rutter scales (McGee et al. 1985, Rutter 1967, Rutter et al. 1970;) or the Child Behavior Checklist (CBCL) (Achenbach, 1991; Achenbach and Edelbrock 1983) and its derivatives, selecting for more intensive evaluation those subjects with high scores and a sample of the remainder, so that the false negative rate of the screening instrument can be estimated. This strategy is highly efficient if the disorder to be studied is rare, a screening test with high specificity and sensitivity is available, and recruitment and screening are inexpensive compared to the cost of diagnosis (Newman et al. 1990). Though it can be argued that only the last of these criteria has applied to the majority of child epidemiological studies, the method has been very popular. The second stage of evaluation has usually included some form of standardized psychiatric interview, commonly highly structured so that it can be administered by lay interviewers, such as the Diagnostic Interview for Children and Adolescents (DICA) (Herjanic and Reich 1982), or the Diagnostic Interview Schedule for Children (DISC) (Costello et al. 1984), but sometimes using a semi-structured instrument, as in the interview used by Rutter in the pioneering Isle of Wight study (Rutter et al. 1970). It has generally been assumed that because such interviews correspond to conventional clinical interviewing, with more structure to improve reliability, validity is assured, but in studies of general population samples, of individuals with no presenting complaints, this assumption may not be warranted (Dohrenwend 1990), and indeed there is evidence that some parts of such interviews may be misunderstood by children (Breslau 1987).

Many studies have used only the first element of this approach, relying exclusively on general psychopathology checklists to give prevalence estimates. This method reduces cost, making it possible to devote more effort to data collection from large samples, at the expense of precision. There is a close relationship between some clinical diagnoses and the relevant factor scales of these instruments (Edelbrock and Costello 1988) but not one close enough to be able to extrapolate from factor scores to clinical diagnosis. Alternatively, one of several self-report scales designed to specifically detect depression can be used, such as the Center for Epidemiological Studies Depression scale (CES-D) (Radloff 1977) or the CDI (Kovacs 1985). It must be remembered that these scales are based on theoretical or empirical views of the nature of depression, and though the content of the scales clearly relates to the conventional diagnosis of depression, they may not accurately reflect the criteria used to make a *DSM-III* diagnosis (Costello and Angold 1988). Surprisingly this strategy may not improve specificity; there is some evidence that such scales detect general rather than specific psychopathology, despite the face validity of the content and the evidence that the sensitivity is good.

In part, this may be because of inappropriate cut-off points, and more recent work (Garrison et al. 1991) suggests that specificity can be improved considerably by the choice of an appropriate cut-off score, though performance is still not much improved over general scales, and the CES-D at least performs just as well as a screen for any psychiatric disorder. An alternative explanation is that these specialized scales are picking up nonspecific psychological distress, aspects of what has been termed *demoralization* (Dohrenwend 1990, Frank 1973). The finding may also reflect errors in the nosology. If syndromes are not truly distinct, an apparently unrelated measure of a different syndrome may serve as well to identify depression, and vice versa, as a measure clearly related to the central concept. High scorers on the CDI, for example, tend to be more anxious (Fundudis et al. 1991), though this may be a relationship dependent on the age of the informant. For 16-year-olds, for example, the Beck Depression Inventory (BDI) (Beck et al. 1961), a closely related instrument, may be a somewhat more specific screen even though it was designed for adults (Roberts et al. 1991).

Some approximation to *DSM-III* diagnoses can be achieved by adding questions to instruments such as the CBCL to cover additional details of symptomatology, which these instruments omit. This strategy has been used in the Ontario Child Health study (Boyle et al. 1987) to cover a variety of disorders, including a depressive syndrome. Obviously, this method cannot obtain all of the detail required for true *DSM-III* or *DSM-III-R* diagnoses, but it is feasible for use with very large samples, a virtue that may outweigh its disadvantages.

None of the strategies discussed so far addresses the problem that many studies have revealed significant numbers of children who display enough symptoms to meet diagnostic criteria for depression or other disorders but who have not sought services and who are not assessed as in need of treatment. It is perhaps inevitable that a nosology based on clinical experience does not provide criteria adequate to distinguish between symptomatic but functional individuals and those cases truly in need of help. Impairment measures may be helpful in making this distinction (Bird et al. 1990, Costello et al. 1988), but as yet few studies have examined the extent to which significant depression is associated with impairments in everyday functioning.

SPECIFIC FINDINGS

Despite this gloomy appraisal of the problems surrounding epidemiological knowledge on childhood depression, some conclusions can still be drawn. Several studies have measured depression in a way that comes close to current clinical practice, and so the findings have some relevance for the practicing child psychiatrist. I do not discuss here many earlier studies that, though important in the development of our current knowledge of the epidemiology of childhood and adolescent depression, are to some extent superseded by more recent studies. Nor do I cover studies of great importance, but that have covered specific symptomatology or constructs of depression very different from those in general use. For more comprehensive reviews, the reader is referred to Angold (1988) and Fleming and Offord (1990). Though this review is organized by age range, the classification can be only approximate because in many studies the sampling was by school grade, and even when this was not the case, no conventions for sampling by age have ever been adopted. Therefore, the overlap of age ranges is considerable.

Preschool Children (Under 4 years)

For preschoolers little information is available. No studies of psychopathology in community samples of this age range have examined or indeed identified a syndrome that corresponds closely to the construct of any affective disorder for older children as described by *DSM-III*, and although the apathy of reactive attachment disorder in infancy has sometimes been equated with later depression, there is little information on its prevalence. Since Kashani and colleagues (1987) found only nine cases of major depression in a sample of 1, 000 children aged 1 to 6, consecutively referred to a child development unit, the rate in the community must be very low indeed.

Prepubertal (4- to 12-Year-Olds)

In the Ontario Child Health Study (Fleming et al. 1989), the instrument was a modified version of the CBCL (Achenbach and Edelbrock 1983, Boyle et al. 1987). A depressive subtype was defined by total scores on items related to depression, using simple algorithms to define cases of high, medium, and low diagnostic certainty. Several measures were used to validate caseness. At the high certainty level, prevalence of depression for 6- to 11-year-olds was 0.6 percent, with almost equal rates for boys and for girls. As the level of diagnostic certainty fell, the rate increased markedly, but without any effect on the sex ratio. Even at the high level of certainty, and though these children were much heavier users of mental health and social services, only about one in five had actually had contact with a service in the preceding 6 months, though teachers or parents thought a third needed professional help for emotional or behavioral problems.

One particularly important set of epidemiological studies is of a group of children born between 1972 and 1973, in one hospital in New Zealand, who have been followed longitudinally. When the children were 9 Kashani and colleagues (1983) used the Rutter scales and the Kiddie Schedule for Affective Disorders and Schizophrenia (Kiddie Epidemiology) (K-SADS-E) for interviewing both parent and child to estimate the prevalence of depression. The point prevalence of current major depression was 1.8 percent ± 1.8, and for minor depression 2.5 percent ± 2.2, with a slight excess of boys over girls. Two years later, on the same sample, Anderson and colleagues (1987), using an early version of the DISC and relying on clinical interpretation rather than computer algorithm to make diagnoses, obtained an overall rate for depressive disorders at the age of 11 of 1.8 percent ± 0.9, with a similar sex difference.

Bird and colleagues (1990), in one of the best-designed recent epidemiological studies of child psychiatric disorder, found that the overall point prevalence rate for children aged 4 to 16 of *DSM-III* depression and dysthymia was 5.9 percent ± 1.1, but if the diagnosis was confined to those with a Child Global Assessment Scale (CGAS) score of at least 61, the rate fell to 2.8 percent ± 0.7. Even with a total (first stage) sample of 2,064 households, the numbers were not large enough to estimate age-specific rates, but the frequency of depression increased with age across the sample. No sex differences were found, but lower-class children were at greater risk for depression. As in other studies, less than one-third of the children with an affective disorder diagnosis received no other diagnosis. Conduct disorders were the most common comorbid condition, but attention deficit disorder and anxiety disorders also were found with depression, though none of the anxious/depressed children also showed conduct problems. Using similar instrumentation in a longitudinal study, Velez and colleagues (1989) found much the same rates in an upstate New York sample, though the majority of their subjects were at or above the prepubertal age range.

In a Spanish sample of 1, 121 children in Barcelona, mainly 9- and 10-year-olds, Ezpeleta and colleagues (1990) used a two-stage design, screening with the CDI and defining caseness by a multiple-informant, multiple-method strategy that appears very close to *DSM-III* criteria. Seventy-six children had a CDI score greater than or equal to 19, and among these, four cases of major depression were found, along with twelve cases of dysthymic disorder. In a sample of 135 of the remainder who scored lower on the CDI, two cases of major depression and twelve cases of dysthymia were identified, so for the whole sample it can be calculated that there would have been nineteen cases of major depression (1.7 percent) and 104 cases of dysthymic disorder (9.3 percent).

For prepubertal school-aged children, the evidence is that the rate of severe handicapping depression is between 0.6 percent and 2.8 percent. The limited number of studies using a methodology that can be compared with clinical diagnostic methods, and the variety of populations studied, do not as yet permit any conclusions about where to place the rate for specific populations within this range. The sex ratio is approximately equal in most studies, and in most children it should be expected that depressive symptomatology is only one aspect of psychopathology to be found.

Adolescents (13- to 18-Year-Olds)

Though suicide attempts cannot be equated with depression, and, though they are very rare before puberty, they are common in adolescents, on the order of 2–4 percent (Garfinkel et al. 1982, Otto 1972, Stanley and Barter 1970). Kienhorst and colleagues (1990) found that a self-rating of depression was by far the best predictor of a suicide attempt.

Garrison and colleagues have mainly depended on the CES-D scale in a series of studies of adolescent depression. In a sample of seventh, eighth, and ninth graders drawn from a single high school (Garrison et al. 1989), about 4.4 percent (30 in a sample of 677) had symptom profiles that approximated to *DSM-III* major depression. The prevalence was highest for black females (11 percent) and lowest in black males (1.67 percent) and white females (4.45 percent), though high symptom scores and persistent symptoms were more common in females than males and more common in black than in white individuals. Since associations with high depression scores and higher absenteeism rates were found, and absenteeism rates were higher in the 11 percent who did not respond, the rates found may be underestimates. Other studies using similar self-report scales have shown that symptomatology is higher among female than male high school students and higher in minorities (Emslie et al 1990, Schoenbach et al. 1982).

Garrison and colleagues (1991) drew a large sample (2,465) of students from the seventh, eighth, and ninth grades in a public school system and used a two-stage procedure with the CES-D as a screen and what presumably was a fairly structured version of the K-SADS, administered by nurse clinicians, for the second stage. This gave a prevalence rate for major depression of 8.21 percent in males and 8.66 percent in females. Surprisingly, not only were the rates of dysthymia lower, but the condition was rarer in females (2.89 percent) than in males (6.78 percent). In this study, it appeared that a lower cut-off point on the CES-D was more appropriate for males, because even depressed boys had much lower scores than were common in girls.

Some indication of the correspondence of BDI scores in a community sample to those found in a clinical population is provided by a Swedish study by Larsson and Melin (1990). In a sample of 547 teenagers (13–18 years) drawn from two schools, they found that 8 percent had moderate scores on the BDI, but only 2 percent had scores as high as those in a small clinic sample. As in other studies, most of the high scorers were girls.

In the Ontario Child Health Study described earlier (Fleming et al. 1989), the rate of severe depression (high diagnostic certainty) increased to 1.8 percent for 12-to 16-year-olds, with a male:female ratio of 1:1.92. As for the younger age group, as the level of diagnostic certainty fell, the rate increased, with preservation of the sex ratio. Though adolescents self-reported more depressive symptoms, there was little agreement between their reports and those of their parents.

Kashani and colleagues (1987) identified seven adolescents (4.7 percent) in a sample of 150 high school students aged 14 to 16, who met criteria for a diagnosis of major depression based on a modified version of the DICA. Five other met diagnostic criteria for *DSM-III* dysthymia, and thirty-three others had significant depressive symptoms but were not assessed as being dysfunctional or in need of treatment. All of those assessed as having a depressive disorder had additional *DSM-III* diagnoses, commonly an anxiety disorder. The majority (ten) of the depressed individuals were girls.

McGee and colleagues (1990) followed up at the age of 13 the children in the Dunedin longitudinal study who had been depressed at 9 years. The instrumentation consisted of a modified DISC-C, parent and teacher ratings using the Rutter scales, and the Revised Behavior Problem Checklist (RBPC) (Quay and Peterson 1983). They found that depression persisted in all the children. The most recent follow-up of this sample was reported by McGee and colleagues (1990) when the members of the sample were 15 years old. Using a further modification of the DISC, McGee and colleagues found a prevalence of current major depression of 1.2 percent ± 0.7, and a prevalence of past major depression of 1.9 percent ± 0.7. Though by this age more girls than boys reported current and past depression, the sex difference was much more marked for past depression. This may be an age-specific reporting effect, as described by Angold and colleagues (1991). In contrast to most other studies, dysthymia was not more common; the prevalence was 1.1 percent ± 0.7, again with an excess of girls. The rate of co-morbidity in this sample was moderate—of the thirty-seven adolescents with a depressive disorder, twenty-four (65 percent) had at least one other major diagnosis, either of anxiety or conduct disorder. Unfortunately, the changes in methodology of this sample from one follow-up to the next make it difficult to attribute much significance to the variation in rates, though it is surprising that the rate in adolescence is not higher, particularly in girls.

RELATED DIAGNOSIS

Kovacs's longitudinal studies of clinic cases (Kovacs et al. 1984a,b, 1989) provide strong support for the belief that it is important to include adjustment disorder with depressed mood, to include dysthymic disorder with minor degrees of depression, and to distinguish between depressive subtypes in future epidemiological studies. Kovacs's data suggest that prognosis may be determined both by severity and by duration of depressive symptoms, and though severity has been considered in epidemiological studies so far, duration has generally not been considered so long as the not very demanding criteria of *DSM-III* or *DSM-III-R* were met.

Finally, on the topic of prevalence, it should be noted that though refinements in methodology may alter our understanding of the epidemiology of depression, at the same time there may be real changes in incidence and prevalence. There is a body of data, convincing though indirect, that rates of depression are increasing, and it is possible that the age of onset is decreasing (Klerman 1988). There is not enough information as yet available to determine if this is an effect peculiar to those born after World War II (the "baby boom" generation), or if subsequent generations now entering adolescence will have a different risk of developing depression in childhood or adolescence.

RISK FACTORS

Though reliable estimates of prevalence are important, and differences in prevalence from one population to another may be important cues to etiology, the most useful contribution of epidemiology is the definition of risk factors. Unfortunately, the epidemiology of depression in childhood and adolescence is still at too primitive a level to give pointers to any but the most obvious risk factors. As has been seen, adolescence is itself a risk factor, though estimates of prevalence are still too variable to be able to assign even an order of magnitude with any certainty. In adolescence, but not in childhood, girls have a higher rate of depression than boys. From Bird's study (Bird et al. 1989), it seems possible that poor academic attainment, family dysfunction, stressful life events, and maternal history of psychiatric disorder are all associated with depression in childhood and adolescence, but though these seem probable risk factors, these findings are not supported by other studies. The difficulties of case determination make any assessment of risk factors speculative at best.

CONCLUSION

From the ground covered in this chapter, it should be evident to the reader that the most basic questions, such as what is the prevalence of depression in childhood, cannot be answered with any confidence. Small changes in the defining criteria, alternative sampling and design strategies, and variations in instrumentation may all make important differences to estimates of prevalence and to associated findings. There is little agreement on which criteria define a true disorder, nor is there clear evidence on which to base a diagnostic procedure that can be applied for every or even any age range or on how to resolve differences between informants. Here it is sufficient to note that those prevalence rates that have been found may soon need to be revised, because there is no consensus on the resolution of the many methodological problems, and the concept of depression in childhood and adolescence is still in flux. At this stage of research development, it is premature to make more than guesses at risk factors that are specific for depression, because the diagnostic entity is still too unstable. Similarly, though epidemiological designs other than population surveys, such as case control studies, which may be used more economically to identify risk factors, have been attempted, we are too uncertain about the diagnostic entity itself to be able to attach much significance to the results.

REFERENCES

Achenbach, T. M. (1991). *Manual for the Child Behavior Checklist/4–18 and 1991 profile*. Burlington, VT: University of Vermont.

Achenbach, T. M., and Edelbrock, C. S. (1983). *Manual for the Child Behavior Checklist and Revised Child Behavior Profile*. Burlington, VT: University of Vermont.

American Psychiatric Association. (1980). *Diagnostic and Statistical Manual of Mental Disorders*. 3rd ed. Washington DC: American Psychiatric Association.

———— (1987). *Diagnostic and Statistical Manual of Mental Disorders*. 3rd ed. — rev. Washington DC: American Psychiatric Association.

Anderson, J., Williams, S., McGee, R., and Silva, P. A. (1987). *DSM-III* disorders in preadolescent children. *Archives of General Psychiatry* 44:69–80.

Angold, A. (1988). Childhood and adolescent depression: I. Epidemiological and aetiological aspects. *British Journal of Psychiatry* 152:601–617.

Angold, A., Weissman, M., John, K., et al. (1991). The effects of age and sex on depression ratings in children and adolescents. *Journal of the American Academy of Child and Adolescent Psychiatry* 30:67–74.

Beck, A. T., Ward, C. H., Mendelsohn, M., et al. (1961). An inventory for measuring depression. *Archives of General Psychiatry* 4:53–63.

Bird, H. R., Gould, M. S., Yager, T., et al. (1989). Risk factors for maladjustment in Puerto Rican children. *Journal of the American Academy of Child and Adolescent Psychiatry* 28:847–850.

Bird, H. R., Yager, T. J., Staghezza, B., et al. (1990). Impairment in the epidemiological measurement of childhood psychopathology in the community. *Journal of the American Academy of Child and Adolescent Psychiatry* 29:796–803.

Blazer, D., Swartz, M., Woodbury, M., et al. (1988). Depressive symptoms and depressive diagnoses in a community population. *Archives of General Psychiatry* 45:1078–1084.

Boyle, M. H., Offord, D. R., Hoffman, H. G., et al. (1987). Ontario Child Health Study: I. Methodology. *Archives of General Psychiatry* 44:826–831.

Breslau, N. (1987). Inquiring about the bizarre: false positives in diagnostic interview schedule for children (DISC) ascertainment of obsessions, compulsions and psychotic symptoms. *Journal of the American Academy of Child and Adolescent Psychiatry* 26:639–644.

Clayton, P. J., Grove, W. M., Coryell, W., et al. (1991). Follow up and family study of anxious depression. *American Journal of Psychiatry* 148:1512–1517.

Cole, D. A. (1990). Relation of social and academic competence to depressive symptoms in childhood. *Journal of Abnormal Psychology* 99:422–429.

Cole, D. A., and Carpentieri, S. (1990). Social status and the comorbidity of child depression and conduct disorder. *Journal of Consulting and Clinical Psychology* 58:748–757.

Costello, E. J. (1991). Married with children: predictors of mental and physical health in middle-aged women. *Psychiatry* 54:292–305.

Costello, E. J., and Angold, A. (1988). Scales to assess child and adolescent depression: checklists, screens and nets. *Journal of the American Academy of Child and Adolescent Psychiatry* 27: 726–737.

Costello, E. J., Costello, A. J., Edelbrock, C., et al. (1988). Psychiatric disorders in pediatric primary care: prevalence and risk factors. *Archives of General Psychiatry* 45:1107–1116.

Costello, E. J., Edelbrock, C., Costello, A. J., et al. (1988). Psychopathology in pediatric primary care: the new hidden morbidity. *Pediatrics* 82:415–424.

Costello, A. J., Edelbrock, C., Dulcan, M. K., et al. (1984). Development and testing of the NIMH Diagnostic Interview Schedule for children in a clinic population. Final report (Contract No. RFP-DB-81-0027). Rockville, MD: Center for Epidemiologic Studies, National Institute of Mental Health.

Dohrenwend, B. P. (1990). The problem of validity in field studies of psychological disorders revisited. *Psychological Medicine* 20:195–208.

Edelbrock, C., and Costello, A. J. (1988). Convergence between statistically derived behavior problem syndromes and child psychiatric diagnoses. *Journal of Abnormal Child Psychology* 16:219–231.

Edelbrock, C., Costello, A. J., Dulcan, M. K., et al. (1985). Age differences in the reliability of the psychiatric interview of the child. *Child Development* 56:265–275.

_____ (1986). Parent–child agreement on child psychiatric symptoms assessed via structured interview. *Journal of Child Psychology and Psychiatry* 27:181–190.

Emslie, G. J., Weinberg, W. A., Rush, A. J., et al. (1990). Depressive symptoms by self-report in adolescence: phase I of the development of a questionnaire for depression by self-report. *Journal of Child Neurology* 5:114–121.

Ezpeleta, L., Polaino, A., Domenech, E., and Domenech, J. M. (1990). Peer nomination inventory of depression: characteristics in a Spanish sample. *Journal of Abnormal Child Psychology* 18:373–391.

Fleming, J., and Offord, D. R. (1990). Epidemiology of childhood depressive disorders: a critical review. *Journal of the American Academy of Child and Adolescent Psychiatry* 29:571–580.

Fleming, J. E., Offord, D. R., and Boyle, M. H. (1989). Prevalence of childhood and adolescent depression in the community Ontario health study. *British Journal of Psychiatry* 155:647–654.

Frank, J. D. (1973). *Persuasion and Healing.* Baltimore: Johns Hopkins University Press.

Fundudis, T., Berney, T. P., Kolvin, I., et al. (1991). Reliability and validity of two self-rating scales in the assessment of childhood depression. *British Journal of Psychiatry* 159:(Suppl. 11) 36–40.

Garfinkel, B. D., Froese, A., and Hood, J. (1982). Suicide attempts in children and adolescents. *American Journal of Psychiatry* 139:1257–1261.

Garrison, C. Z., Addy, C., Kirby, L., et al. (1991). The CES-D as a screen for depression and other psychiatric disorders in adolescents. *Journal of the American Academy of Child and Adolescent Psychiatry* 30:636–641.

Garrison, C. Z., Schluchter, M. D., Schoenbach, W. J., and Kaplan, B. K. (1989). Epidemiology of depressive symptoms in young adolescents. *Journal of the American Academy of Child and Adolescent Psychiatry* 28:343–351.

Golding, J., and Lipton, R. I. (1990). Depressed mood and major depressive disorder in two ethnic groups. *Journal of Psychiatric Research* 24:65–82.

Hagnell, O., Lanke, J., Rorsman, B., and Ojesjö, L. (1982). Are we entering an age of melancholy? Depressive illness in a prospective epidemiologic study over 25 years: the Lundby Study, Sweden. *Psychological Medicine* 12:279–289.

Herjanic, B. and Reich, W. (1982). Development of a structural psychiatric interview for children. Part 1: Agreement between child and parent on individual symptoms. *Journal of Abnormal Child Psychiatry* 10:370–424.

Kaplan, G. A., Roberts, R. E., Camacho, T. C., and Coyne, J. C. (1987). Psychosocial predictors of depression. *American Journal of Epidemiology* 125:206–220.

Kashani, J. H., Carlson, G. A., Beck, N. C., et al. (1987). Depression, depressive symptoms, and depressed mood among a community sample of adolescents. *American Journal of Psychiatry* 144:931–934.

Kashani, J. H., McGee, R. O., Clarckson, S. E., et al. (1983). Depression in a sample of 9-year-old children: prevalence and associated characteristics. *Archives of General Psychiatry* 40:1217–1223.

Kashani, J. H., Rosenberg, T. K., and Reid, J. C. (1989). Developmental perspectives in child and adolescent depressive symptoms in a community sample. *American Journal of Psychiatry* 146: 871–875.

Kienhorst, C. W., deWilde, E. J., Van den Bout, J., et al. (1990). Characteristics of suicide attempters in a population-based sample of Dutch adolescents. *British Journal of Psychiatry* 156: 243–248.

Klerman, G. L. (1988). The current age of youthful melancholia. Evidence for increase in depression among adolescents and young adults. *British Journal of Psychiatry* 152:4–14.

Kovacs, M. (1985). The Children's Depression Inventory. *Psychopharmacology Bulletin* 21: 995–998.

Kovacs, M., Feinberg, T. L., Crouse-Novak, M. A., et al. (1984a). Depressive disorders in childhood. *Archives of General Psychiatry* 41:229–237.

———— (1984b). Depressive disorders in childhood: II. A longitudinal study of the risk for a subsequent major depression. *Archives of General Psychiatry* 41:643–649.

Kovacs, M., Gatsonis, C., Paulauskas, S. L., and Richards, C. (1989). Depressive disorders in childhood: IV. A longitudinal study of comorbidity with and risk for anxiety disorders. *Archives of General Psychiatry* 46:776–782.

Larson, R., Richards, M., Raffaelli, M., et al. (1990). Ecology of depression in late childhood and early adolescence: a profile of daily states and activities. *Journal of Abnormal Psychology* 99:92–102.

Larsson, B., and Melin, L. (1990). Depressive symptoms in Swedish adolescents. *Journal of Abnormal Child Psychology* 18:91–103.

Leaf, P. J., Bruce, M. L., Tischler, G. L., et al. (1988). Factors affecting the utilization of specialty and general medical health services. *Medical Care* 26:9–26.

Leon, R. G., Kendall, P. C., and Garber, J. (1982). Depression in children: parent, teacher and child perspectives. *Journal of Abnormal Child Psychology* 10:307–324.

Links, P. S., Boyle, M. H., and Offord, D. R. (1989). The prevalence of emotional disorder in children. *Journal of Nervous and Mental Disease* 177:85–91.

McGee, R., Feehan, M., William, S., et al. (1990). *DSM-III* disorders in a large sample of adolescents. *Journal of the American Academy of Child and Adolescent Psychiatry* 29:611–619.

McGee, R., Williams, S., Bradshaw, J., et al. (1985). The Rutter Scale for completion by teachers: factor structure and relationships with cognitive abilities and family adversity for a sample of New Zealand children. *Journal of Child Psychology and Psychiatry* 26:727–739.

Murphy, J. M., Olivier, D. C., Monson, R. R., et al. (1988). Incidence of depression and anxiety: The Stirling County Study. *American Journal of Public Health* 78:534–540.

Newman, S. C., Shrout, P. E., and Bland, R. C. (1990). The efficiency of two-phase designs in prevalence surveys of mental disorders. *Psychological Medicine* 20:183–193.

Orvaschel, H., Puig-Antich, J., Chambers, W., et al. (1982). Retrospective assessment of prepubertal major depression with the K-Sads-E. *Journal of the American Academy of Child Psychiatry* 21: 392–397.

Otto, U. (1972). Suicidal acts by children and adolescents. *Acta Psychiatrica Scandinavica Supplement* 233:7–123.

Puig-Antich, J., Perel, J., Lupatkin, W. et al. (1987). Imipramine in prepubertal major depressive disorders. *Archives of General Psychiatry* 44:81–89.

Quay, H. C., and Peterson, D. R. (1983). Manual for the revised behavior problem checklist. Unpublished manuscript.

Radloff, L. S. (1977). The CES-D scale: a self-report depression scale for research in the general population. *Applied Psychological Measurement* 1:385–401.

Regier, D. A., Boyd, J. H., Burke, J. D., et al. (1988). One-month prevalence of mental disorders in the United States based on five epidemiologic catchment areas. *Archives of General Psychiatry* 45:977–986.

Richman, N. (1974). The effect of housing on pre-school children and their mothers. *Developmental Medicine and Child Neurology* 16:53–58.

Roberts, R., Lewinsohn, P., and Seeley, J. (1991). Screening for adolescent depression: a comparison of depression scales. *Journal of the American Academy of Child and Adolescent Psychiatry* 30:58–66.

Robins, L. N. (1985). Epidemiology: reflections on testing the validity of psychiatric interviews. *Archives of General Psychiatry* 42:918–924.

Rutter, M. (1967). A children's behavior questionnaire for completion by teachers: preliminary findings. *Journal of Child Psychology and Psychiatry* 8:1–11.

Rutter, M., Tizard, J., and Whitmore, K. (1970). *Education, Health and Behavior*. London: Longman.

Ryan, N. D., Puig-Antich, J., Ambrosini, P., et al. (1987). The clinical picture of major depression in children and adolescents. *Archives of General Psychiatry* 44:854–861.

Ryan, N. D., Puig-Antich, J., and Cooper, T. (1986). Imipramine in adolescent major depression: plasma level and clinical response. *Acta Psychiatrica Scandinavica* 73:289–294.

Ryan, N. D., Puig-Antich, J., Rabinovich, H., et al., (1988). MAOIs in adolescent major depression unresponsive to tricyclic antidepressants. *Journal of the American Academy of Child and Adolescent Psychiatry* 27:755–758.

Schoenbach, V. J., Kaplan B. H., Grimson R. C., and Wagner E. H. (1982). Use of a symptom scale to study the prevalence of a depressive syndrome in young adolescents. *American Journal of Epidemiology* 116:791–800.

Schulterbrandt, J. G., and Raskin, A., eds. (1977). *Depression in Children: Diagnosis, Treatment and Conceptual Models*. New York: Raven.

Stanley, E. J., and Barter, J. T. (1970). Adolescent suicidal behavior. *American Journal of Orthopsychiatry* 40:87–96.

Sussman, L. K., Robins, L. N., and Earls, F. (1987). Treatment seeking for depression by black and white Americans. *Social Science and Medicine* 24:187–196.

Velez, C. N., Johnson, J., and Cohen, P. (1989). A longitudinal analysis of selected risk factors for childhood psychopathology. *Journal of the American Academy of Child and Adolescent Psychiatry* 28:681–864.

Weinstein, S., Stone, K., Noam, G. G., et al. (1989). Comparison of

DISC with clinicians' *DSM-III* diagnoses in psychiatric inpatients. *Journal of the American Academy of Child and Adolescent Psychiatry* 28:53-60.

Weissman, M. M. (1987). Advances in psychiatric epidemiology: rates and risks for major depression. *American Journal of Public Health* 77:445-451.

Weissman, M. M., Leaf, P. J., Tischler, G. L., et al. (1988). Affective disorders in five United States communities. *Psychological Medicine* 18:141-153.

Weissman, M. M., Wickramaratne, P., Warner, V., et al. (1987). Assessing psychiatric disorders in children: discrepancies between mother's and children's reports. *Archives of General Psychiatry* 44:747-753.

Weller E. B., Weller R. A., Preskorn S. H., and Glotzbach, R. (1982). Steady-state plasma imipramine levels in prepubertal depressed children. *American Journal of Psychiatry* 139:506-508.

Wickramaratne, P. J., Weissman, M. M., Leaf, P. J., and Holford, T. R. (1989). Age, period and cohort effects on the risk of major depression: results from five United States communities. *Journal of Clinical Epidemiology* 42:333-343.

6: THE FAMILY TRANSMISSION OF DEPRESSION

Linda Schwoeri, M. A., M. F. T.
G. Pirooz Sholevar, M. D.

INTRODUCTION

Interest in depression and families of depressed persons has burgeoned in the past two decades and is analogous to the extensive research of the 1950s and 1960s in studying schizophrenic families. Research focusing on the children of depressed parents has made tremendous leaps. The newer, more systematic and sophisticated studies indicate an outpouring of interest from many interrelated disciplines such as infant and child psychiatry, developmental psychology, and family psychiatry, as well as psychobiology.

The study of the etiology, onset, transmission, and treatment of depression in children, adolescents, and adults has been supported and encouraged by the development of clearer, specific diagnostic criteria in the *DSM-III* (1980) and *DSM-III-R* (1987). More systematic use of the research diagnostic criteria (RDC) and structured interview formats such as the Renard Diagnostic Interview (RDI) and the Schedule for Affective Disorders and Schizophrenia (SADS) have helped lessen the methodological problems in data collection and interpretation. Heightened research interest in the biological correlates of depression, especially the dexamethasone suppression test (DST) and other potential biological markers, has helped identify and interrupt the onset and course of depression that could last for months, disrupt all facets of the patient's life, and possibly result in suicide. Recent developments in psychopharmacology and new developments in treatment manuals specific for the treatment of depression utilizing an interpersonal approach (Klerman et al. 1984) and cognitive therapy (Beck 1963) have proven to be effective in reducing hopelessness and depressive symptoms.

This chapter reviews a number of selected studies on the transmission of depression because of the high incidence of depression among children of depressed parents. The studies selected represent the more recent trends in understanding the interactional and familial aspects of depression. Reviews of the early research findings from the high-risk studies and research on risk factors are presented in an effort to emphasize the importance of accurate diagnosis and appropriate research methods. The chapter also proposes an integration of some of the views expressed in the literature regarding the transmission of depression through the interaction of the child with a depressed parent within a family.

INFLUENCE OF *DSM-III* AND *DSM-III-R* CRITERIA ON DIAGNOSIS AND RESEARCH

Similar to the investigations of the transmission of schizophrenia in the family, research in the past two decades has confirmed the risk of transmission of depression within the family (Beardslee et al. 1988, Decina et al. 1983, McKnew et al. 1979, Orvaschel et al. 1988; Rutter and Quinton 1984; Trad 1986, Weissman et al. 1984, Weissman et al. 1987, Welner and Rice 1988). In these studies, rates of affective disorder vary between 11 percent and 50 percent (Lee and Gotlib 1989, Rutter 1990, Waters 1987) in contrast to control families in which the rates range between 11 percent and 24 percent (Beardslee et al. 1986, Merikangas et al. 1988, Weissman et al. 1987).

As indicated in the Downey and Coyne (1990) review, the children of depressed parents initially served as controls in high-risk research on the offspring of schizophrenic parents. These children were considered an ideal control group because depression and schizophrenia were viewed as equally severe but genetically distinct disorders (Kendler et al. 1981, Rosenthal 1970). These control-group children were used as a comparison group to test the hypothesis that the problems of children with schizophrenic parents were due to schizophrenia per se and not to the correlates of the psychiatric disturbance, namely stress, life events, and marital problems. In the course of the research, it was found that emotional disturbance of these children was equal to that of the children of schizophrenic parents, and that their problems were multidetermined as were those of the children of depressed parents. The early findings that the children of depressed and schizophrenic parents exhibited similar adjustment problems were due to the presence of parents in the schizophrenic sample who would now be diagnosed with an affective disorder.

It is common for depression to be associated with other psychiatric problems such as alcoholism, drug dependence, and personality disorder (Rutter and Quinton 1984). These associated problems may create the larger risk to the children according to Rutter (1990). A parent who is depressed and alcoholic will undoubtedly expose the child to more stress, and the risk of conduct disorder as well, than one who is diagnosed with only a major depression. Family risk factors such as parent–child discord, low family cohesion, and divorce were all significantly associated with conduct disorder (Rutter 1990). Axis II diagnoses are often associated with an earlier onset of depression, poorer recovery, and more frequent suicide attempts. All of these affect the children (Black et al. 1988 Phofl et al. 1984).

The *DSM-III* improved the diagnostic criteria used in research; however, the question of etiology due to genetic factors and psychosocial variables, including marital discord and impaired parenting, persists. Likewise the interaction among these variables continues to challenge researchers. Newer studies suggest that depression in children and adolescents is very similar to that experienced by adults. Research has also moved in the direction of viewing the interaction among different family-environmental factors in the transmission of depression.

OVERVIEW OF THE RISKS FOR CHILDREN OF DEPRESSED PARENTS

Family-Environmental Risk Factors

Children of depressed parents are at risk for a full range of psychological problems. A family history of depression appears to be the major risk factor for depression in children (Merikangas et al. 1988).

Having at least one parent with an affective disorder significantly increases the rate of depression and other psychopathology in children, compared with children whose parents have no history of affective illness (Beardslee et al. 1983, Weissman et al. 1984). Prospective follow-up studies of children diagnosed as having a major depression found that these episodes are usually of long duration (Kovacs et al. 1984a) with high rates of relapse after recovery (Kovacs et al. 1984b).

Reviews of the literature have shown high rates of symptomatology and impairment in offspring of probands with major depression (Beardslee et al. 1983, McKnew et al. 1979, Orvaschel et al. 1980). The rates of any *DSM-III* diagnoses in children of depressed parents range from 11 percent to 73 percent as opposed to 52 percent to 65 percent in control families (Keitner and Miller 1990, Keller et al. 1986, Merikangas et al. 1988, Rutter 1990, Weissman et al. 1987). In their review of the literature, Downey and Coyne (1990) indicate that the rate of depression for children of depressed parents is six times that of controls. A longitudinal study by Hammen and colleagues (1990) found that 80 percent of the children of unipolar depressed mothers received a major psychiatric diagnosis by age 18.

There has been variance in the reported rates of disturbance in the children of depressed parents (both unipolar and bipolar); however, a number of studies addressing this clinical issue arrive at a similar conclusion. Children of depressed parents have a higher rate of psychiatric and psychological disturbance than children whose parents are without psychiatric problems (Orvaschel et al. 1988). Negative environmental factors such as family discord, instability, and disruption are consistently reported in retrospective studies of depressed adults and in studies of children with depression (Orvaschel et al. 1980). Different studies have attempted to sort out the importance and impact of different risk factors for the children. Results of the studies may vary; however, they point out the need to look at the total family context in understanding the links between depression in parents and risks to children. For example, recently, Fendrick and colleagues (1990) assessed the importance of multiple risk factors on psychopathology in children of depressed and nondepressed parents. They reported that the presence of depressed parents may constitute an environmental risk to children above and beyond that identified by any single risk factor included in the study (p. 49). They found that parental depression was consistently more important as a predictor of major depression and anxiety disorders than any diagnosis in offspring. However, both parental depression and family risk factors were consistently more important as risk factors for conduct disorder than for any other disorders.

It is becoming apparent that living with a depressed person and coping on a daily basis with the manifestations of depression are associated with a great deal of family strain and disruption. Coyne and colleagues (1987) found that over 40 percent of adults living with a patient in a depressive episode were distressed themselves to the point of meeting criteria for needing therapeutic intervention. Family members feel the burden of the patient's depression through the patient's lack of interest in social life, fatigue, feelings of hopelessness, and constant worrying (Keitner et al. 1990).

Depression is a realistic threat to children living with a depressed parent. Affective disorders in children and adolescents appear to be more common than previously believed. It has been reported that 2 percent of children in the general population, 7 percent of pediatric inpatients, and 30 percent to 60 percent of child psychiatry outpatients meet *DSM-III-R* criteria for depression (Weller and Weller 1986).

In a longitudinal study, Radke-Yarrow and colleagues (1988) found that by middle and late childhood significantly more children of affectively ill mothers had depressive and disruptive problems and multiple behavior problems. The offspring of unipolar mothers developed problems earlier, and siblings were likely to have behavior problems. Hammen and colleagues (1987) also found that children of unipolar mothers fared worse than bipolar or medically ill mothers. By later childhood, the rates of problems in the offspring of both bipolar and unipolar groups were 61 percent and 68 percent, respectively (Radke-Yarrow et al. 1988). This relatively high rate of overall problem behavior seems to reflect that middle to later childhood is a time of increased risk in the co-morbidity of children's problems. It is indicative of the stresses imposed on vulnerable children as adolescence advances.

Beardslee and colleagues (1985) have emphasized the heightened risk and the increased episodes of major depression during adolescence. Hammen and colleagues (1990), in a longitudinal study of diagnoses in children and adolescents whose mothers have bipolar or unipolar depression, report that by age 18, approximately 80 percent of the children will receive a major psychiatric diagnosis. In earlier studies, as many as 40–50 percent of the children of a depressed parent were given psychiatric diagnoses (Cytryn et al. 1982, Decina et al. 1983).

In terms of family interactions, it appears that hostility becomes more pronounced when depressed mothers interact with school-aged children. The mother's behavior is more irritable and critical and less task-focused or positive while attempting to resolve tasks with her child (Gordon et al. 1989, Hammen et al. 1987). Panaccione and Wahler (1986) found a strong association between the mother's depressive symptoms and hostile child-directed behavior, which included shouting and slapping.

Families of depressed patients report significant dysfunction in family communications, problem solving, and the capacity of individual family members to experience appropriate affect over a range of stimuli (Keitner et al. 1990). They feel less able to show love or affection for each other and are concerned about the lack of emotional responsiveness in family members. Family rules and regulations are problematic because expectations are unclear, and members are unable to discuss feelings. Miller and colleagues (1986) reported that families of patients with major depression consistently showed the most impaired family functioning (75 percent reported disturbances) when compared with families of patients with alcohol dependence, adjustment disorders, schizophrenia, or bipolar disorder.

Beardslee and colleagues (1985) reported on the impact of specific indexes of severity and chronicity of parental depression, measures of familial discord, and demographic variables as predictors of impaired adaptive function and psychopathology in seventy-two children and their mothers. At least one biological parent in each of the thirty-seven families had a depressive disorder but not a history of mania, schizophrenia, or schizoaffective disorder. There was impaired adaptation and the presence of DSM-III-diagnosed disorder in the children and an associated increase in discord among married or separated parents. There was association of impairment in children's adaptive functioning and a history of DSM-III diagnosis seen in married and separated parents. The association suggests that if the biological parents have a poor relationship with each other, then their children will have impaired adaptation. This finding in the divorced families is further evidence for the deleterious effects on children of the parents' poor relationship when they separate or divorce.

Current family and marital problems frequently are cited as correlates of depression (Merikangas et al. 1985). It has been shown that marital dysfunction exists both before and after an acute episode of depression (Weissman 1979). Studies indicate that depression-prone women are more likely to be married to men with a history of psychological difficulties that make the men less available for an intimate relationship in the marriage. This intimate relationship could help reduce the woman's experience of depression (Coyne 1990). It has also been shown that depressed women tend to be married to men with personality disorders (Merikangas and Speker 1982, Negri et al. 1979), thereby further increasing the risk factors in the marriage and to the children of that relationship.

Marital distress makes problem-solving interactions around parenting more difficult. There is more dysphoric affect in the interactions (Hops et al. 1987); there is more aggressive behavior during interactions with spouses (Biglan et al. 1988); and coercive behaviors become part of the family's interactional style as they are initiated and reciprocated within the family (Patterson 1982). These studies show an increasing trend toward viewing depression within the family context. They indicate the need to assess the total family situation as well as the individual pathology reported.

Although there is no definitive research on the temporal order between the onset of the parent's and child's illness, an association has been established. In the sample reported on by Beardslee and colleagues (1985), the first episode of major depression in the children who became depressed always followed an episode of depression in at least one parent. This was true of the first episode of any *DSM-III* disorder in 97 percent of the seventy-two children in the study. In establishing an association between indexes of parental illness and psychopathology in the children, a first step was taken in predicting a deficit in the adaptive functioning capacity of the children.

The clinical relevance of this for the clinician is that he or she must be aware that children of affectively ill parents are at high risk for developing psychopathology and impaired adaptive functioning in close proximity to that of the parents. The development of childhood disorder should be identified rapidly. The association of poor marital relations and childhood psychopathology should alert clinicians to the risks involved for children of separated or divorced families. Above all, a careful family history of both parents for affective disorder should be taken. If there is a history of severe and chronic parental depression, special attention should be paid to detecting the early development of impaired adaptation, general psychopathology, and depression in the children (Beardslee et al. 1985). Guidelines for diagnosing childhood depression in the *DSM-III* and *DSM-III-R* are now more specific in this area.

Biological/Genetic Risk Factors

Puig-Antich (1986) has attempted to isolate biological correlates to depression. He defines biological markers as "characteristics that have been shown to be specifically associated with the disorder in question, during an episode, during the symptom-free intervals, or both" (p. 342). Trad (1986) notes the differentiation between *state markers* and *trait markers*. *State markers* show abnormalities associated with the onset of the disorder and subside during symptom-free periods. True *trait markers* measure persistent abnormalities in fully recovered patients and predate the onset of morbidity. Some prominent biological markers for affective disorders include sleep EEG abnormalities and abnormalities in biogenic amines such as dopamine, norepinephrine, and serotonin, which are involved in the regulation of neurotransmitter functions.

The DST has been useful in measuring cortisol levels associated with depression. Puig-Antich (1986) refers to cortisol as a state marker because cortisol hypersecretion occurs only during a depressive episode and returns to normal on recovery. The DST has not been used as extensively with children as with adults. However, its ability to discriminate among different subtypes of depression is noted as somewhat comparable for children and adults (Trad 1986, p. 30).

There is more current research suggesting that depression is a familial disorder, and that genetic and/or biochemical variables play a pathogenic role in the development of a depressive disorder (Papolas and Papolas 1987). Investigations are attempting to sort out the possible contributions of biochemical and genetic factors. Family aggregation studies demonstrate that relatives of depressed patients have higher rates of affective illness than normal controls (Weissman and Akiskal 1984, Winokur et al. 1978). Biochemical studies include research related to neurotransmitter studies (Anisman and Zacharko 1982), neuroendocrine studies (Carroll et al. 1981), and studies of pharmacologic treatments (Charney and Menher 1981). Although the full extent of the influence of genetic and/or biological vulnerabilities to depression is at best still speculative, research is progressing in this direction (Holder and Anderson 1990). (A comprehensive review of the biological disturbances associated with childhood depression is included in Chapter 8.)

The interactive effects among genetic vulnerability, impaired parenting skills, and family-environmental stress all contribute to the psychopathology of children of depressed parents. Research has suggested that, as with other life stressors, individual variations exist among the children of parents with mental illness. However, the children are less likely to be affected adversely if the parental disorder is (a) mild; (b) of short duration; (c) unassociated with family discord, conflict, and disorganization; (d) unaccompanied by impaired parenting; and (e) does not result in family break-up (Cohler 1987, Rutter in press).

TRANSMISSION OF DEPRESSION THROUGH PARENT–CHILD INTERACTION

The transmission of depression through parent–child interaction has been studied by researchers from different orientations and perspectives. Some of the concepts relevant to discussing this transmission include:

1. The influence of the child's temperament and gender on the interactions between parent and child
2. The role of maternal affect communication in the transmission of depression and the child's duplication of the mother's affect
3. How the mother's depression interferes with attachment behavior
4. The social learning of coercive processes in interactions with a depressed mother

Together these perspectives form a matrix for studying the life of the children faced with a depressed parent.

Temperament and Gender Differences

A factor of prime consideration is the child's individual personality and temperament. Thomas and Chess (1984) feel that temperament, which is viewed as an inherently genetically determined characteristic, is mediated by the environment. The child is affected by the parent's depression while also having a strong effect on the parent's depression. Thomas and Chess also suggest that coping with a temperamentally difficult child may present overwhelming difficulties for an already depressed mother or parent. The child who presents fewer difficulties might receive more positive affect from the mother, engage in less problematic interactions with the mother, and possibly form a more positive attachment to her. Attempting to soothe and comfort a fussy, irritable infant can be a most unrewarding experience for any mother. When the mother is depressed, feeling incompetent in dealing with the child and frustrated by her attempts, the mixture of child temperament and maternal depression makes for a disturbing interaction. The experience further highlights her feelings of inadequacy and worthlessness and thereby adds to her depressed mood.

Rothbard and Derryberry (1982) have advanced a general view of temperament that also argues for the innate components of temperament, but they stress that these elements are shaped by the physical and social environment. This suggests a somewhat flexible and fluid quality to the concept of temperament. According to this view, the child interacts with his environment based on his innate difference and responds to the affective stimuli in it to form his own affective range of behavior. This view is more interactive and less critical of the mother and child and their respective personality traits as contributions to the interaction.

Rutter (1990) also emphasizes and cautions that individual differences in children must be considered when discussing the transmission of depression. Parents interact with their children, at least in part, based on the stimuli provided by the children. Furthermore, studies have shown that temperamental qualities and gender differences influence this interaction. Temperamentally difficult children are more likely to be the target of parental irritability and criticism (Rutter and Quinton 1984).

Some mothers seek comfort from their daughters, which draws them into the mother's own distress and unhappiness. This is described as a type of prolonged physical affection with the daughters and as a kind of "security blanket" (Radke-Yarrow et al. 1988, p. 59). Radke-Yarrow (1990) also has found that in interactions with her son, the depressed mother shows anger and unhappiness in the face of aggression and less joyfulness when he exhibits shyness. Shyness in boys tends to be associated with negative social interactions, whereas in girls, shyness is associated with positive interaction (Radke-Yarrow 1990, Simson and Stevenson-Hinde 1985). Depression in the parent is reflected in difficulties in parenting. There are reciprocal influences of children on parents and parents on children necessitating a comprehensive view of the family context.

Coercive Exchanges between Mother and Child

Research supports a bidirectional relationship between hostile, irritable, and negative parenting by a depressed mother and child maladjustment (Hammen et al. 1990, Patterson 1982, Patterson and Forgatch 1990, Radke-Yarrow et al. 1988). Because of this bidirectionality, it is difficult to disentangle causal factors. The question remains whether the interactions are the result of the child's reaction to the mother's depressed, irritable mood, or if the mother is responding to a predisposition in the child. Most importantly, the interactions establish a complex pattern that becomes learned through its circularity and repetition. This pattern becomes internalized by the child and is then transferred to interactions beyond the mother–child dyad.

The work of Patterson and Forgatch (1990) notes that maternal irritability and depressed mood are concomitant reactions to stress and loss of support for single mothers, and that together they set the stage for the coercive exchanges. Children of depressed mothers become active participants in a coercive cycle that serves to relieve the mother's depression as well as to provide respite from its effects. The child consequently learns the benefits of coercive behavior, and the mother learns how to disengage from the child's aversive behaviors. (The process described here is fully elaborated in Chapter 6 by Schwoeri and Sholevar.)

Maternal Affect During Interaction and the Child's Duplication of It

Observational studies of depressed mothers in face-to-face interactions with their children 3–61 months of age present a picture of the dampening effect of depression. These mothers express little positive affect and respond more slowly and less consistently to the children, without the exaggerated intonation characteristic of playful speech. Their reduced energy levels and self-absorption are characteristic of depressive symptomatology (Bettes 1988, Cohn et al. 1990, Field 1984, Field et al. 1985, 1988, Fleming et al. 1988). Studies have reported that depressed mothers are more irritable toward their infants than are control mothers, and that maternal irritability and hostility increase under stress (Field et al. 1990, Lyons-Ruth et al. 1986, Rutter 1990, Patterson 1990).

As the child and mother interact, they share respective affective states. Stern (1985) calls this process *mirroring*, a form of empathy between the child and mother. Because early interactions or exchanges provide the important nonverbal building blocks of affective communication, they help inform the infant of his success in communicating feelings and interpreting those of the mother. The mother's depressed affect will have a profound impact on the child's sense of self and may contribute to his or her vulnerability to depression. These mother–child interactions essentially become part of the child's view of the world as perhaps a less than happy place to be.

One striking example of the impact of maternal affect is Field's (1984) observations of mother–infant dyads. Field compared the interactions of dyads with depressed and nondepressed mothers and found that changes in the mother's behavior elicited changes in the infant's behavior, while continuity in the mother's affective behavior predicted continuity in the infant's affective behavior. When nondepressed mothers simulate depressed affect, their infants react with protest to the change. The infants of depressed mothers, however, appear undisturbed by the behavior. They have, in effect, become accustomed to this affect and habituate to it.

Impact of Maternal Depression on Attachment Behavior

Studies of attachment behavior provide a context for further possible explanations of the transmission of depression in the interactions between a child and depressed mother. Depressed mothers who are helpless, irritable, unresponsive, and unaffectionate (Weissman et al. 1972) in caring for their children make parent–child attachments difficult. Children of depressed parents present different attachment behaviors than those of nondepressed parents. Radke-Yarrow and colleagues (1985) found that twice as many children of mothers with major depression had insecure attachments as compared with children of clinically normal parents or of those with only mild depression. Zahn-Waxler and colleagues (1984) found children of bipolar parents were also insecurely attached. These insecure attachments correspond to the avoidant and ambivalent attachment described by Ainsworth and colleagues (1978). According to Ainsworth's work, secure children use their attachment figures or caretakers as a secure base from which to explore the new and unfamiliar environment. The Strange Situation Procedure has been used to observe this. Children who are securely attached seek to establish contact and interaction, and thereby comfort, upon the return of the caretaker to the room. In contrast, the infant who appears undistressed by the caregiver's departure, and avoids her or him on return—preferring to play with toys, for example—is classified with avoidant attachment. Ambivalent attachment refers to ambivalent reactions upon the caretaker's return—demanding attention and yet resisting it.

Role of the Other Parent

Another factor to consider is the role played by the other, nondepressed parent. The effect of having one depressed parent who is emotionally unavailable and often reactive to his or her child's everyday ups and downs can be worsened if the other parent is likewise depressed, detached, or feeling overwhelmed. The marital relationship is a major factor in the child's vulnerability to depression. As studies have shown, the mother who lacks an intimate relationship fares much worse and, therefore, her child is placed at greater risk. It would be crucial to involve both parents or significant relationships in the assessment of the child's depression in order to determine what family and parental resources are available in the treatment of the child and subsequently in the assessment of the improvement of the child's condition.

A nondepressed parent can mitigate the effects of compromised parenting and provide the nurturing that is often lost to the effects of depression in the parent. If the nondepressed parent has his or her own share of healthy adaptation to the depression, the child can better tolerate any losses he or she may have to endure through the family's struggle with the symptoms of depression.

INTEGRATION OF VIEWS OF FAMILY TRANSMISSION OF DEPRESSION

The transmission of depression or the predisposition to depression occurs through a number of routes. Several have been discussed briefly. These routes have a common focus that is the formation of the child's pattern of behavior as well as his or her internal model for relationships. Because of this, the child is at risk not only for depression but also for a wide range of psychopathology based on daily interactions with the depressed parent. The child who is living with an aggressive or abusive parent will undoubtedly develop and refine his or her coercive skills during interactions with the parent and ultimately, although unconsciously, transfer this interactional sequence to his or her own children. Likewise, a child exposed to daily interactions with a depressed, passive, or irritable mother will incorporate this style of affective behavior and behave toward others in a similar manner.

Understanding and treating children of depressed parents present a challenge to the clinician, who must look at the child and never ignore the family environment in which the child dwells. Depression imposes itself cruelly on the lives of children. Their interactional and affective lives are always compromised by the effects of the illness.

David Reiss (1988) has described two theoretical perspectives that help explain the transmission of these interactional patterns through the generations. The first perspective is the *practicing family perspective*. It describes the transactional patterns or microchains of interactional sequences that have been studied by social learning theorists such as Patterson (1982, 1990). On a descriptive behavioral level, the child and parent become involved in a continuing pattern in which the child and parent mutually coerce and reinforce each other's behavior. Reiss also describes how internal objects and self-object representations are formed and concretized during repetitions of these interactions between the child and the parent. He calls this the *represented family perspective*. This perspective discusses how through the continued practiced behaviors the child's internal structures stabilize and are then transmitted across time throughout the generations. The child exposed to depression and aggression or violence will have this organizing feature in relationships with his or her own children.

The concepts of practicing and represented family perspectives help explain how depressed parents transfer their depressed, irritable, angry moods. The practicing family perspective is essentially the social learning interactional sequences described by Patterson and his colleagues at the Oregon Social Learning Center (OSLC). The represented family perspective is essentially an object relations description of the internalization of these transactions across time. Together they form a picture of the child's external and internal world when living with a depressed parent. Essentially, these two perspectives demonstrate the interrelationship between the behavioral manifestations of depression and the internal representations of the child–parent relationship. This dynamic interaction between inner and outer reality underscores the need for research in the interactions between parent and child when the child lives in a family with a depressed parent(s).

CONCLUSION

The high rate of psychopathology in the children of depressed parents has become a well-known and alarming finding. The plight of children of depressed parents, particularly depressed mothers, poses a major challenge to the preventive and therapeutic programs for depression. The rate of psychopathology in children of depressed parents varies in different studies depending upon the characteristics of the sample population and level of depression in the parents. The estimated rate of diagnosable illnesses (mostly affective in nature) ranges from 11 percent to 73 percent for children of depressed parents. The paramount factors determining the transmission of depression and psychopathology from the parents to the children are the severity and chronicity of depression in the parents, the emotional status of the nondepressed parent, the health and functionality of other familial and nonfamilial support systems, and the age of the child at the onset of depression. Maternal depression has more profound impact than depression of the father. The marital strife between the parents can enhance the psychopathogenic impact of parental depression in multiple ways. The role of genetic and family interactional factors in the transmission of depression and psychopathology to children is well established, although a detailed delineation of the exact mechanisms awaits new investigation.

The transmission of depression does not occur through one particular medium, nor is there one causal link involved. The transmission of depression involves a complex interaction among repeated behavior patterns, differences in temperament of the child and affect in the mother, and the internal representations of those factors within the child exposed to the depressed parent. The biological and genetic factors come to bear also, and in view of such, depression represents a multidimensional psychiatric problem.

Preventive programs to protect children from the ill effects of parental depression are currently in existence, but they are infrequently used in clinical settings. These programs are psychoeducational in nature and inform all family members, including the children, of the nature of depression, its symptomatology, therapeutic principles, and the impact of the illness on the familial environment. The preliminary investigation of the impact of preventive programs on the children is encouraging.

Future investigation in this field should search for the factors that determine the form of the psychopathology, depressive or nondepressive, in the children as well as the exact factors enhancing the resiliency of some of the children in the face of parental depression.

REFERENCES

Ainsworth, D., Blehar, W., and Walters, E. (1978). *Patterns of Attachment.* Hillsdale, NJ: Lawrence Erlbaum.

Anisman, H., and Zacharko, R. M. (1982). Depression: The predisposing influence of stress. *Behavioral and Brain Sciences* 55:89–137.

Beardslee, W., Bemporad, J., Keller, M. B., et al. (1983). Children of parents with major affective disorder: a review. *American Journal of Psychiatry* 140:825-832.

Beardslee, W., Keller, M., Lavori, P. et al. (1988). Psychiatric disorder in adolescent offspring of parents with affective disorders in a non-referred sample. *Journal of Affective Disorders* 15:313-322.

Beardslee, W., Klerman, G., Keller, M., et al. (1985) But are they cases? Validity of *DSM-III* major depression in children identified in family study. *American Journal of Psychiatry* 142:687-691.

Beck, A. (1963). Thinking and depression idiosyncratic content and cognitive distortions. *Archives of General Psychiatry* 9:36-45.

Bettes, B. (1988). Maternal depression and motherese. Temporal and intonational features. *Child Development* 59:1089-1096.

Biglan, A., Hops, H., Sherman, L., et al. (1988). Problem-solving interactions of depressed women and their husbands. *Behavior Therapy* 16:431-451.

Black, D. W., Bell, S., Hulbert, J., and Nasrallah, T. (1988). The importance of Axis II disorders in patients with major depression: a controlled study. *Journal of Affective Disorders* 14:115-122.

Carroll, B. H., Feinberg, M., Greden, J. F., et al. (1981). A specific laboratory test for the diagnosis of melancholia: standardization, validation, and clinical utility. *Archives of General Psychiatry* 38:15-22.

Charney, D. S., and Menher, D. B. (1981). Receptor sensitivity and the mechanism of action of antidepressant treatment: implications for the etiology and therapy of depression. *Archives of General Psychiatry* 38:1160-1175.

Cohler, B. J. (1987). Adversity, resilience and the study of lives. In *The Invulnerable Child*, ed. E. J. Anthony and B. J. Cohler, pp. 363-424. New York: Guilford.

Cohn, J. E., Campbell, S. B., and Matias, R. (1990). Face to face interactions of postpartum depressed and non-depressed mother-infant pairs at two months. *Developmental Psychology* 26:15-23.

Coyne, J., Kahn, J., and Gotlib, I. H. (1989). *Depression in Family Interaction and Psychotherapy*, ed. T. Jacob. New York: Plenum.

Coyne, J. (1990). Interpersonal processes in depression. In *Depression and Families: Impact and Treatment*, ed. G. Keitner. Washington DC: APPI Press.

Coyne, J., Kessler, R., Tol, M., et al. (1987). Living with a depressed person: burden and psychological distress. *Journal of Consulting and Clinical Psychology* 55:347-352.

Cytryn, L., McKnew, D. H., Bartho, J., et al. (1982). Offspring of patients with affective disorders II. *American Academy of Child Psychiatry* 21:389-391.

Decina, P., Kestenbaum, C. J., Farber, S., et al. (1983). Clinical and psychological assessment of children of bipolar probands. *American Journal of Psychiatry* 140:548–555.

Downey, G., and Coyne, J. C. (1990). Children of depressed parents: an integrative review. *Psychology Bulletin* 108:50–76.

Fendrick, M., Warner, V., and Weissman, M. (1990). Family risk factors parental depression and psychopathology in offspring. *Developmental Psychology* 26:40–50.

Field, T. M. (1984). Early interactions between infants and their postpartum depressed mothers. *Infant Behavior and Development* 7:517–522.

Field, T. M., Healy, B., Goldstein, S., and Gethertz, M. (1990). Behavior state matching and synchrony in mother–infant interactions of non-depressed versus depressed dyads. *Developmental Psychology* 26:7–14.

Field, T. M., Healy, B., Goldstein, S., et al. (1988). Infants of depressed mothers show "depressed" behavior even with non-depressed adults. *Child Development* 60:1569–1579.

Field, T. M., Sandberg, D., Garcia, R., et al. (1985). Pregnancy problems, postpartum depression and early mother–infant interaction. *Developmental Psychology* 21:1152–1156.

Fleming, A., Ruble, D., Flett, G., and Shaul, D. (1988). Postpartum adjustment in first time mothers: relations between mood, maternal attitudes and mother–infant interactions. *Developmental Psychology* 24:71–81.

Gordon, D., Burger, D., Hammen, C., et al. (1989). Observations of interactions of depressed women with their children. *American Journal of Psychiatry* 146:50–55.

Hammen, C., Burge, D., and Stansbury, K. (1990). Relationship of mother and child variables to child outcomes in a high risk sample: a causal modeling analysis. *Developmental Psychology* 26:24–30.

Hammen, C., Gordon, D., Burge, D., et al. (1987). Maternal affective disorder, illness, and stress: risk for children's psychopathology. *American Journal of Psychiatry* 144:736–741.

Holder, D., and Anderson, C. (1990). Psychoeducational family intervention for depressed patients and their families. In *Depression and Families: Impact and Treatment*, ed. G. Keitner, pp. 159–184. Washington, DC: APPI.

Hops, M., Biglan, A., Sherman, L., et al. (1987): Home observations of family interactions of depressed women. *Journal of Consulting and Clinical Psychology* 55:341–346.

Keitner, G., and Miller, I. (1990). Family functioning and major depression: an overview. *American Journal of Psychiatry* 147:1128–1137.

Keitner, G., Miller, I., Epstein, N., et al. (1990). The functioning of families of patients with major depression. *International Journal of Family Psychiatry* 7:11–16.

Keller, M. B., Beardslee, W. R., Dorer, D. J., et al. (1986). Impact of severity and chronicity of parental affective illness on adaptive functioning and psychopathology in their children. *Archives of General Psychiatry* 43:930–937.

Kendler, K., Gruenberg, A., and Strauss, J. (1981). An independent analysis of the Copenhagen sample of the Danish adoption study of schizophrenia. *Archives of General Psychiatry* 38:973–990.

Klerman, G. L., Weissman, M. M., and Rounsaville, B. J. (1984). *Interpersonal Psychotherapy of Depression*. New York: Basic Books.

Kovacs, M., Feinberg, T. L., Crouse-Novak, M. A., et al. (1984a). Depressive disorders in childhood: I. A. longitudinal prospective study of characteristics and recovery. *Archives of General Psychiatry* 41:229–237.

——— (1984b). Depressive disorders in childhood: II. A longitudinal study of the risk for a subsequent major depression. *Archives of General Psychiatry* 41:643–649.

Lee, C., and Gotlib, I. (1989). Clinical status and emotional adjustment of children of depressed mothers. *American Journal of Psychiatry* 146:478–483.

Lyons-Ruth, K., Zoll, D., Connell, D., and Greenbaum, H. (1986). The depressed mother and her one-year-old infant. Environment, interaction, attachment, and infant development. In *Maternal Depression and Infant Disturbance*, ed. E. Tronech and T. Fields, pp. 61–82. San Francisco: Jossey-Bass.

McKnew, D. H., Cytryn, L., Efron, A. M., et al. (1979). Offspring of patients with affective disorders. *British Journal of Psychiatry* 134:148–152.

Merikangas, K. R., and Speker, D. G. (1982). Assortive mating among inpatients with primary affective disorder. *Psychological Medicine* 12:753–764.

Merikangas, K. R., Prusoff, B. A., Kupfer, D., et al. (1985). Marital adjustment in major depression. *Journal of Affective Disorders* 9:5–11.

Merikangas, K. R., Prusoff, B. A., and Weissman, M. M. (1988). Parental concordance for affective disorders: psychopathology in offspring. *Journal of Affective Disorders* 15:279–290.

Miller, I. W., Kabacoff, R., Keitner, G., et al. (1986). Family functioning in the families of psychiatric patients. *Comprehensive Psychiatry* 27:302–312.

Negri, F., Melica, A. M., Zubiani, R., et al. (1979). Assortive mating and affective disorders. *Journal of Affective Disorders* 1:247–253.

Orvaschel, H., Weissman, M. M., and Kidd, K. K. (1980). Children —

depression: the children of depressed parents, the childhood of depressed patients, depression in children. *Journal of Affective Disorders* 2:1-16.

Orvaschel, H., Walsh-Allis G., and Weijar, Y. (1988). Psychopathology in children of parents with recurrent depression. *Journal of Abnormal Child Psychology* 16:17-28.

Panaccione, V. F., and Wahler, R. G. (1986). Child behavior, maternal depression, and social coercion as factors in the quality of child care. *Journal of Abnormal Child Psychology* 14:263-278.

Papolas, D. F., and Papolas, J. (1987). *Overcoming Depression*. New York: Harper & Row.

Patterson, G. (1982). *A Social Learning Approach to Family Intervention: Vol. 3. Coercive Family Process*. Eugene, OR: Castalia.

_____ (1990). *Depression and Aggression in Family Interaction*. Hillsdale, NJ: Lawrence Erlbaum.

Patterson, G., and Forgatch, M. (1990). Initiation and maintenance of process disrupting single-mother families. In *Depression and Aggression in Family Interaction*, ed. G. Patterson, pp. 209-244. Hillsdale, NJ: Lawrence Erlbaum Associates.

Phofl, B., Stangl, D., and Zimmerman, M. (1984). The implications of *DSM-III-R* personality disorders for patients with major depression. *Journal of Affective Disorders* 7:309-318.

Puig-Antich, J. (1986). Psychobiological markers: effects of age and puberty. In *Depression In Young People*, ed. M. Rutter, E. E. Izard, and P. B. Read, pp. 341-382. New York: Guilford.

Radke-Yarrow, M. (1990). Family environments of depressed and well parents and their children: issues of research methods. In *Depression and Aggression in Family Interaction* ed. G. Patterson, pp. 169-184. Hillsdale, NJ: Lawrence Erlbaum Associates.

Radke-Yarrow, M., Cummings, E., Kuczynski L., and Chapman, M. (1985). Patterns of attachment in two- and three-year-olds in normal families with parental depression. *Child Development* 56:884-893.

Radke-Yarrow, M., Richters, J., and Wilson, E. (1988). Child development in the network of relationships. In *Relationships within Families: Mutual Influences*, ed. R. A. Hinde and J. Stevenson-Hinde, pp. 48-67. Oxford, England: Clarendon.

Reiss, D. (1988). The represented and practicing family. Contrasting visions of family continuity. In *Early Relationship Disorders*, ed. A. J. Sameroff and R. N. Emde. New York: Basic Books.

Rosenthal, D. (1970). *Genetic Theory and Abnormal Behavior*. New York: McGraw-Hill.

Rothbard M. K., and Derryberry, D. (1982). Theoretical issues in temperament. In *Developmental Disabilities: Theory, Assessment, and*

Intervention, ed. M. Lewis and L. T. Taft, pp. 383–400. New York: S. P. Medical and Scientific Books.

Rutter, M. (1990). Commentary. Some focus and process considerations regarding effects of parental depression on children. *Developmental Psychology* 26:60–67.

Rutter, M. (in press). A fresh look at "maternal deprivation." In *The Development and Interpretation of Behavior*, ed. P. Bateson and P. Marler. Cambridge, England: Cambridge Press.

Rutter, M., and Quinton, D. (1984). Parental psychiatric disorder: effects on children. *Psychological Medicine* 14:853–880.

Simson, A. E., and Stevenson-Hinde, J. (1985). Temperamental characteristics of 3- and 4-year-old boys and girls and child–family interactions. *Journal of Child Psychology and Psychiatry* 26:43–53.

Stern, D. (1985). *The Interpersonal World of the Infant*. New York: Basic Books.

Thomas, A., and Chess, S. (1984). Genesis and evaluation of behavior disorders: from infancy to early adult life. *American Journal of Psychiatry* 141:1–9.

Trad, P. W. (1986). *Infant Depression, Paradigm and Paradoxes*. New York: Springer-Verlag.

Wallerstein, J. S., and Kelly, J. B. (1990). *Surviving the Breakup: How Parents and Children Cope with Divorce*. New York: Basic Books.

Waters, B. (1987). Psychiatric disorders in the offspring of parents with affective disorder: a review. *Journal of Preventive Psychiatry* 3:191–206.

Weintraub, S. (1987). Risk factors in schizophrenia. The Stony Brook High-Risk Project. *Schizophrenia Bulletin* 13:439–449.

Weissman, M. M., and Akiskal, H. S. (1984). The role of psychotherapy in chronic depression: a proposal. *Comprehensive Psychiatry* 25:23–31.

Weissman, M. M., Gammen, G. D., Merikangas, K. R., et al. (1987). Children of depressed parents: increased psychopathology and early onset of major depression. *Archives of General Psychiatry* 44:847–853.

Weissman, M. M., Paykel, E., and Klerman, G. (1972). The depressed woman as mother. *Social Psychiatry* 7:98–108.

Weissman, M. M., and Pickle, E. (1974). *The Depressed Woman. A Study of Social Relations*. Chicago: University of Chicago Press.

Weissman, M. M., Prusoff, B. A., Gammen, G. D., et al. (1984). Psychopathology in children (ages 6-18) of depressed and normal persons. *Journal of the American Academy of Child Psychiatry* 23:78–84.

Weissman, M. M., Prusoff, B. A., DiMascio, A., et al. (1979). The efficacy of drugs and psychotherapy in the treatment of acute depressive episodes. *American Journal of Psychiatry* 136:555–558.

Weller, E., and Weller, R. (1986). Assessing depression in pre-pubertal children. *Hillside Journal of Clinical Psychiatry* 2:Fall/Winter.

Welner, Z., and Rice, J. (1988). School-aged children of a blind and controlled study. *Journal of Affective Disorder* 15:291–302.

Winocur, G., Behar, D., and Van Valkenburg. (1978). Is a familial definition of depression both feasible and valid? *Journal of Nervous and Mental Disorders* 166:764–768.

Zahn-Waxler, C., Cummings E., McKnew, D., and Radke-Yarrow, M. (1984). Altruism, aggression, and social interactions in young children with a manic-depressive parent. *Child Development* 55:112–122.

7: A SOCIAL LEARNING FAMILY MODEL OF DEPRESSION AND AGGRESSION: FOCUS ON THE SINGLE MOTHER

Linda Schwoeri, M.A., M.F.T.
G. Pirooz Sholevar, M.D.

INTRODUCTION

For more than two decades, Gerald Patterson and his colleagues at the Oregon Social Learning Center (OSLC) have studied family process and interaction with a special emphasis on the behavior of antisocial children. Consistent with a social learning approach, the research group maintains that poor parenting practices lead to an increase in antisocial behavior as the child learns to use increasingly disruptive (coercive) behavior, which, in turn, increases parental stress, making it more difficult to parent effectively. This interactive, reciprocal exchange is ongoing, resulting in an amplification of the stress and further disruption in the parenting.

There are different contextual variables influencing the relationship between parenting practices and child adjustment. The two main variables that are discussed in this chapter are the mother's depression and her recent marital separation. The work of Patterson and Forgatch (1990)* on depression in single mothers provides a

*The authors wish to thank Marion Forgatch, Ph.D., for her tireless and critical editorial assistance in enhancing the quality of this chapter. Part of the data for this chapter was supported by Grant MH #38318.

structure for describing the disruption that occurs during the first year of marital separation. The disruption takes on a cyclical nature. The mother's mood disruptions and irritability and the child's aggressiveness mutually interact and affect each other within a type of feedback loop. As shown in Figure 7–1, contextual factors, such as parental depression, affect the mother's management practices and problem solving, which, in turn, affect the child's adjustment. As the child reacts with aggressiveness, the mother's management of the child becomes less effective, and this occurs within the context of many stressors in her life. Stress produces dramatic increases in negative behaviors during social interactions (Patterson 1983, Wahler and Dumas 1983). Stress amplifies existing irritability, and the Patterson and Forgatch (1990) study indicates that the levels of stress, irritability, and depressed mood remain high during the first year of marital separation.

Some important clinical questions that must be considered in understanding the relationship between maternal depression and child aggression are What is the mechanism of transmission? Why do some mothers become entrenched in this coercive interactive process? How do other mothers escape?

The Parent Skills Mediator Model (see Figure 7–1, Forgatch and Stoolmiller 1991) illustrates that parenting skills mediate the effect of harsh contextual factors, such as maternal depression and single parenting, on child adjustment. The model suggests a bidirectional relationship, such that the child adjustment problems create more stress, diminishing parental effectiveness. The degree to which the stressors result in aggressive behaviors clearly depends on the degree to which parenting practices are employed by the mother. Studies have shown that teaching parenting skills is effective in changing antisocial child behavior (Forgatch 1991b, Patterson 1985, Patterson et al. 1982). Treatment and intervention outcomes are discussed briefly.

THE PARENT SKILLS MEDIATOR MODEL

Description

The Parent Skills Mediator Model (Forgatch and Stoolmiller 1991) puts into perspective one explanation of the mechanism of trans-

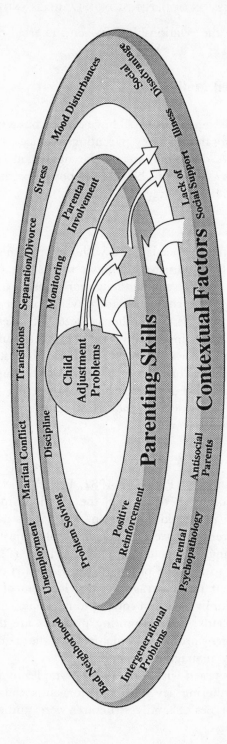

FIGURE 7-1. Parent Skills Mediator Model. From Gerald R. Patterson, John B. Reid, and Thomas J. Dishion, 1992, *Antisocial Boys*. Eugene, OR: Castalia Publishing Company. The authors acknowledge Grant # MH 38318. Used by permission.

mission involved in the relationship between maternal depression and child aggression.

Studies of Depressed Mothers

Patterson and his colleagues at OSLC have carried out a number of studies demonstrating that two key parenting practices, poor monitoring and ineffective discipline, account for significant variance in multiagent measures of antisocial behavior in boys (Forgatch 1991b, Patterson and Bank 1987, Patterson et al. 1992).

Contextual Variables

The recently separated mother is faced with the problems inherent in a transition in marital status: the high stress of single parenting, financial problems, moves to other neighborhoods, loss of social supports, and the many psychological and physical problems related to being depressed. Because the mother is faced with these contextual stressors, her parenting ability will inevitably suffer. The conjoint occurrence of these problems increases her stress, and stress disrupts discipline (Forgatch et al. 1988). The composite is a possible explanation of the relationship between the separated mother's continued depressed psychological state and the child's increasingly aggressive behavior.

Parenting Practices

Patterson's coercion model (Patterson 1982, Patterson et al. 1992) provides a framework for discussing the relationship between maternal depression and child aggression. Patterson's model proposes a set of key parenting practices crucial to child adjustment: (1) monitoring the youngster's behavior and activities, (2) effective discipline strategies to manage problem behaviors, (3) contingent positive reinforcement to encourage the development of prosocial behaviors, and (4) family problem solving to negotiate conflict and resolve family problems. Poor parenting practices are thought to lead to child adjustment problems, which make it more difficult for parents to effectively manage their children.

This model was tested with three OSLC samples in a study by Forgatch (1991b).Differing levels of risk for antisocial child behavior and varying types of family structures were studied.

1. In the Oregon Divorce Study (ODS) there were 197 single-parent, mother-head-of-household families. The subsample of 96 families with boys in grades three to six was employed in the analysis under discussion.
2. In the Oregon Youth Study (OYS), there were 200 families with grade four boys at risk for delinquency.
3. In the clinical sample, there were seventy-one boys and girls between ages 6 and 12 who were referred for serious conduct problems.

All studies employed multiagent, multimethod measurement. Constructs in the models were formed with multiagent indicators similar in each sample. Structural Equation Modeling (SEM) was used to test the a priori model for all three samples. There was a good fit between the model and the data. The hypothesized path coefficients from poor monitoring and inept discipline to antisocial behavior problems were significant, and the models accounted for between 30 percent and 52 percent of the variance in antisocial behavior problems. These findings provide strong evidence that the model generalizes nicely in samples of families with children at risk and referred for behavior problems. The model also generalizes across samples of single-parent and two-parent families.

The model was tested in two independent samples: the ODS and the OYS. The samples included one-third each of three family types: single mother, mixed family types, and intact families. (Intact families were defined as both parents being the child's biological parents and living together.) Data was available for 141 families in the ODS sample and 165 families in the OYS sample. Within the OYS sample, there were 65 intact families, and a separate analysis was conducted with the subsample. Three assessments using the same measure over a 4-year period were employed using latent growth curve modeling. Latent growth curve modeling is an extension of repeated measures analysis of variance that permits an examination of individual differences in growth as well as growth in group mean level, which partials out the effects of measurement error.

Forgatch and Stoolmiller (1991) tested an aspect of the Parent Skills Mediator Model. Their hypothesis stated that maternal depressed mood leads to troubled parenting in terms of harsh discipline and uninvolved monitoring. Depressed mood was assessed with the Center for Epidemiological Studies Depression Scale (CES-D) (Radloff 1977) and telephone interview ratings of mood collected six times over a 3-week period at each assessment. Discipline was measured from a questionnaire filled out by mothers and from interviewers' ratings following an interview asking parents about their parenting practices. Monitoring was assessed from telephone interviews and interviewer ratings.

The hypothesis was supported for the relationship between depressed mood and harsh discipline for all samples (ODS, OYS). The variance ranged from 10 percent to 53 percent. Individual differences in the course of maternal depressed mood over time were associated with individual differences in harsh discipline. Mothers who showed diminishing depressed mood over the 4 years displayed less harsh discipline practices; mothers whose mood worsened over time displayed more harsh discipline practices; and mothers who remained the same in mood over time remained relatively the same in harsh discipline.

The findings for the relationship between depressed mood and uninvolved monitoring were somewhat different. The expected relationship was found for the single-mother sample (ODS) only, accounting for 18 percent of the variance. A relationship was not obtained for the OYS sample, either for the mixed family types or for the intact subsample.

Taken together, the findings strongly support an association between maternal depressed mood and harsh discipline practices. This relationship generalized across single-parent and two-parent families. The relationship between socioeconomic status, stress/ distress, and parental psychopathology is seen as affecting child adjustment, but primarily to the extent that all three factors disrupt parenting practices. Most importantly, an analysis within the clinical treatment sample showed that families who improved their monitoring and discipline practices during treatment had children who showed commensurate decreases in antisocial behavior by termination of treatment.

THE CRISIS YEAR FOR THE SINGLE MOTHER AND HER CHILD

Description of the Problem

Patterson and Forgatch (1990), in studying the first year of marital separation, describe it as a crisis year. During this time, the mothers are more stressed than are mothers from intact families (Forgatch et al. 1988, Hetherington 1980, Hetherington et al. 1978, 1979, Zill 1978). Marital separation marks a sudden increment in levels of maternal stress (Bloom et al. 1978; Wallerstein and Kelly 1980).

Marital separation also sets in motion a series of situations that disrupt the mother's social interaction with friends, relatives, and children and entrap her in a state of depression that may be long-lasting (Patterson and Forgatch 1990). The increased rates of irritable and sad behaviors and exchanges with friends serve to push people away, leaving her without needed supports. As she becomes more isolated and unidimensional in reaction to her depression, her supports tend to drop away. If she selects a confidante who is likewise depressed or irritable, she will find that her efforts to problem solve are less effective, which relates to future high levels of stress. As she becomes more isolated, she becomes more irritable and depressed. This further colors her interactions with her children. As the child reacts to the mother's level of stress, adding his or her own contribution based on temperament and personal needs, increasingly frequent coercive exchanges occur, especially during disciplinary confrontations. Antisocial behaviors become reinforced and, over time, contribute to the maintenance of the mother's stress and depression. The process becomes circular, making it difficult to identify which contributes more to the disruptiveness.

The disrupting influence of stress is supported by empirical studies (Biglan et al. 1990, Gottman 1990, Patterson 1983, Radke-Yarrow 1990, Wahler and Dumas 1986). Single mothers feel overwhelmed by the demands placed on them because of the marital separation, and some continue to struggle with these problems and with their children some years after the separation (Hetherington et al. 1989).

The extensive work of Brown and Harris (1978), which identified family and social variables common to women who were severely depressed, underscores the difficulties discussed in this chapter in relation to the single mother. Four classes of variables were identified, with three referring to current life events. They found:

1. The women had suffered a severe adverse event usually involving an important personal loss or disappointment within the year prior to the onset of their depression.
2. There was an absence of a companion in whom to confide.

3. They lived in chronically financially difficult situations and were responsible for the care of a number of children under the age of 14.

The Course of Self-reported Depression

Figure 7-2 indicates the course of self-reported depression over a 4-year period in a sample of 138 mothers based on CES-D ratings of depression (Radloff 1977). People in the depressed group obtained a score of sixteen or more on the CES-D, the cutting score usually indicating depression. The breakdown of seventy depressed and sixty-eight nondepressed at t_1 (3-12 months) indicates that nearly half the mothers report symptoms of depression. Those who are asymptomatic at the initial period remained largely so throughout the 4-year period. In fact, 51 percent remained nondepressed by t_4 (39-48 months).

Those who were symptomatic for the first two assessments seem to have become entrapped in a process that continued for at least 2 years. There is some drop in the number by t_3 (15-24 months), but only for 27 percent of the mothers. There is also some movement from nondepressed to depressed by t_2 and t_3; however, the total number of women who were nondepressed at first but became depressed was sixteen (24 percent).

It seems possible to predict that if a mother begins the separation year in a depressed state, her chances are slightly less than 50 percent that she will still be depressed by the end of a year. However, if she starts nondepressed, her chances are less than 30 percent that she will become depressed a year later. Overall, Figure 7-2 shows that those who start out in the process as depressed remain in it, and that those who are nondepressed remain so.

Stress and Depression

Based on a social learning perspective, the longer the depressed mother is engaged in the process, the more likely she is to move on to more extreme manifestations of the disruption process. The study of the disruption process involves two phases. The first phase addresses changes in the level of support and stress experienced by the mothers over the first year. The second phase describes the

Figure 1. The Course of CES-D Reported Depression.

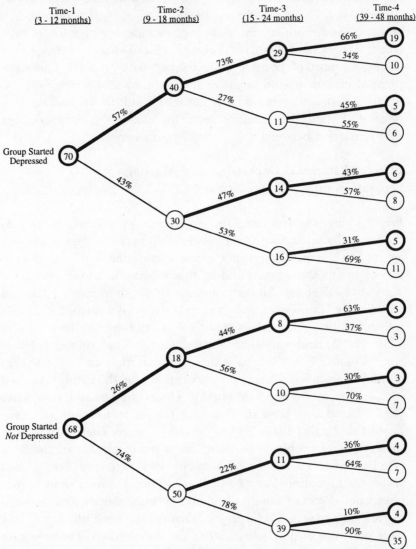

FIGURE 7-2.   The course of CES-D Reported Depression.

Marion S. Forgatch, Ph.D., and Mike Stoolmiller, Ph.D. (April 1991). The relationship between maternal depression and parenting practices. In H. Hops (Chair), *Contextual relationships and parenting predictors of child/adolescent adjustment; Multiagent/Multimethod Approaches.* Symposium conducted at the biennial meeting of the Society for Research in Child Development, Seattle, WA. Used by permission.

reaction of the social environment to her depression. The intervals studied are t_1 (3–12 months), t_2 (9–18 months), t_3 (15–24 months), and t_4 (39–48 months). Stress factors include negative life events, recent hassles, and financial problems. Social support refers to the mother's report of positive daily contact with friends. There are slight decreases in the negative life events and hassles, whereas financial problems remain fairly constant until the 51- to 60-month interval. Financial difficulties seem to subside for those mothers who remarried between the 3- and 5-year interval.

Effects of Parental Depression and Marital Separation on Child Adjustment

When a parent is depressed and experiencing a marital separation, the factors contributing to the relationship between depression and aggression intensify and potentiate each other. A number of investigations converge in finding that separation and divorce have a negative effect on child adjustment. In the short term, separated and divorced families seem to have more negative outcomes than do intact families. Clinical longitudinal studies by Wallerstein and Kelly (1980) and empirically based longitudinal studies (Hetherington et al. 1979, 1985) have shown that the first and second years of marital separation represent a crisis point for the family. As cited in Capaldi and Patterson (1991), Hetherington and colleagues (1979) found that boys in particular tended to be more noncompliant during this time. Follow-up data 6 years later showed that these types of problems persisted for a small number of the boys (Hetherington et al. 1987). Capaldi and Patterson (1991) also reviewed the national survey (Zill et al. 1982), which showed that boys from divorced families had significantly more problems with aggression and school adjustment. Divorce has been implicated in a wide spectrum of psychiatric difficulties for children (Hetherington et al., 1985, Rutter et al. 1970, Zill 1983).

DISRUPTION-AMPLIFICATION PROCESS

The Stress Model

A process is set in motion during the first year of the marital separation, which places both mothers and children at risk for the perpetuation of disruptions in family process. These disruptions serve to increase the aggressive interactions between the mother and child and increase the mother's depression. Living with aggressive, difficult children increases the likelihood of depression among the mothers by virtue of the constant exposure to conflict, criticism, and blame from the neighbors or family. The mother is hassled by interactions with the authorities (school, correction agencies) as the behavior becomes increasingly unmanageable. This undermines the parent's already weakened sense of competence in relation to the child and lowers her self-esteem as a parent. This contributes to her depressed and irritable mood. Lacking the parenting skills needed to interrupt the coercive exchanges, she adds to the problems inherent in the already difficult situation.

The Disruption Process

The mother's depression makes interactions quite burdensome for the children as well as her social friends because there are also increases in irritable and/or depressive words, sad facial expressions, and sad voice tones, as well as negative attributions.

Forgatch and Stoolmiller (1991) examine the relationship between maternal depression and maternal monitoring over time. The mother's dysphoric mood may escalate from one that lasts several days to one that continues over weeks until symptoms characteristic of a diagnosable clinical depression prevail. As this happens, her ability to monitor and discipline her child's behavior and influence it in a responsible and effective manner is diminished (Forgatch and Stoolmiller 1991). Stress greatly impairs how she thinks and acts. Mother and child affect each other in their interactions around discipline and monitoring practices, and they can quickly move into a disruption process that contributes to the mother's depression and the child's aggressive behavior.

Rearing even normal children provides a mother with a relatively high rate of aversive events that may be accompanied by temporary or periodic depression and dysphoria. However, antisocial or aggressive children will perform aversive acts, such as whining and crying, humiliating and teasing others, and destroying property, more than twice as frequently as nonproblem children. Having aggressive children is associated with a higher incidence of depression (Patterson 1974a). Mothers of aggressive children have been found to be less effective in performing parenting skills and use more coercive means in disciplining children than mothers of nonaggressive children (Patterson 1974b). Because there are constitutional differences among children, these will affect the interactions and parenting practices of the mothers. Sameroff and Seifer (1983) and Werner and Smith (1977) found that the combination of difficult child temperament and marginally skilled parents places the child at significant risk for later antisocial behavior.

When the mother is depressed and irritable, these interactions will take on a different nature than when she is not depressed. For example, a depressed mother who is faced with an extremely active child who presents more difficult child management problems will experience far greater levels of stress than the mother of a child who is not as active. As has been seen by Forgatch, younger children are especially stressful to mothers, especially those between the ages of 2 and 3. Forgatch (personal communication 1992) notes that when a child is young, the direction of the depression-aggression relationship is strongly from the mother to the child. One possible explanation is that when the child is young and as yet unable to spend more than brief periods of time in solitary and focused play, the mother is continually stressed by the need to interact with the child. More interactions usually necessitate more disciplinary confrontations. Wessman and Ricks (1966) have noted the covariation of the mother's mood and aversive events. They suggest that on days when the mother describes herself as dysphoric, the child is more likely to perform coercive behaviors at high rates. Failure by parents to effectively punish coercive behaviors sets into motion interaction sequences that are the basis for training in aggression. The process involves family members in patterned exchanges of aversive behaviors that reinforce each other and become increasingly aversive. Patterson (1982) labeled this process *coercion* because in the presence of relatively trivial behaviors such as noncompliance, whining, teasing, yelling, and disapproval, there is a learning structure for increasingly aggressive behaviors. The movement from these trivial behaviors to more aggressive ones is determined by reinforcers supplied by the family members in their exchanges (Patterson 1982).

The single depressed mother experiences a variety of stresses that place her at great risk for coercive interactions. Through negative reinforcement or escape-avoidant conditioning, the mother's depressed behavior becomes an effective aversive tool that contributes to the coercive process. She may learn that her irritable behavior elicits soothing reactions from her daughters and compliance from her son. Her irritable outbursts and shouting commands can work in her favor, at least temporarily. Her behavior coerces the child into stopping his deviant/aggressive behavior in the short run. In the long run, the child will continue the aversive pattern, as will the mother. Increasing frequency and heightened levels of aversiveness are the results of these interactions (Patterson 1982).

The study by Patterson and Forgatch (1990) showed that on any given day during the first 12 months, 58 percent to 61 percent of the mothers report being both irritable and depressed, whereas 11 percent to 15 percent report being only irritable, and 4 percent to 7 percent report being only depressed. The combined factors of irritability and depression over an extended period of time serve to maintain maternal depression while contributing to future high levels of stress. It has been indicated that the irritable behavior of highly stressed single mothers covaries with disciplinary confrontations. The irritable exchanges with the son during discipline tend to increase the child's use of coercive tactics and the disruptions in mother–confidante social exchanges brought on by stress. These factors point out the many contingencies involved in the maternal depression–child aggression exchanges.

THE HETHERINGTON EFFECT

Based on the work of Hetherington (Hetherington, 1980, Hetherington et al. 1978, 1979, 1989), the OSLC labeled a resulting model the *Hetherington effect* (Forgatch et al. 1988). It examines the relationship among single-parent stress, disrupted discipline, and the antisocial behavior of boys of single parents. Patterson (1980), found that in disciplinary confrontations, parents of problem children threaten, nag, scold, and natter but seldom follow through on their threats. (*Nattering* refers to the mother's irritability while interacting with the son, regardless of what he is doing.) *Explosive discipline* or *explosiveness* referred to the mother's abusive reactions, including threats, humiliations, and hitting. Not following through was part of the failure pattern. The 1980 study of adolescent boys by Olweus, based on mothers' retrospective accounts of their children's temperament during the preschool years, supports this. Olweus found that permissive parenting and explosive discipline, as well as the child's temperament, contribute to antisocial behavior. Glueck and Glueck (1959) have noted that at least one half of their sample of adolescent delinquents established a recognizable antisocial pattern prior to the fourth grade. In their review of findings from longitudinal studies, Greenwood and Zimring (1985) found that 36 percent to 70 percent of the offending delinquent adolescents continue on to become criminals.

INTERVENTION AND TREATMENT

Overview of the Parent Training Therapy (PTT) Approach

Over the past two decades, the work of Patterson and his colleagues at the OSLC has focused on the management and treatment of antisocial, aggressive children. They saw the need to address this group because at least one half of the referrals for treatment involved problems with children's aggression. They soon noted that when other forms of externalizing problems, such as hyperactivity, were considered, then referrals in this category mounted to more on the order of 75 percent (Patterson et al. in press).

Until the mid-1950s, the treatment of choice in clinics for antisocial, aggressive children was primarily psychodynamic. Although this approach remains a dominant one, the 1960s and 1970s saw a rise in the number of innovations in the treatment of antisocial children. One of the most profound influences on innovative approaches was that of B. F. Skinner. His efforts focused on what came to be known as a contingency theory of children's aggression (Patterson et al. 1992). Also, in the 1970s there was a shift toward looking at the bidirectional nature of these children's problems. The work of Bandura and Walters (1963) on social learning theory was compatible with that of Skinner and added to the question of context for contingencies. It was seen that the social environment produced and reinforced the contingencies that led to the aggressive behavior in question. This shifted the focus off the child and onto the social/family environment in which the child learns aggressive behaviors through modeled behavior and reinforcement. This shift in focus led Patterson and his group to look at aversive events in the natural environment. This was an innovation because it emphasized the extent to which negative events affect the family.

As family therapy began to move more into clinical prominence, and as the need to find alternatives to the original child-guidance approach gained recognition, the clinical community was ready to look at different approaches to treating aggressive children. Patterson and his group initiated home-based observation as well as laboratory studies of aggressive children. Their work showed that certain settings produced the reinforcers for aggression. One of the earliest works reflecting this was the work of Patterson and Reid (1970) on the coercion process. Later, the coercion process was described and detailed in *A Social Learning Approach to Family Intervention: Vol. 3, Coercive Family Process* (Patterson 1982). Throughout this work, Patterson and colleagues at the OSLC have emphasized that family management skills control the contingencies that govern antisocial behavior. Ineffective parental discipline and monitoring practice are thought to control the reinforcers available for antisocial behavior. They assumed that measures of parental discipline and monitoring practices should account for much of the variance in measures of child antisocial behavior (Patterson et al. 1992). It is with this assumption firmly in mind that research on parenting practices was conducted and through which Parent Training Therapy (PTT) was established. PTT exists in various forms depending on the age of the child and whether home- (foster, family, or community) or school-based intervention is indicated. The main focus is teaching and enhancing effective parenting.

PTT includes a mixture of contingency contracting, time out, privilege removal and restitution through chores, positive reinforcement for prosocial behavior, and sanctions for problem behavior. (For a more extensive discussion of treatment and outcome studies, see Patterson et al. in press.) The research presents encouraging data on the effectiveness of this approach, especially when used in combination with other forms of behavioral training, such as SST (Social Skill Training), FST (Family Systems Therapy), and CST (Cognitive Skills Training).

Outcome Studies of Younger Children

The outcome studies reviewed by Patterson and colleagues (1992) evaluate the contribution of cognitive and social skills training components. The studies use random comparison designs and include pre- and posttreatment measures such as court records, observation, or teacher ratings. Reviews of the literature on the treatment of conduct problems (Dumas 1989, Kazdin 1987, McMahon and Wells 1990) have indicated that PTT produces the most consistent positive treatment effects for antisocial children (Patterson et al. in press). Patterson further states that younger children are probably easier to treat than older problem children, due to the older child's longer history of defeating the parents' attempts at discipline. When comparing younger with older children, 63.2 percent of the younger and 26.9 percent of the older children showed clinically significant improvement. Furthermore, the longer the history, the more the parent is likely to avoid attempts to confront or control the child. Parents of older problem children (11 to 12 years) had worse discipline practices during base-line observation and failed to show any improvement during the course of treatment. (See Patterson et al. 1992 for details of all age groups studied.)

In treatment outcomes for younger antisocial children, Forehand and colleagues (1980) have documented in programmatic studies the effectiveness of PTT. These studies were of mildly disturbed children ages 6 to 8 from essentially middle-class families. Families were assigned to a PTT group that included self-help materials in addition to videotapes or included only videotape materials; the groups were then compared to a wait-list control group. Both experimental groups showed significant changes in parent and child behavior on the observation data, whereas the control group did not show these changes.

This major contribution to the field was replicated in a study of young disturbed children ages 3 to 8 (mean age 4.5) referred to a university clinic because of oppositional problems (Webster-Stratton et al. 1989). Eighty families were randomly assigned to three experimental groups (self-administered videotape-based, group discussion plus videotape materials, or group discussion alone) and a wait-list control condition. As before, the videotape and self-help materials detailed the PTT procedures. The pre- and posttreatment comparison data from the observations showed significant changes for all three experimental groups compared with the wait-list control group. There were no significant differences among the experimental groups. The replicated findings strongly underscore the utility of self-administered parent-training materials. These effects were maintained for two-thirds of the sample in a 1-year follow-up study (Webster-Stratton et al. 1989), and the 1990 follow-up further strengthened the results.

One significant and relevant finding was that the children who remained maladjusted tended to be from single-parent, lower-socioeconomic-status families in which there were increased maternal depression and a family history of alcoholism and drug abuse (Patterson et al. 1992).

CONCLUSION

The recent work of Patterson and Forgatch on depression in families of children with disruptive and antisocial behavior is a major contribution to the understanding of the phenomenon of depression and aggressive conduct behaviors. It builds upon the superstructure of the work of Patterson and his group, which correlates poor parenting practices with increased antisocial behavior in the children. The disruptive and coercive behavior of the child results in increased environmental and parental stress. The parental stress, in turn, decreases the parental effectiveness, which results in the perpetuation of this vicious cycle.

The recent work of Patterson and Forgatch, described in this chapter, addresses two variables that influence parenting practices, namely, maternal depression and recent marital separation. The first year of marital separation is particularly stressful for the parent, resulting in maternal mood disruption, irritability, and depression. The mother's depression affects her management practices, resulting in maladjusted behavior on the part of the child. This, in turn, increases parental stress. The stress and irritability result in depressed mood, which entraps a sizeable number of recently separated mothers. Some mothers, however escape this coercive interactive process.

Through the Parent Skills Mediator Model, it becomes clear that the parenting skills of the mother mediate the effect of the maternal depression on the child's adjustment. The depressed mood of the mother results in uninvolved parenting, poor monitoring of the child's behavior, and periodic harsh discipline. The marital separation also disrupts maternal/social interaction, which further entraps her in a state of depression. The selection of a depressive confidante is an important contributor to the continuation and perpetuation of maternal depression. The bidirectional relationship addressed in the Parent Skills Mediator Model offers one explanation of the process in which maternal depression and child aggression reciprocally affect each other. The total context of the mother's and child's life, however, must be considered if an understanding of depression and its interactional manifestations is sought.

REFERENCES

Bandura, A., and Walters, R. (1963). *Social Learning and Personality Development*. New York: Holt, Rinehart and Winston.

Biglan, A., Lewis, L., and Hops, H. (1990). A contextual approach to the problem of aversive practices in families. In *Depression and Aggression in Family Interaction*, ed. G. Patterson. Hillsdale, NJ: Lawrence Erlbaum.

Bloom, B. L., Asher, S. J., and White, S. W. (1978). Marital disruption as a stressor: a review and analysis. *Psychological Bulletin* 85:867–894.

Brown, G. W., and Harris, T. (1978). *The Social Origins of Depression*. London: Tavistock.

Capaldi, D., and Patterson, G. (1991). The relationship of parental transition to boy's adjustment problems. I. A linear hypothesis and II. Mothers at risk for transitions and unskilled parenting. *Developmental Psychology* 27:489–504

Dumas, J. E. (1989). Treating antisocial behavior in children: child and family approaches. *Clinical Psychology Review* 9:197–222.

Forehand, R., Wells, K. C., and Griest, D. L. (1980). An examination of the social validity of a parent training program. *Behavior Therapy* 11:488–502.

Forgatch, M. S. (1991a). *Families in the Divorce Process: Theory and Intervention*. NIMH Monograph Grant #MH38318. Washington, D.C.

——— (1991b). The clinical science vortex: treatment as an experimental manipulation. In *The Development and Treatment of Childhood Aggression*, ed. D. Peplar and K. Rubin, pp. 291–315. Hillsdale, NJ: Lawrence Erlbaum.

Forgatch, M. S., Patterson, G. R., and Skinner, M. (1988). A mediational model for the effect of divorce on antisocial behavior in boys. In *Impact of Divorce, Single Parenting, and Step-Parenting on Children*, ed. E. M. Hetherington and J. D. Arasteh, pp. 135–154. Hillsdale, NJ: Lawrence Erlbaum.

Forgatch, M. S., and Stoolmiller, M. (1991). The relationship between maternal depression and parenting practices. *Contextual Relationships Parenting Predictors of Child/Adolescent Adjustment: Multiagent/Multimethod*

Approaches. Symposium conducted at the biennial meeting of the Society for Research in Child Development, Seattle, WA, April.

Glueck, S., and Glueck, E. (1959). *Unraveling Juvenile Delinquency.* Cambridge, MA: Harvard University Press.

Gottman, J. M. (1990). How marriages change. In *Depression and Aggression in Family Interaction,* ed. G. Patterson, pp. 77–101. Hillsdale, NJ: Lawrence Erlbaum Associates.

Greenwood, P. W., and Zimring, F. E. (1985). *One More Chance. The Pursuit of Promising Intervention Strategies for Chronic Juvenile Offenders.* Santa Monica, CA: Rand.

Hetherington, E. M. (1980). Children and divorce. In *Parent Child Interaction: Theory, Research and Prospect,* ed. R. Henderson. New York: Academic.

Hetherington, E. M., Cox, M., and Cox, R. (1978). The aftermath of divorce. In *Mother/Child, Father/Child Relationships,* ed. J. H. Stevens and M. Mathews. Washington, DC: National Association for the Education of Young Children.

_____ (1979). Family interaction and the social, emotional, and cognitive development of children following divorce. In *The Family: Setting Priorities,* ed. V. Vaughn and T. Brazelton, pp. 89–128. New York: Science and Medicine.

_____ (1985). Long-term effects of divorce and remarriage on parents and children. *Journal of the American Academy of Psychology* 24(5): 518–530.

_____ (1987). Divorce and remarriage. Paper presented at the second annual Family Consortium Conference, *Understanding Family Life Transitions,* Santa Fe, NM, June.

Hetherington, E. M., Stanley-Hagan, M., and Anderson, E. R. (1989). Marital transitions: a child's perspective. *American Psychologist* 44:302–312.

Kazdin, A. (1987), Conduct disorders. In *International Handbook of Behavior Modification and Therapy,* 2nd ed., ed. A. Bellack, A. Hersen, and A. Kazdin, pp. 669–706. New York: Plenum.

McMahon, R., and Wells, K. (1989). Conduct disorder. In *Treatment of Childhood Disorders,* ed. E. J. Mach and R. A. Barkley, pp. 73–132. New York: Guilford.

Olweus, D. (1980). The consistency issue in personality, psychology revisited — with special reference to aggression. *British Journal of Social and Clinical Psychology* 19:377–390.

Patterson, G. (1974a). Interventions for boys with conduct problems. Multiple settings, treatments, and criteria. *Journal of Consulting and Clinical Psychology* 42:471–481.

_____ (1974b). Retraining of aggressive boys by their parents: review of recent literature and follow-up evaluation. *Canadian Psychiatric Association Journal* 19:142–161.

_____ (1980). Mothers: the unacknowledged victims. *Monographs of the Society for Research in Child Development* 45:(5 Serial No. 186).

_____ (1982). *A Social Learning Approach to Family Intervention*: Vol. 3. *Coercive Family Process*. Eugene, OR: Castalia.

_____ (1983). Stress: a change agent for family process. In *Stress, Coping and Development in Children*, ed. N. Garmezy and M. Rutter, pp. 235–264. New York: McGraw-Hill.

_____ (1985). Beyond technology: the next stage in developing an empirical base for parent training. In *Handbook of Family Psychology and Therapy*. *II*. Ed. L. L'Abate, pp. 1344–1379. Illinois: Dorsey.

_____ (1986). Performance models for antisocial boys. *American Psychologist* 41:432–444.

_____ (1990). *Depression and Aggression in Family Interaction*. Hillsdale, NJ: Lawrence Erlbaum.

Patterson, G. R., and Bank, (1987). When is a nomological network a construct? In *Assessment for Decision*, ed. D. R. Peterson and D. B. Fishman, pp. 49–73. New Brunswick, NJ: Rutgers University Press.

Patterson, G., Chamberlain, P., and Reid, J. (1982). A comparative evaluation of a parent-training program. *Behavior Therapy* 13:638–650.

Patterson, G. R., Dishion, T. J., and Chamberlain, P. (in press). Outcomes and methodological issues relating to treatment of antisocial children. *Effective Psychotherapy: A Handbook of Comparatives Research*, ed. T. R. Giles. New York: Plenum.

Patterson, G., and Forgatch, M. (1990). Initiation and maintenance of process disrupting single-mother families. In *Depression and Aggression in Family Interaction*, ed. G. Patterson, pp. 209–245. Hillsdale, NJ: Lawrence Erlbaum.

Patterson, G. R., and Reid, J. D. (1970). Reciprocity and coercion: two facets of social systems. In *Behavior Modification in Clinical Psychology*, ed. C. Neuringer and J. Michael, pp. 133–177. New York: Appleton-Century-Croft.

Patterson, G., Reid, J., and Dishion, T. J. (1992). *Antisocial Boys*. Eugene, OR: Castalia.

Radke-Yarrow, M. (1990). Family environments of depressed and well parents and their children: issues of research methods. In *Depression and Aggression in Family Interaction*, ed. G. Patterson, Hillsdale, NJ: Lawrence Erlbaum Associates.

Radloff, L. S. (1977). The CES-D Scale: a self-report depression scale for research in the general population. *Applied Psychological Measurement* 1:385–401.

Rutter, M. (1979). Maternal depression. *Child Development* 50:282–305.

Rutter, M., Tizard, J., and Whitemore, K. (1970). *Education, Health and*

Behavior: Psychological and Medical Study of Childhood Development. New York: Wiley.

Sameroff, A., and Seifer, R. (1983). Sources of continuity in parent/child relations. Paper presented at the meeting of the Society for Research in Child Development, Detroit, MI.

Wahler, R. G., and Dumas, J. E. (1986). Maintenance factors in coercive mother–child interactions: the compliance and predictability hypothesis. *Journal of Applied Behavioral Analysis* 19:13–22.

Wallerstein, J. and Kelly, J. B. (1980). *Surviving the Breakup: How Children and Parents Cope with Divorce*. New York: Basic Books.

Webster-Stratton, C., Hollinsworth, T., and Kolpacoff, M. (1989). The long-term effectiveness and clinical significance of three cost-effective training programs for families with conduct-problem children. *Journal of Consulting and Clinical Psychology* 57:550–553.

Werner, E., and Smith, R. (1977). *Kauai's Children Come of Age*. Honolulu, HI: University of Hawaii Press.

Wessman, A. E., and Ricks, D. F. (1966). *Mood and Personality*. New York: Holt, Rinehart and Winston.

Zill, N. (1978). Divorce, marital happiness, and the mental health of children: findings from the FCD National Survey of Children. Paper presented at the NIMH workshop, Divorce and Children. Bethesda, MD, February.

——— (1983). *Happy, Healthy and Insecure*. New York: Doubleday.

Zill, N., Sigal, H., and Brim, O. G. (1982). Development of childhood social indicators. In *America's Unfinished Business: Child and Family Policy*, ed. E. Zigler, S. L. Kagan, and E. Klugman. New York: Cambridge University Press.

8: NEUROBIOLOGY IN MAJOR DEPRESSION IN CHILDREN AND ADOLESCENTS

Shahnour Yaylayan, M.D.
Elizabeth B. Weller, M.D.
Jacquelyn Miller Zavodnick, M.D.

INTRODUCTION

According to the *Diagnostic and Statistical Manual of Mental Disorders, Third Edition, Revised (DSM-III-R)* (American Psychiatric Association 1987), the core symptoms of a major depressive episode in children and adolescents are the same as those in adults. There are, however, age-specific associated features for different age and developmental levels. In depressed adolescents, negative and antisocial behavior, grouchiness, and withdrawal from social activities can occur. In prepubertal children, the age-specific features of depression include somatic complaints, mood-congruent hallucinations, psychomotor agitation, moodiness, and irritability.

Epidemiological studies have reported widely varying rates of major depressive disorder in children. There are several reasons for these apparent discrepancies in prevalence rates. Different sex ratios, different age ranges, different patient populations (e.g., inpatient vs. outpatient, general population vs. psychiatric population), use or nonuse of structured interviews, and different criteria used to diagnose major depression may all contribute to variations in reported rates of depression. Kashani and Sherman (1988), looking at a series of epidemiological studies, reported a 0.3 percent prevalence of depression in preschoolers from the general population, 1.8 percent in a prepubertal nonreferred sample, and 4.7 percent in a community sample of adolescents aged 14 to 16 years.

The basic phenomenology of major depression may be the same for school-aged children as well as for adolescents and adults (Carlson and Cantwell 1980, Poznanski 1982, Puig-Antich et al. 1978, Strober et al. 1982). Not as much is known about the phenomenology of depression in children younger than 6 years. If the basic phenomenology of depressive disorder is the same across different age groups, this suggests the possibility that the same neurobiological parameters shown to be associated with adult major depressive disorder may also be associated with depression in children and adolescents.

The neurobiological parameters that have been studied in adults and children with major depressive disorder include polysomnographic variables; growth hormone levels; thyroid-stimulating hormone (TSH) levels; cortisol secretion; a positive dexamethasone suppression test (DST); neurotransmitters and metabolites in blood, cerebrospinal fluid (CSF), and urine; and drug responsiveness as correlated with theoretical brain mechanisms.

NEUROCHEMISTRY

Since the norepinephrine hypothesis of Schildkraut (1965) appeared in the sixties, the importance of monamine pathways in depression has been underlined while new discoveries every day complexify our understanding of neurochemistry. Monamine systems are best known and many psychotropic drugs depend on our understanding of these systems. In understanding depression in children, the sequence of the development of these systems in the brain may be important. The developmental sequence may also influence the relative efficacy of our interventions (Anderson and Cohen 1991).

Norepinephrine (NE) axons originate in cells in the pontine and medullary reticular formation. Cells in the locus ceruleus and lateral tegmentum are rather differentially targeted toward the thalamus and cortex in the former and the brainstem-hypothalamus in the latter. Although epinephrine provides a very small concentration in the central nervous system (CNS) compared with NE, epinephrine neurons have been identified in the medulla oblongata, providing terminals to almost all of the forebrain. The terminals are found in the amygdala, hypothalamus, ventral thalamus, and central (grey) brainstem as well as the dorsal vagal complex, and locus ceruleus.

Serotonin cells originate in the raphe nuclei in the brainstem, which extend from the rostral end of the mesencephalon down into the caudal medulla along the midline. Cells send terminals to widely different areas of the forebrain by collaterals from single axons. Raphe nuclei also send terminals to the cerebellum.

Research has shown that metabolites of neurotransmitters are at their peaks in the neonatal period and decline with age. 5-Hydroxyindole acetic acid (5-HIAA) and homovanillic acid (HVA) decline over the years. In contrast, 3 methoxy-4 hydroxyphenylglycol (MHPG) values decline until 2–5 years of age and then stabilize. Blood concentration and urinary excretion rate of the catabolamines and their metabolites also decline over childhood. There may be decreased synthesis and increased catabolism. Blood levels of 5-hydroxytryptamine (5-HT), however, if expressed as a ration to platelets, remain constant throughout childhood because they are dependent on platelet uptake and storage that are fully developed. Depression is a very rare and controversial disease below age 6, is rare in childhood and more common in adolescents, but peaks in early adult life. This appearance of classical depressive symptoms may depend on neurotransmitter system maturation.

Looking in depth at the role of neurotransmitters is more difficult due to the lack of access to the brain in live subjects. When looking at neurotransmitters in blood, one is looking at both CNS and peripheral sources of these neurotransmitters. In the example of serotonin, the contribution of CNS serotonin is small compared to the peripheral contribution. Accessing CSF values is difficult in children, but data is available with adults.

In general, CSF HIAA and plasma and platelet 5HT serotonin are diminished in depression. Interestingly, they are also diminished in violent subjects and certain retardation conditions. Schildkraut's original hypothesis of decreased functional NE activity was supported by low urinary MHPG (Schildkraut 1965). Recently, the focus has been on dysfunction of the NE peripheral system because of studies showing derangement of peripheral NE, epinephrine, and their metabolites in a subgroup of depressives (Davis et al. 1988, Maas et al. 1968).

Because the norepinephrine–epinephrine and serotonin systems are important considerations in depression, a biochemical review of the knowledge of these systems follows. But the story does not end with these systems, so a review of our limited knowledge of neurotransmission will help illuminate the overwhelming complexities of brain chemistry, which make understandable our often contradictory findings in depression. This complexity also promises potential new avenues for treatment and understanding of depression.

MONOAMINE NEUROTRANSMITTERS

The metabolism of the monoamine neurotransmitters is discussed first, followed by a review of their known receptor sites. Finally, the other possible neurotransmitters and peptides that may influence depression are discussed (Barabon and Coyle 1989).

Serotonin is influenced by the tryptophan levels in blood and brain, which are influenced by dietary tryptophan and other tryptophan sources. Tryptophan hydroxylase in the initial and rate limiting step to 5HT is not saturated by the ambient levels of tryptophan. Thus, tryptophan-containing food causes mild sedation by increasing brain serotonin synthesis. 5HT is decarboxylated to serotonin. Serotonin released into the synapse is then uptaken (reuptaken) by the serotonergic nerve terminal unless inhibited by uptake inhibitors. Intracellular serotonin not in vesicular storage is catabolized by monoamine-oxidase-A to 5-HIAA (MAO-A).

Serotonergic receptors have been partially differentiated. Hallucinogens appear to act at $5\text{-}HT_2$ receptors, which are, interestingly, selectively located in the cerebral cortex. Recently, some researchers suggest that $5HT_2$ may be important in aggression. Previously, $5HT_{1B}$ in rats was specifically correlated with aggression, but this is not replicated in human models. $5\text{-}HT_{1A}$ receptors have been implicated in many disorders including depression, anxiety, and obsessive-compulsive disorder.

Catecholamine pathways are tightly regulated entirely within the nerve terminal. This ensures a stable amount of NE at the nerve terminal regardless of activity level. In contrast to the serotonin pathway, the synthesis of NE is at the end of a series of steps in which the first step, from tyrosine to L-dopa, is at a low velocity, and the tyrosine hydroxylase is saturated by the precursor L-tyrosine. When L-dopa is converted to dopamine, the amount is regulated, because when it exceeds the vesicle storage capacity, it inhibits tyrosine hydroxylase. Noradrenergic neurons contain the enzyme dopamine-β-hydroxylase, which converts dopamine to NE. Inactivation of NE is through reuptake by a gradient across the neuronal membrane. Norpramin selectively inhibits this uptake, which may form a basis for its action against depression.

Enzymatic degradation of NE occurs with MAO-A in the nerve terminal. New catecholamine synthesis is protected from this mechanism by being stored in vesicles by an energy-dependent pump. Reserpine inhibits this pump leading to deamination of catecholamine by MAO. Catecholamine O-methyltransferase inactivates catecholamine that has gone beyond the synaptic cleft. Degrading enzymes have broad distribution, whereas synthesizing enzymes are restricted to the neurons. This protects people from dietary excesses of tyramines and catecholamines. This protection is currently lost when MAO-I drugs are used in depression. NE is further catabolized to epinephrine in certain areas of the brain.

Adrenergic receptors in the brain include β_1-receptors localized to neurons and β_2-receptors in glia and blood vessels. NE and epinephrine serve as agonists for β_1-receptors, while β_2-receptors are more sensitive to epinephrine than NE. α_1-receptors are peripheral, while α_2-receptors for catecholamines cause decreases in peripheral and central noradrenergic activity.

The role of the other important monamine neurotransmitter, dopamine, in depression is not well understood, although its importance in psychosis is well known.

Despite all the studies of catecholamines and serotonin in depression, the monamine neurons (serotonin, NE, epinephrine, dopamine) account for less than 1 percent of CNS neurons. Thus, amino acid neurotransmitter neuropeptides and second and third messengers may have more importance in depression than we currently can acknowledge (Worley et al. 1987).

The roles of the amino acid neurotransmitters in general are only barely understood, while their role in depression is unknown. The association of GABA$_\alpha$ receptors with anxiety states is well known. The role of the more recently discovered GABA$_\beta$ is less well defined. The relation of GABA to depression may be mediated through anxiety or by mechanisms we do not yet understand.

Excitatory amino acids such as glutamate are more closely linked with seizure activity. The roles of glutamate and its receptors

N-methyl-D-asastic acid (NMDA, quisquelate, and kainate) are not linked to depression as of yet.

Neuropeptides present another barely explored area of brain chemistry that is linked directly to the role of hormones in the CNS. The list of peptides from neural and endocrine sources is almost endless and grows daily. For example, somatostatin is extremely widespread in the brain. Neurotension is also widespread and may have potent effects on dopamine systems. Corticotropin releasing factor is involved with hormonal response to stress. The many examples of colocalization of transmitters and neuropeptides lead to theories of cotransmission instead of the traditional idea of one transmitter to one neuron. Examples include colocalization of NE and enkephalin in various brain sites, localization of NE with neuropeptide Y in the medulla, and colocalization of serotonin with TRH with enkephalon or substance P in the medulla. If cotransmission is a result of colocalization, then our understanding of neurotransmission changes and renders our inconsistent results with "proven" treatment of depression less difficult to understand (Worley et al. 1987).

There is, however, much more to the neurotransmission story. For example, what might be the role of opioid receptors in depression through the linking concept of self-inflicted harm? Might they have a role in why very depressed people don't have the energy to kill themselves, whereas recovering depressives are often at risk? The opiate active peptides are produced from three precursors: proenkephalin, prodynorphin/neoendorphin, and POMC. They act at three known receptors: delta, kappa, and mu, respectively. The mu receptor is associated with analgesic effects, while kappa receptor activation is known to produce hallucinations and, more importantly, dysphoria. Different precursors can produce different peptides, which are then capable of acting at several receptor sites. Thus, the one transmitter–one neuron hypothesis is overturned. In addition, POMC, as an example, can be cleaved into several active peptide forms depending on its location. These peptides can then be further modified, so that, for example, there can be six possible beta-endorphin forms. Peptide processing can thus be quite flexible and probably results in wide variation of the activity of the end product. The cellular responses of peptide systems involve responses to both local and distant stimuli and can cause rapid or long-term changes. Thus, the state of these systems could depend on length of a stress or may be a factor in creating a short or long illness. This may be an important idea in depression, which has so many different outcomes.

Lithium ions block inositol-1-phosphatase, an enzyme involved in IP3 (inisotol 1,4,5 triphosphate) recycling. IP3 is one of two active phospholipid second messengers. Theoretically, lithium could make cells less responsive to second messengers.

Second messenger systems such as cyclic nucleotides (cAMP, cGMP), calcium ions, and phospholipid metabolites are interrelated in neurons. They are of increasing psychopharmacologic interest. These second messenger systems often create the intraneuronal effects of the monoamine, amino acid, and peptide neurotransmitters that are not coupled directly with ion channels. Even ion channels, another area of interesting research, are often regulated by second messengers. Calcium channel blockers are of some interest because psychotropic drugs and some antipsychotics have effects on calcium.

G-proteins are a group of membrane proteins that link receptor proteins that bind first messengers (e.g., neurotransmitters) to effector proteins such as ion channels or enzymes. Thus, G-proteins increase and make specific the neuronal response to the first messengers. They are abundant compared to receptor proteins and act essentially as amplifiers of the second messenger signal. Because there are a number of different G-proteins, a single neurotransmitter could activate many second messenger systems in different neurons, depending on the G-protein present. Thus, G-proteins could affect drug action. They could also lead to disease states if they are too high or too low in amount (Grebb and Browning 1989).

Proteins do the work of the cell. Protein kinases are abundant in the brain, and phosphorylation is a major way to regulate protein function. The phosphates act as possible switches to turn the proteins on or off. Kinases are clearly involved with neurotransmitter synthesis and release as well as cell metabolism. There is evidence that first messengers are mediated by protein kinase activation. Thus, phosphoproteins might be third messengers. At least seventy brain phosphoproteins have been identified. There are generalized brain phosphoprotein, regional phosphoprotein, and local phosphoprotein types. Examples of known phosphoproteins are those from phosphorylation of tyrosine hydroxylase, the rate limiting enzyme in the synthesis of catecholamine. This phosphorylation then increases the synthesis of catecholamines. Thus, there is a clear role for understanding protein kinases in understanding disorders like depression.

HORMONAL AND OTHER STUDIES

Depression may also depend on environmental factors mediated through brain changes. The model for this is shown in Harlow's monkeys and the anaclitic depression of Spitz's orphans. Biological models of studies of infant stress have primarily looked at hormonal mediation of brain activity and development. These studies show that such stress leads to brain changes. However, the effects studied are immediate and explain disorders like failure to thrive, psychosocial dwarfism, and global brain problems. This may not be a mechanism to explain a late appearing disorder like depression unless a milder insult or a major insult with mediating positive influences is postulated. It is of interest that the sex ratio of depression changes from prepuberty to adulthood; whereas boys equal girls or even slightly exceed girls in depression prepubertally, females rapidly become excessive carriers of depression by adult life. While this may reflect something hormonal, it may also reflect a basic fact that an overwhelming majority of childhood behavioral and brain disorders are found in males. Thus, the implication is that depression is much less likely to be a child disorder and much more likely a late developmental disease or a disorder related to environmental influences on the brain. These influences could be mediated through neurohormonal mechanisms.

Most of the current biological investigations of depression look at the neurohormonal axis. This is, in part, due to easier access than to brain chemistry per se. Neuroendocrine studies in depressed adults have shown a definite overactivity of the hypothalamus-pituitary-adrenal (HPA) axis in major depression. There is hypersecretion of cortisol, alteration in corticosteroid feedback as demonstrated by dexamethasone suppression, sleep alteration of adrenocorticotropic hormone (ACTH)/cortisol rhythms, evidence of increased brain cortisol releasing factor (CRF), and some evidence of decreased CRF receptors in the brains of suicides. Since these changes are often normalized with recovery, maladaption to stress may be the pathological process. These findings have been inconsistent in adults but are even more inconsistent in children. The

HPA axis may be less sensitive to stress in prepubertal children (Harger and Irwin 1991), except in children in the neonatal period.

Abnormal growth hormone (GH) patterns are seen in adult depressives. As demonstrated by Puig-Antich (1984a,b), the pattern is also abnormal in depressed children, but in a different manner than in adults. GH secretion may be a trait marker of depression unlike HPA-axis findings, which appear to be state markers.

Early separation produces changes in processes regulated by the hypothalamus, such as temperature and sleep. Thus, sleep studies are utilized (Hofer 1984).

Beyond postulated hormonal changes, there is also evidence of immunological changes induced by stress. Monkeys that are separated from their mothers demonstrate lymphocyte reduction. Certain adult depressives (not all) may have reductions of natural killer cells (Harger and Irwin 1991, Irwin and Gillin 1987). Similar work has not been done in children.

To understand the discussion that follows, the difference between state and trait markers should be defined. A state marker is only abnormal during the depressive episode and disappears or returns to normal when the patient recovers from the depressive episode. A state marker is also absent prior to the depressive episode. Thus, a state marker is potentially useful in determining duration of treatment of depression, evaluating treatment response, or predicting relapse. A trait marker for depression is an abnormality that is present before, during, and after a depressive episode. A trait marker does not return to normal after recovery and may best serve as a sensitive indicator of a child's predisposition to develop a future depressive episode.

Polysomnographic Studies

Depression in adults has been associated with reduced slow-wave sleep (stages 3 and 4), shortened rapid eye movement (REM) latency, and increased REM density (Goodwin and Guze 1989). Evidence in adults for occurrence of these polysomnographic markers during a major depressive episode appears fairly strong. Some sleep studies of depressed children, however, have failed to demonstrate these findings, whereas others found abnormalities of sleep architecture in depressed children that are similar to those findings in depressed adults. Young and colleagues (1982) compared the EEG sleep records of prepubertal depressed children to those of nondepressed psychiatric controls and normal children. There were no significant differences between prepubertal children and controls. Similarly, Puig-Antich and colleagues (1982) reported no significant polysomnographic differences between prepubertal children during an episode of major depressive disorder and nondepressed psychiatric controls and normal controls.

Goetz and colleagues (1987) did polysomnographic studies in forty-nine depressed adolescents compared with controls ($N=40$). Depressed groups had significantly longer sleep latencies ($p=.03$) and lower sleep efficiency ($p=.01$) than nondepressed groups. No group differences were present in the sleep architecture of REM sleep measurements, including REM activity and density. All groups showed similar sleep EEG characteristics. The authors hypothesized that sleep EEG correlates of major depression observed in adults are likely to result from an interaction between age and depression.

Lahmeyer and colleagues (1983) found significantly shorter REM latency ($p=.01$) and significantly increased REM density in the depressed adolescents ($N=13$) compared with age-matched controls ($N=13$).

Emslie and colleagues (1987) compared the data from their patients aged 12 or 13 years ($N=10$) to published data for normal control subjects aged 12 or 13 years ($N=27$) (Coble et al. 1984). Analysis found depressed prepubertal subjects had significantly shorter REM latency than normal controls and more REM density, which was similar to adults. Finally, Emslie and colleagues (1990) again showed that depressed children and adolescent subjects had reduced REM latencies when compared to age-matched controls. Thus, polysomnographic studies in children and adolescents have been minimal and have had contradictory findings.

Melatonin

Melatonin is a biologically active indole amine produced by the pineal gland (Tamarkin et al. 1979). Melatonin is of interest because it has a prominent circadian rhythm to its serum levels (Tamarkin et al. 1979). Also, melatonin has an important inhibitory influence on both the pituitary gland and the adrenal cortex (Urry and Ellis 1975). Acutely depressed adults have lower peak melatonin concentrations during the night than either normal subjects or unipolar and bipolar patients who are in remission (Beck-Friis et al. 1984).

Cavallo and colleagues (1987) studied nine RDC and *DSM-III* depressed male subjects aged 7 to 13 years. Controls were ten age-matched males who were not depressed. All had the typical 24-hour plasma melatonin profile, that is, low daytime concentrations and a gradual increase to a period of highest concentration during the night, followed by a gradual decrease. However, the mean 24-hour melatonin-integrated concentrations were significantly lower in the depressed patients $(30.5 + 9.4$ pg/ml) than in controls $(47.0 + 12.0$ pg/ml). Melatonin secretion is also decreased in depressed adults (Beck-Friis et al. 1984).

Thyroid-Stimulating Hormone (TSH) Response to Thyrotropin-Releasing Hormone (TRH)

The thyroid-releasing hormone (TRH) test has been studied in several samples of depressed adults. Of fifty-five studies involving about 1, 200 patients, the TRH-induced response was blunted in about 24 percent of depressed adult subjects (Loosen and Prange 1982). Puig-Antich (1987) measured TSH response to TRH stimulation in depressed prepubertal children and matched controls. There were no significant differences between the two groups in TSH response to TRH. Khan (1987) studied the biochemical profile of thirty-three depressed adolescents and fifty-one nondepressed psychiatric controls. There was no significant difference with regard to TRH stimulation test results. Greenberg and colleagues (1985) also reported negative findings.

Growth Hormone

Growth hormone (GH) is a polypeptide hormone produced by the anterior pituitary. GH secretion is stimulated by exercise, stress, hypoglycemia, insulin, and certain medications, such as amphetamine, apomorphine, L-dopa, desmethylimipramine (DMI), and clonidine. GH secretion is also stimulated by dopamine, NE, and serotonin (Brown et al. 1978).

Depressed adults show reduced GH response to clonidine Charney et al. 1982, Glass et al. 1982) and to insulin (Casper et al.

1977). GH secretion is also reduced in depressed adults (Jarrett et al. 1990).

Meyer and colleagues (1985) measured the GH levels in depressed children and compared them to three groups: nondepressed normal, short, and delayed-growth pubertal children. The 24-hour integrated GH concentration was significantly lower in the depressed subjects compared with the controls. This finding is similar to that found in depressed adults. Meyer and colleagues (1985) in the same study, measured glucose concentrations after insulin administration. The children with major depressive episode had blunted GH response to insulin-induced hypoglycemia.

Puig-Antich and colleagues (1984a) carried out insulin tolerance tests (ITT) on forty-six prepubertal drug-free children aged 6 to 12 years with severe emotional disorders. Thirty subjects met RDC for major depressive episode (thirteen had endogenous subtype and seventeen had nonendogenous subtype). Controls included sixteen children who fit *DSM-III* criteria for nondepressed neurotic disorders. Children with endogenous subtype of depression had significantly more hyposecretion of GH in response to insulin-induced hypoglycemia than nonendogenously depressed children and nondepressed neurotic controls.

Puig-Antich and colleagues (1984b) determined GH concentrations in seventy-one prepubertal children: twenty-two with endogenous subtype of depression, twenty with nonendogenous subtype of depression, twenty-one with nondepressed neurotic disorders, and eight normals. Both depressed groups secreted significantly more GH during sleep than the control group.

Kutcher and colleagues (1988) measured nocturnal GH secretion in nine depressed adolescents and nine matched controls. The depressed adolescents showed significantly greater secretory amplitude compared with controls.

Puig-Antich and colleagues (1984c) performed ITTs in eighteen drug-free prepubertal children aged 6 to 12 years. These children had had a major depressive episode but had been in sustained recovery for at least 4 months at the time of the study. Eleven children had endogenous subtype of depression, and seven had nonendogenous subtype. Controls were sixteen nondepressed prepubertal children with neurotic disorders. Recovered subjects with endogenous depression had hyposecretion of GH during ITT when compared with recovered subjects with nonendogenous depression and nondepressed neurotic controls. Thus, prepubertal children with endogenous major depression continued to have hyposecretion of GH in response to ITTs even in a recovered state. The authors concluded that this neuroendocrine marker was a trait marker of endogenous depression. This was confirmed in another study (Puig-Antich et al. 1984a). In addition, depressed subjects had a blunted GH response to apomorphine, but a normal GH response to 5-hydroxytryptophan. Finally, the average amount of GH secretion following stimulation with L-dopa showed no difference between depressed and normal children.

Jensen and Garfinkel (1990) measured GH response to stimulation with clonidine and L-dopa in fourteen boys (six prepubertal and eight pubertal) with major depression and fifteen normal boys. The six depressed children who were prepubertal or at early puberty had a significantly lower GH peak and area under the GH curve in response to both clonidine and L-dopa, compared with ten normal subjects. However, the eight depressed subjects who were Tanner stage III, IV, and V did not significantly differ from five normal subjects who were Tanner stage III, IV, and V on any of the measures of GH secretion. This findings is the opposite of results one might expect based on depressed adults who have a blunted response.

Ryan and colleagues (1987) studied GH response to 75 mg of desmethylimipramine (DMI) in fifteen depressed adolescents (six suicidal and nine nonsuicidal) and eighteen normal controls. Depressed adolescents had significantly lower mean GH secretion following DMI administration. The depressed suicidal group had significantly lower GH levels than depressed nonsuicidal and normal subjects.

Growth hormone studies in children and adolescents have small sample sizes, and the results to date are mixed. Replication of these studies with larger numbers of subjects are needed to clarify the relation of GH secretion to childhood depression. Although some studies show results similar to those in adults, not all studies do so. The distinction of endogenous versus nonendogenous adds confusion to earlier studies.

Cortisol Secretion

About 50 percent of adults with endogenous subtype of depression hypersecrete cortisol during the depressive episode. This cortisol hypersecretion returns to normal upon recovery from the depressive episode (Sachar 1975, Sachar et al. 1973). In a preliminary report, Puig-Antich and colleagues, (1978) found cortisol hypersecretion in two out of four medically healthy prepubertal children who met RDC for major depressive disorder, endogenous subtype. In a later study, Puig-Antich (1987) carried out 24-hour studies in twenty prepubertal children with RDC for major depressive disorder. Fifteen had endogenous subtype of depression and five had nonendogenous subtype. None in the nonendogenous group hypersecreted cortisol.

Endogenous/nonendogenous distinctions are rarely, if ever, used today, especially since the epidemiological catchment area (ECA) study (Weisman 1984). Instead, the current criteria for major depressive disorder are RDC, *DSM-III*, or *DSM-III-R* criteria.

Weller and colleagues (1985) studied fifty hospitalized prepubertal children who met *DSM-III* criteria for major depressive episode, eighteen nonhospitalized normal controls, and eighteen hospitalized psychiatric controls. Depressed prepubertal subjects had significantly higher baseline cortisol levels at 4:00 P.M. than psychiatric and normal controls ($p = .005$).

Meyer and colleagues (1985) measured 24-hour integrated cortisol levels in five boys aged 7 to 13 who met RDC for a major depressive episode. There was a nonsignificant trend toward increased baseline cortisol levels in the depressed subjects. Thus, the studies of cortisol, as with adults, yield variable results.

The Dexamethasone Suppression Test (DST)

Dexamethasone is a synthetic glucocorticoid that produces suppression of serum cortisol for at least 24 hours when given to normal subjects (Evans and Golden 1987). The DST was originally seen as a specific laboratory test for the diagnosis of so-called endogenous depression (melancholia) (Carroll et al. 1981a). In adults, the test consists of administering a 1-mg oral dose of dexamethasone at night. An abnormal test result is defined as a serum cortisol concentration of greater than 5 ug/dl at a defined time.

In order to interpret studies of the DST, it will be helpful to define some statistical terms. The *sensitivity* of a test refers to the frequency of positive test results (true positive rate) in a population of subjects who have the condition that the test is trying to identify. The *specificity* of a test refers to the frequency of negative test results (true negative rate) in a population of subjects who do not have the condition that the test is trying to identify (Evans and Golden 1987). *Predictive value* refers to the percentage of positive/negative test results that are true positives/negatives, that is, the percentage of subjects that a test correctly classifies (Evans and Golden 1987).

The following are clinical guidelines that have been suggested for the use of DST (Arana et al. 1985, Carroll 1985). The DST may be used to confirm the diagnosis of major depressive episode, but the diagnosis cannot be determined by DST results. In order to avoid false positive and false negative results in using the DST, the patient should be medically healthy, physiologically stable, and medication-free. Patients should be off of anticonvulsants and barbiturates for at least 3 weeks before taking the DST. The DST is affected by the stress of hospitalization leading to false negatives due to the rise of glucocorticoids. A positive DST may confirm the diagnosis of major depressive episode, but a negative DST does not rule out the diagnosis of major depressive disorder. Repeating the DST may be useful in predicting relapse of major depressive episode.

Arana and Mossman (1988) reviewed the literature on the use of the DST in adult psychiatric patients. The 150 studies reviewed all used *DSM-III* criteria to make psychiatric diagnoses. In general, studies used a cortisol level of at least 5 ug/dl (rarely 4 or 6 ug/dl) to define nonsuppression and a dose of dexamethasone of 1 mg (rarely 2 mg). Most studies obtained blood samples at 4:00 P.M. and 11:00 P.M. the day after dexamethasone administration, but several studies included an 8:00 A.M. sample or used only a single sampling time. More than 4, 400 patients with major depressive episode were reviewed. The overall sensitivity of the DST was 43 percent. However, there were variations at different age groups. Thus, the sensitivity was higher in patients over 60 years of age with major depressive episode (64.5 percent) than all adult subjects (43 percent) or patients younger than 18 years (34 percent). The authors did not specify if prepubertal children were included or if only adolescents were studied. The specificity was calculated by including normal controls as well as patients with psychiatric disorders other than major depression (2,000 cases). The specificity of the DST was 86.5 percent.

Arana and Mossman (1988) reviewed studies using the DST to assess short-term treatment response in adults. There were eight studies with more than 319 depressed patients who had a positive DST and were treated with antidepressants or electroconvulsive therapy (ECT). The difference in treatment response rates between DST supressors and nonsuppressors was not statistically significant. There were also at least thirteen uncontrolled studies with 144 depressed subjects. Depressed nonsuppressors who subsequently converted to suppressor status and maintained normal cortisol suppression had a good clinical response; only 19 percent had poor clinical outcome (Arana and Mossman 1988).

In a similar review of the use of the DST in prepubertal and adolescent psychiatric patients, Casat and colleagues (1989) analyzed DST results from thirteen prospective studies on the use of the DST in children and adolescents. All studies used a cortisol level of 5 ug/dl to define nonsuppression. Four of the five prepubertal studies reported administrating 0.5 mg of dexamethasone. The fifth study used a cortisol dose of 20 ug/kg, which resulted in a mean dose of 0.64 mg of dexamethasone. All eight adolescent studies used 1.0 mg of dexamethasone. Most studies included serum cortisol levels at 4:00 P.M. and 11:00 P.M. on the day after administration of dexamethasone. Several studies also included 8:00 A.M. cortisol levels. Of the seventy-nine prepubertal children with major depressive disorder, fifty-five were nonsuppressors yielding a DST sensitivity of 70 percent and a specificity of 70 percent with a predictive value of 74 percent. Of the 157 adolescents with major depressive disorder, seventy-four failed to suppress, yielding a sensitivity of 47 percent and a specificity of 80 percent, with a predictive value of 54 percent. It was not reported if these differences were statistically significant. There were several metabolic variations between the different studies, which included the time of sampling, cortisol assay method, patient status, diagnostic methods, and criteria. Some of the differences may account for some of the variation that was observed in the severity and specificity of the DST.

CASAT'S SUMMARY WORK

Casat's summary work demonstrates marked variability in study results. The methods for studying children below 18 remain the same as above: the diagnosis of depression remains a clinical one. DST at this point is a research study, not a diagnostic tool.

DST and Suicide

Because suicide is a serious risk in depressed patients, a biological marker that could predict suicide would be extremely valuable. In regard to the DST, some adult studies (Carroll et al. 1981b, Lopez-Ibor et al. 1985, Yehuda et al. 1988) found DST nonsuppressors are more likely to attempt and complete suicide at a later time. However, other studies did not find this association (Brown et al. 1986, Secunda et al. 1986).

In order to investigate the DST and suicidality in adolescents, Robbins and Alessi (1985) studied forty-five adolescents aged 13 to 18 years who were psychiatrically hospitalized. Suicide attempts and ideation were evaluated. Of the forty-five adolescents, twenty-three had attempted suicide. All six of those with DST nonsuppression attempted suicide prior to admission, while seventeen of the twenty-two with normal DSTs had not attempted suicide. The association between suicide attempts and DST nonsuppression was significant. Of those who attempted suicide, four of the six nonsuppressors made medically dangerous or lethal attempts, whereas none of the seventeen DST suppressors made such a severe attempt. The authors suggested additional research was necessary to establish the clinical applications of the DST in adolescents.

Chabrol and colleagues (1983) studied twenty adolescents aged 13 to 18 years who had been consecutively referred to a clinic for attempted suicide. None of the twenty met the *DSM-III* criteria for major depressive episode. Of the twenty adolescents, four had DST nonsuppression. In Klee and Garfinkel's study (1984), in which the DST was administered to thirty-three children and adolescents aged 11 to 17 years, there was no difference in suicidal ideation between the depressed DST nonsuppressors (n $=8$) and the depressed DST suppressors (n $= 12$). Similarly, Emslie and colleagues (1987) did not find any association between the DST and suicidal behavior in ninety-four child and adolescent psychiatric inpatients. Recently, Pfeffer and colleagues, (1991) evaluated forty-nine prepubertal psychiatric inpatients aged 6 to 12 years. Cortisol levels were measured pre- and post-dexamethasone. The sample was divided into four groups based on suicidality: nonsuicidal children (n $= 10$), children with suicidal ideations (n$= 14$), children who had threatened suicide (n = 12), and children who had made mild suicide attempts (n = 13). Children with major depression had higher suicidal behavior ratings than children without major depression. There was no association between suicidal behavior at admission versus 7 weeks later in postdexamethasone cortisol suppression. Children with continuing suicidal behavior had significantly higher predexamethasone cortisol levels at 4:00 P.M. than children who did not have persistent suicidal behavior, both at admission and 7 weeks later.

DST Plus Treatment Response

Preskorn and colleagues (1987) did a double-blind, randomly assigned, placebo-controlled trial of imipramine in twenty-two hospitalized prepubertal children aged 6 to 12 years, all meeting *DSM-III* criteria for major depressive disorder. The DST nonsuppressors had the best response to imipramine and the poorest response to placebo.

Weller and colleagues (1986) studied twenty-eight hospitalized prepubertal children aged 6 to 12 years who met *DSM-III* criteria for major depressive disorder and had positive DSTs. All were moderately to severely depressed. All subjects were treated and were given repeat DSTs at 6 weeks and 5 months. After 6 weeks of treatment, clinical remission had occurred in nine of the twenty-one patients (43 percent) retested. Of the nine in remission, four (44 percent) had normal DSTs; 50 percent of the twelve subjects who remained clinically depressed had normal DSTs. At 5 months, six of the fourteen subjects (43 percent) tested had clinical remissions; all six had normal DSTs. Of the eight whose depression had not remitted, only one had a normal DST. Thus, DST results were significantly correlated with clinical status at 5 months but not at 6 weeks. In contrast, Targum and colleagues (1983) presented data at the American Psychiatric Association's annual meeting in 1985 on adolescents with abnormal DSTs who were matched with adolescents with normal DSTs. There were no differences between the two groups as to the rate of rehospitalization or ongoing treatment after 12 to 15 months.

In comparing DST findings across different age groups, there appear to be some age-related trends in the DST specificity from childhood to old age. Thus, Arana and Mossman (1988) reported the highest DST sensitivity (65 percent) in elderly subjects (more than 60 years) compared with adults (43 percent) and patients under the age of eighteen (34 percent). However, they do not specify if prepubertal children are included in the latter group. On the other hand, Casat and colleagues (1989), in a review of DST studies in children and adolescents, found the DST sensitivity to be highest among prepubertal depressed children (70 percent) compared with adolescents (47 percent). Combining these two literature reviews, it appears that at the extremes of age groups (prepubertal and elderly), the DST has the highest sensitivity. It is difficult to draw any generalizations, however, in view of the varied methodological approaches in all these studies with respect to the dose of the dexamethasone, the time it had been administered, sampling time of cortisol, various methods of cortisol assay, and methods of assessment. DST has been disappointing as a diagnostic instrument but still holds some promise in research understanding.

SUMMARY

The essential features of major depressive disorder in adults are present in children and adolescents. However, opinions are divided about how similar or different childhood and adult depressive syndromes are.

Most studies in childhood depression are done in the areas of neuroendocrinology, polysomnography, and biochemical changes. The DST has been the most extensively studied biological marker. The sensitivity of the DST is highest in depressed children (70 percent) and adolescents (47 percent) have a DST sensitivity comparable to that of adults (43 percent). The specificity of the DST in depressed children (70 percent) was lower than in adolescents (80 percent) or adults (87 percent).

The results of GH studies are varied and need replication. Sleep EEG results are also mixed.

Overall, these studies are considered preliminary and need replication with larger numbers of subjects.

REFERENCES

American Psychiatric Association (1987). *Diagnostic and Statistical Manual of Mental Disorders* 3rd ed. – rev. Washington, DC: American Psychiatric Association.

Anderson, G. M., and Cohen, D. J. (1991). The neurobiology of childhood neuropsychiatric disorders. In *Child and Adolescent Psychiatry: A Comprehensive Textbook*, pp. 28–38. Baltimore: Williams & Wilkins.

Arana, G. W., Baldessarini, R. J., and Ornsteen, M. (1985). The dexamethasone suppression test for diagnosis and prognosis in psychiatry. *Archives of General Psychiatry* 42:1193–1204.

Arana, G. W., and Mossman, D. (1988). The dexamethasone suppression test and depression: approaches to the use of a laboratory test in psychiatry. *Neurology Clinics of North America* 6:21–39.

Barabon, J. M., and Coyle, J. T. (1989). Receptors, monamines, and amino acids. In *Comprehensive Textbook of Psychiatry*, vols. I/V, ed. H. Kaplan and B. Sadock, pp. 45–52. Baltimore: Williams & Wilkins.

Beck-Friis, J., Von Rosen, D., and Kjellman, B. F. (1984). Melatonin in relation to body measures, sex, age, season, and the use of drugs in patients with major affective disorders and healthy subjects. *Psychoneuroendocrinology* 9:261–277.

Brown, G. M., Seggie, J. A., and Chambers, J. W. (1978). Psychoendocrinology and growth hormone: a review. *Psychoneuroendocrinology* 3(2):131–153.

Brown, R. B., Mason, B., and Stoll, P. (1986). Adrenocortical function and suicidal behavior in depressive disorders. *Psychiatry Research* 17:317–323.

Carlson, G. A., and Cantwell (1980). Unmasking masked depression in children and adolescents. *American Journal of Psychiatry* 137:445–449.

Carroll, B. J. (1985). Dexamethasone suppression test: a review of contemporary confusion. *Journal of Clinical Psychiatry* 46:13–24.

Carroll, B. J., Feinberg, M., and Greden, J. F. (1981). A specific laboratory test for the diagnosis of melancholia. *Archives of General Psychiatry* 38:15–22.

Carroll, B. J., Greden, J. R., and Feinberg, M. (1981). Suicide, neuroendocrine dysfunction and CSF 5-HIAA concentration in depression. In *Recent Advances in Neuropsychopharmacology*, ed. B.C Angiest. New York: Pergamon.

Casat, C. D., Arana, G. W., and Powell, G. (1989). The DST in children and adolescents with major depressive disorder. *American Journal of Psychiatry* 146:503–507.

Casper, R. C., Davis, J. M., and Pannday, G. N. (1977). Neuroendocrine and amine studies in affective illness. *Psychoneuroendocrinology* 2(2):105–113.

Cavallo, A., Holt, K., Hejaji, M., et al. (1987). Melatonin circadian rhythm in childhood depression. *Journal of the American Academy of Child and Adolescent Psychiatry* 26:395–399.

Chabrol, H., Chaverie, J., and Moron, P. (1983). DST, TRH test and adolescent suicide attempts. *American Journal of Psychiatry* 140(2):265.

Chambers, J. W., and Brown, G. M. (1976). Neurotransmitter regulation of growth hormone and ACTH in the rhesus monkey: effects of biogenic amines. *Endocrinology* 98:420-428.

Charney, D. S., Heninger, G. R., and Sternberg, D. E. (1982). Adrenergic receptor sensitivity in depression. Effects of Clonidine in depressed patients and healthy subjects. *Archives of General Psychiatry* 39(3): 290-294.

Coble, P. A., Kupfer, D. I., and Taska, L. S. (1984). EEG sleep of normal healthy children. Part I: Findings using standard measurement methods. *Sleep* 7:289-303.

Davis, J., Koslow, S., and Gibbon, R. (1988). Cerebrospinal fluid and urinary biogenic amines in depressed patients and healthy controls. *Archives of General Psychiatry* 45:705-717.

Emslie, G. H., Roffwarg, H. P., and Rush, J. (1987). Sleep EEG findings in depressed children and adolescents. *American Journal of Psychiatry* 144:668-670.

Emslie, G. H., Rush, J., and Weinberg, W. A. (1990). Children with major depression show reduced rapid eye movement latencies. *Archives of General Psychiatry* 47:119-124.

Emslie, G., Weinberg, W. A. and Rush, A. J. (1987). Depression and dexamethasone suppression testing in children and adolescents. *Journal of Child Neurology* 2:31-36.

Evans, D. L., and Golden, R. N. (1987). The dexamethasone suppression test: a review in *Handbook of Clinical Psychoneuroendocrinology*. Ed. C. B. Nemeroff and P. T. Loosen, pp. 313-335. New York: Guilford.

Glass, I. B., Checkley, S. A., and Shur, E. (1982). The effect of desipramine upon central adrenergic function in depressed patients. *British Journal of Psychiatry* 141:372-376.

Goetz, R. R., Puig-Antich, J., and Ryan, N. (1987). Electroencephalographic sleep of adolescents with major depression and normal controls. *Archives of General Psychiatry* 44:61-68.

Goodwin, D. W., and Guze, S. B., eds. (1989). *Affective Disorders in Psychiatric Diagnosis*. Ed. D. W. Goodwin and S. B. Guze, pp. 3-42. New York: Oxford University Press.

Grebb, J., and Browning, M. (1989). Intraneuronal biochemical signals. *Comprehensive Textbook of Psychiatry /V*. Vol. 1. Ed. H. Kaplan and B. Sadock. Baltimore: Williams & Wilkins.

Greenberg, R., Rosenberg, G., and Weisberg, L. (1985). The dexamethasone suppression test and the thyrotropin-releasing hormone test in adolescent major depressive disorder (abs). Proceedings for papers and new research presented at the 32nd Annual Meeting of the American Academy of Child Psychiatry, San Antonio, TX. Washington DC: American Academy of Child & Adolescent Psychiatry 42.

Harger, R., and Irwin, M. (1991). *Developmental Aspects of Psychoneuroendo-*

crinology. *Child and Adolescent Psychiatry: A Comprehensive Textbook.* Baltimore Williams & Wilkins.

Hofer, M. A. (1984). Relationships as regulators: a psychobiologic perspective on bereavement. *Psychosomatic Medicine* 46:183–197.

Irwin, M., and Gillen, J. (1987). Impaired natural killer cell activity among depressed patients. *Psychiatry Research* 20:181–182.

Irwin, M., and Harger, R. L. (1991). *Developmental Aspects of Psychoneuroimmunology. Child and Adolescent Psychiatry: A Comprehensive Textbook.* Ed. M. Lewis. Baltimore: Williams & Wilkins.

Jarrett, D. B., Miewald, J. M., and Kupfer, D. J. (1990). Recurrent depression is associated with a persistent reduction in sleep-related growth hormone secretion. *Archives of General Psychiatry* 47:113–118.

Jensen, J. B., and Garfinkel, B. D. (1990). Growth hormone dysregulation in children with major depressive disorder. *Journal of the American Academy of Child and Adolescent Psychiatry* 29:295–301.

Kashani, J. H., and Sherman, D. D. (1988). Childhood depression: epidemiology, etiological models and treatment implications. *Integrative Psychiatry* 6(1):1–8.

Khan, A. V. (1987). Biochemical profile of depressed adolescents. *Journal of the American Academy of Child and Adolescent Psychiatry* 6:873–878.

Klee, S. J., and Garfinkel, B. D. (1984). Identification of depression in children and adolescents: the role of dexamethasone suppression test. *Journal of the American Academy of Child and Adolescent Psychiatry* 23:410–415.

Kutcher, S. P., Williamson, P., and Silverberg, J. (1988). Nocturnal growth hormone secretion in depressed older adolescents. *Journal of the American Academy of Child and Adolescent Psychiatry* 6:751–754.

Lahmeyer, H. W., Poznanski, E. O., and Bellur, S. N. (1983). EEG sleep in depressed adolescents. *American Journal of Psychiatry* 140:1150–1153.

Loosen, P. T., and Prange, A. J., Jr. (1982). The serum thyrotropin (TSH) response to thyrotropin-releasing hormone (TRH) in depression: a review. *American Journal of Psychiatry* 139:405–416.

Lopez-Ibor, J. J., Jr., Saiz-Ruiz, J., and de Los Lobos, J. C. P. (1985). Biological correlations of suicide and aggressivity in major depression (with melancholia): 5-hydroxyindoleacetic acid and cortisol in central spinal fluid, dexamethasone suppression test and therapeutic response to 5-hydroxytryptophan. *Neuropsychobiology* 14: 67–74.

Maas, J., Fawcett, H., and DeKirmenjian, H. (1968). 3 Methoxy 4 - Hydroxyphenylglycol (MHPG) excretion in depressive states. *Archives of General Psychiatry* 19:129–134.

Meyer, W. J., Richards, G. E., and Cavallo, A. (1985). Growth hormone and cortisol secretion dynamics in children with major depressive disorder. Presentation at the Annual Meeting of the American Academy of Child Psychiatry, San Antonio, Texas, October.

Pfeffer, C. R., Stokes, P., and Shindledecker, R. (1991). Suicidal behavior and hypothalamic-pituitary-adrenocortical axis indices in child psychiatry inpatients. *Biological Psychiatry* 29:909–917.

Poznanski, E. O. (1982). The clinical characteristics of childhood depression In *Psychiatry '82 Annual Review*, ed. L. Grinspoon. Washington, DC: American Psychiatric Association.

Preskorn, S. H., Weller, E. B., and Hughes, C. W. (1987). Depression in prepubertal children: dexamethasone nonsuppression predicts differential response to imipramine v. placebo. *Psychopharmacology Bulletin* 23:128–133.

Puig-Antich, J. (1987). Affective disorder in children and adolescents: diagnosis, validity and psychobiology. In *Psychopharmacology, the Third Generation of Progress*, ed. H. Y. Meltzer, pp. 843–857. New York: Raven.

Puig-Antich, J., Blau, S., and Marx, N. (1978). Prepubertal major depressive disorder. A pilot study. *Journal of the American Academy of Child Psychiatry* 17:695–707.

Puig-Antich, J., Goetz, R., and Davies, M. (1984b). Growth hormone secretion in prepubertal children with major depression, II. Sleep-related plasma concentrations during a depressive episode. *Archives of General Psychiatry* 41:463–466.

———— (1984c). Growth hormone secretion in prepubertal children with major depression. IV: sleep related plasma concentrations in a drug-free fully recovered clinical state. *Archives of General Psychiatry* 41:479–483.

Puig-Antich, J., Goetz, R., and Hanlon, C. (1982). Sleep architecture and REM sleep measures in prepubertal children with depression: a controlled study. *Archives of General Psychiatry* 39:932–939.

Puig-Antich, J., Novacenko, H., and Davies, M. (1984a). Growth hormone secretion in prepubertal children with major depression, I. Final report on response to insulin-induced hypoglycemia during a depressive episode. *Archives of General Psychiatry* 41:455–460.

Robbins, D. R., and Alessi, N. E. (1985). Suicide and the dexamethasone suppression test in adolescents. *Biological Psychiatry* 20:107–110.

Ryan, N. D., Puig-Antich, J., and Meyer, V. (1987). Growth hormone secretion during sleep in depressed adolescents. Presentation at the Consortium on Affective Disorders in Children, Boston, September.

Sachar, E. J. (1975). Neuroendocrine abnormalities in depressive illness. In *Topics in Psychoneuroendocrinology*, pp. 135–156. New York: Grune & Stratton.

Sachar, E. J., Hellman, L., and Roffwarg, H. P. (1973). Disrupted 24-hour patterns of cortisol secretion in psychotic depression. *Archives of General Psychiatry* 28:19–24.

Schildkraut, J. (1965). The catecholamine hypothesis of affective disorders: a review of supporting evidence. *American Journal of Psychiatry* 122:509-522.

Secunda, S. K., Cross, C. K., and Koslow, S. (1986). Biochemistry and suicidal behavior in depressed patients. *Biological Psychiatry* 21:756.

Strober, M., Green, J., and Carlson, G. (1982). Phenomenology and subtypes of major depressive disorder in adolescents. *Journal of Affective Disorders*. 3:281-290.

Tamarkin, L., Reppert, S. M., and Klein, D. C. (1979). Regulation of pineal melatonin of the syrian hamster. *Endocrinology* 104:385-389.

Targum, S. D., Capodanno, A., and Unger S. (1983). The DST in adolescents: a matched follow-up study. Paper presented at the annual meeting of the American Psychiatric Association, New York, May.

Targum, S. D., Rosen, L., and Capodanno, A. E. (1983). The dexamethasone suppression test in suicidal patients with unipolar depression. *American Journal of Psychiatry* 140:877-879.

Urry, R. L., and Ellis, L. C. (1975). Monoamine oxidase activity of the hypothalamus and pituitary. Alterations after pinealectomy, changes in photoperiod or additional of melatonin in vitro. *Experientia* 31:891-892.

Weisman, M. M. (1984). Depression and anxiety disorders in parents and children: results from the Yale Family Study Archives. *Archives of General Psychiatry* 41:845-852.

Weller, E. B., Weller, R. A., and Fristad, M. A. (1986). Dexamethasone suppression test and clinical outcome in prepubertal depressed children. *American Journal of Psychiatry* 143:1469-1470.

Weller, E. B., Weller, R. A., Fristad, M. A., et al. (1985). The dexamethasone suppression test in prepubertal children. *Journal of Clinical Psychiatry* 46:511-513.

Worley, P., Baraban, J., and Snyder, S. (1987). Beyond receptors: multiple second messenger system in brain. *Annuals of Neurology* 21:217.

Yehuda, R., Southwick, S. M., Ostroff, R. B., et al. (1988). Neuroendocrine aspects of suicidal behavior. *Endocrinology and Metabolism Clinics of North America* 17, 1:83-102.

Young, W., Knowles, J. B., and Maclean, A. W. (1982). The sleep of childhood depressives: comparison with age matched controls. *Biological Psychiatry* 17:1163-1168.

INTERVENTION
Section II

9: TREATMENT OF DEPRESSION WITHIN A FAMILY CONTEXT

James Coyne, Ph.D.
Linda Schwoeri, M.A., M.F.T.
G. Pirooz Sholevar, M.D.

INTRODUCTION

Depression frequently arises in the context of conflictful and unsupportive relationships and stressful life events requiring long-term adjustment. Many of these stressful events impinge upon the rest of the family (Brown and Harris 1978, Coyne et al. in press, Keitner and Miller 1990). Depressed persons are likely to be involved in interpersonal struggles, particularly with their spouses and children. Moreover, depression tends to be a marker for families with other serious difficulties. Stresses on the family and the personal vulnerabilities of family members may predate and contribute to the identified patient's condition; yet living with a depressed person also takes a toll on family life and the well-being of other family members. The nature of the connections between depression and its family context is thus likely to be complex and variable among patients and their families. Understanding and renegotiating the family relationships of depressed persons may be crucial in the recovery of the depressed patient, the reduction of associated family problems, and the prevention of depression relapse in the patient, regardless of how the patterning occurs.

By the time that a patient is diagnosed or seeks treatment for depression, the routines and emotional life of the family are likely to be disrupted. Coyne, Downey, and Boergers (in press) have characterized the family system of depressed persons as *emotionally dysregulated*, that is, family members may be unable to repair negative interactions, resolve disagreements, or resist the contagiousness of each other's negative affect. Rather than eliciting support and efforts at understanding, displays of despair or sadness may be met with anger and hostility. There may be little opportunity for negative affect to be transformed into positive affect. Indeed, depressed persons and their family members may be involved in a cycle in which unsuccessful efforts to resolve differences by discussion or confrontation lead to longer periods of withdrawal and avoidance, during which there is a further accumulation of negative affect, misunderstanding, and misgivings about each other (Kahn et al. 1985). The cumulative effects of stalemates overwhelm family members when they again attempt to settle specific differences. This further increases their pessimism about the possibility of improving their relationships and strengthens their tendencies to deal with each other in a hostile and expedient manner.

For the individual adult depressed patient, family and marital problems predict a reduced response to medication, longer time for recovery, and greater risk of relapse. A focus on the family context of depression might thus be adopted as part of a commitment to the more narrow goal of the recovery and improvement in social functioning of the depressed patient. Depression is frequently associated with serious marital problems. Furthermore, the children of a depressed parent are at considerable risk for psychological disturbance, and depression in a parent suggests the possibility of otherwise undetected and untreated depression in a child. Adoption of a family systems perspective on depression, which includes assessment and intervention with other family members along with the depressed patient, may therefore be undertaken with the broader goals of improving the functioning of the marital unit or family as a whole, thereby reducing the impairment of other family members. This is likely to provide a direct benefit to the depressed patient as well. Depressed patients often have staked their well-being on the resolution of their family problems. They may be engaged in destructive exchanges with their spouses and incapacitated by guilt over the problems of their children. The goal of improving the functioning of the family is in no way inconsistent with a commitment to the individual depressed patient. Finally, there is no evidence of any incompatibility between psychopharmacological treatment and family intervention.

As we have construed it here, a family systems perspective is a way of thinking about the treatment of depression, expanding our range of considerations from individual depressed patients to their involvement in family relationships and their larger family contexts. It is not a rigid commitment requiring all family members to attend all sessions, and such sessions may actually be the exception rather than the rule. The kinds of marital and family problems associated with depression may be such that conventional family therapy with the whole family present is neither conducive to progress nor acceptable to key family members.

For instance, Watzlawick and Coyne (1980) described the brief family treatment of a depressed stroke victim. In a pretreatment interview, the man indicated that his family could seek therapy, but that he would not participate. A subsequent five sessions of family therapy were conducted in his absence and focused on redirecting his family's well-meant but inappropriate efforts to assist his recovery. Much can also be done to reduce family members' personalization of a severely depressed patient's symptoms and their use of hostile criticism as a strategy of influence before the patient is even able to participate in psychotherapy. Also, many spouses of depressed persons might reject conventional marital therapy because of the implication that the problem is to be construed as a bad marriage causing depression rather than as the patient's depression disrupting their marital harmony. The level of marital discord may also be such that a conjoint session would only prove destructive. Yet, in adopting a family systems perspective, a therapist might avoid the issue of the locus of the problem — one does not have to be part of the problem to be part of the solution. In meeting with the patient and spouse separately, the therapist helps identify how each suffers in the current circumstances and engages in a bit of shuttle diplomacy before attempting to bring the couple together. Finally, many children of depressed parents suffer from exposure to their parents' marital conflict. Even when child-rearing issues are primary, excluding children from sessions may be an effective way of allowing parents to confront their differences without involving the children and arriving at an effective collaborative strategy for parenting.

Working with the families of depressed persons can be challenging. It requires a flexibility and even a fluidity in conceptualization, assessment, and intervention. The therapist needs to track not only how depressed patients' involvement in family life may explain some of their difficulties but also how family members' perspectives may radically differ. The therapist needs to assess how depressed persons may participate in, even generate, the marital distress and the more pervasive emotional dysregulation that characterizes their families. Strategic therapy can provide a framework for organizing these concerns.

DEFINITION OF STRATEGIC THERAPY AND ITS APPLICATION TO THE TREATMENT OF DEPRESSION

Strategic therapy is pragmatic, goal-oriented, and relatively short-term, typically entailing no more than ten to fifteen sessions. It evolved as a form of family therapy, but it is a highly flexible and broadly applicable approach to work with individuals, couples, and larger systems. Indeed, it breaks down a sense of rigid distinctions between individual, marital, and family therapy. Even when the focus is on larger systems, attention is often centered on promoting small but crucial changes in the actions of one of a few persons as a way of influencing the broader interpersonal context. Thus, strategic marital therapy is typically conducted with the sessions split between the spouses. In work with families, a major portion of time is spent with the parents in the absence of the rest of the family. As with other forms of psychotherapy, strategic therapy can be seen as an effort to affect how persons conduct their lives in order to relieve their distress or improve their functioning and well-being. However, it is generally more focused on modifying what people do in their everyday lives than are more conventional approaches to psychotherapy. Strategic therapy relies more heavily on *direct* and *indirect suggestions* and the *assignment of extratherapy tasks*, often of a paradoxical nature.

Guided and informed by the innovative thinking of the Mental Research Institute (MRI) group, this model focuses on how the miscarried coping efforts of depressed persons and key persons in their lives are perpetuating their problems. Watzlawick and colleagues (Watzlawick 1978, Watzlawick et al. 1974) emphasized the irony in that the solutions people bring to a problem actually contribute to the persistence or exacerbation of that same problem. In strategic therapy, the task is to break into the repetitive and unproductive but self-perpetuating cycle and redirect the efforts of those involved. In a sense, it is the *coping efforts* — what the patient and family members are doing about the depression — rather than the depression per se that is the focus of intervention. The focus is on what they are doing to cope with a life in a family in which they cannot resolve differences, renegotiate relationships, or even safely and effectively express feelings, rather than on the family's general state of emotional dysregulation.

Interventions involve deliberate attempts to prevent the occurrence of problem-maintaining behavior, typically by reframing or redefining problems so that the existing beliefs and values of those involved can lead to a very different behavior. Strategic therapy is consistent with Harry Stack Sullivan's view of personality (1956) as the pattern of recurring events that characterize a person's life. Strategic therapy focuses on the patterning of contemporary relationships rather than those in the past, and on perceptions and feelings in their interactional context, rather than as manifestations of psychodynamic processes. This approach defines the therapist as one who directly intervenes to modify the contexts, complex feedback processes, and characteristic responses of others that maintain the depression.

A critical task for the therapist is to assist the depressed persons and families to feel empowered. Often, all family members feel powerless and neglected, and this arises from their well-meant but inept and ill-timed efforts to influence their life in the family. Much of their sense of powerlessness comes from efforts to change aspects of the family and its members that they cannot directly or immediately change. For instance, family members cannot by sheer effort cheer up depressed persons or coerce them into feeling better or functioning effectively. Trying too hard to do so, they become frustrated, unsympathetic, and angry, leaving both the depressed persons and themselves feeling bad. Consequently, they unilaterally seek to implement solutions without enlisting other members, are thwarted, and are left feeling isolated, misunderstood, and unsupported.

Empowering refers to the therapeutic task of helping individuals view their situation in terms of its being manageable and for which they have the necessary resources, and as affording the possibility of a positive outcome. A key part of this is to block or discourage the patient and family members from taking responsibility for what they cannot change and to instead focus on what they *can* do. Thus, and perhaps paradoxically, they may have more influence on the quality of family life if they take responsibility for their own behavior rather than for what others think or feel. As they do this, they rediscover the personal and family resources that have been misapplied or gone unrecognized.

RATIONALE FOR WORKING WITH FAMILY MEMBERS SEPARATELY

It may appear odd for family therapists to see members of a family separately; however, depressed persons and their spouses or family members may not share a commitment to therapy or a common perspective. They also may not agree on the continuation of the marriage or the resolution of family problems. They may, in fact, benefit more from therapy if they feel the therapist grasps their unique perspectives, and that they are working toward a personally relevant goal, with progress that can be marked with observable accomplishments. Therefore, in keeping with a systems orientation, the therapist does not need to require that both patient and the spouse or the entire family be present at all times in therapeutic sessions. A systems perspective encourages consideration of how strategic changes in a subsystem can produce changes in the patterning of the whole system.

Another reason for interviewing the subsystems separately is that it facilitates the gathering of detailed information about how, from each person's perspective, problems are occurring in everyday life and how these problems are being approached. This information is a prerequisite to any reframings or homework assignments. Also, when interviewed together, the family or couple may lapse into their characteristic pattern of outbursts and accusations or, alternatively, into inhibition and withdrawal. These interactions interfere with the therapist's ability to obtain a picture of what happens outside of therapy. Such patterns of interaction are, of course, relevant to therapy, but a brief report of their occurrence is as useful as a drawn-out enactment of it in the therapy room.

Furthermore, there is a concern that conflict enacted in the session may reflect the artificiality of the setting and, in particular, the presence of the therapist as a possible ally, referee, or commentator. Such exchanges not only may be unrepresentative of what occurs outside of therapy but may leave the individuals less prepared to undertake any initiative for change.

Finally, and especially in regard to spouses, depressed persons tend to behave less dysfunctionally in the absence of their family members (Hinchcliffe et al. 1978), and everyone may prove to be less defensive and more flexible and compromising when seen alone. They will also often privately agree to initiate small positive changes that they would reject as unacceptable if they were in the presence of the other. Interviewed together, they may face difficult choices between agreeing to a positive change and resisting the appearance of having made a concession to a hostile and coercive family member. Of great importance with this approach is whether disclosure of a plan for change will induce a debilitating preoccupation with the threat of failure.

INITIAL INTERVIEWING: FOCUS OF INTERVIEW

Some of the essentials in the interview involve gathering information on what the person sees as the problem, how it is a problem, how it interferes with daily life, and why therapy for the problem has been sought now rather than previously or later. Finally and quite importantly, an attempt is made to formulate some concrete, minimal goal for treatment, with answers to the question, "What would it take to indicate to you that you were on the right path, even if you were not out of the woods?" Or another example could be: "There is a lot of difficulty and uncertainty in your life, and we cannot expect to take care of it all. Is there one problem such that if we were able to make some small progress in dealing with it, you would feel a bit more able to cope with everything else?" The focus here is on repeated reference to the time-limited nature of therapy and helping the individuals to think in terms of small, observable changes.

The therapy session is viewed as a staging area for small but strategic changes in how depressed persons tackle their problems and how they interact with key persons, particularly spouses. Therapy is explicitly time-limited, with either a preset number of sessions or a contracting for subsequent sessions based on the demonstration of progress. Thus, the therapist may contract with a depressed person to work on a particular problem, and if progress can be seen in six sessions, a new goal will be set and an additional six sessions offered to pursue it. The typical marital session tends to involve 20 to 25 minutes with each spouse and a briefer wrap-up meeting, at the end of which the therapist makes summary comments and provides extratherapy tasks.

Goals are typically small, and strategic changes in behavior are of a more general nature. Achievement of goals is operationalized in terms of the occurrence of specific observable events that would indicate progress was being made, not necessarily resolution of the problems.

INTERVENTION

General Plan

In meeting with depressed persons and family members, the therapist seeks to gather the particulars of what is most upsetting to them, why it is upsetting, and what they are doing to cope with or resolve their situation. With this information, the therapist attempts to identify some small changes that would indicate significant progress was being made if they occurred and to secure agreement that therapy should focus on the attainment of these changes. One principle in the selection of goals and interventions is that they should be attuned to what would leave key persons feeling *empowered* (Coyne 1988). This implies that they are facing manageable difficulties, that the immediate coping tasks facing them afford some opportunity to observe progress, and that they are challenged rather than threatened with the prospect of another failure. A second principle is that goals and interventions should be *ecological*. This refers to being attuned to what are viable changes in particular situations, what opportunities and constraints on change exist, and how key persons are likely to react.

The strategic therapist thus construes the problem-solving efforts of depressed persons and the key persons in their lives in interactional terms, which are sensitive to the efforts of key persons and the perceptions held of these efforts. For the purposes of intervention, the therapist may think *linearly*, in terms of how the actions of particular persons can be isolated and targeted for change. Therefore, it is useful to distinguish among interventions targeting (1) the depressed person, (2) the spouse (or other significant person), (3) the couple (or the relationship), and (4) the whole family. Issues such as parenting, the children's experience, and the parents' role in the depressed child's interactional experience of depression are among the problems addressed.

Specific Strategic Interventions

Working with Depressed Persons

One of the first themes in the interventions with depressed persons is *identifying dignity and achievement in things not being worse*. This strategy relates to empowering the person to see the task ahead as manageable and one for which he or she has the skills and opportunities to effect a positive outcome. For example, in eliciting descriptions of depressed persons' problems, the therapist is careful to communicate an awareness that things are indeed difficult and that they have good reason to be depressed or else they would not be. The most basic rule in working with depressed persons is to never dispute their right and privilege to be depressed. When depressed persons seem particularly sensitive about accusations — perhaps from spouses — that they are getting something out of being depressed, the therapist might comment that one would lose a depression if one became happy with it. At some point, it is generally useful to turn the discussion to the topic of why, given that so much is wrong, someone should not be even more depressed? In this way, many depressed persons are better able to identify their resources than if directly asked to do so. Often, persons who have suffered a catastrophic change in their lives have already been surprised by the discovery that they have not been annihilated by it, and they can readily find pride in their ability to continue to cope with the mundane tasks of everyday life.

Another important intervention is to redefine the depressed person's coping task or *redirecting his or her efforts*. This is an attempt to insulate the depressed person from insolvable tasks and other sources of failure. For example, a woman had been trying unsuccessfully to convince her elderly mother that surgery had rendered the mother incapable of working and that she needed to start making plans for retirement. The more the daughter attempted to reason with her, the more insistent and unrealistic the mother became. The therapist agreed with the woman that her mother was difficult and suggested she needed all the support she could get. It was suggested that the woman should not allow her mother to irritate her and damage their relationship. Instead, she should leave it to the mother and her physicians to discuss whether a return to work was possible and then be prepared to assist her when the inevitable decision was reached.

In relinquishing responsibility for an outcome that is beyond their control, people may experience a resurgence of morale and energy and sometimes a renewal of their relationships. All too often, in attempting to cope with the depressed partner, the spouse gets trapped into destructive and frustrating interactions because he or she is so committed to helping and making a difference.

Haley (1973) has noted that strategic therapists do not typically point out or interpret fears. They look for positive aspects in behavior. The therapist will acknowledge that given the depressed person's circumstances, his or her fears are quite understandable, yet he or she has been able to do quite well. The therapist does not minimize the difficulties but looks for the positive forces active in the person. The focus of the intervention is on bringing about change and expanding the depressed person's world, not on educating the person about his or her inadequacies. Therefore, it is important to allow dignity and defenses rather than to require submission and confession.

Often depressed persons, particularly women, need encouragement to focus more directly on what they need to do for themselves, rather than having to tackle family problems that they are too depressed to manage. They are more likely to accept this shift if it is construed as their becoming more effective in order to tackle the family's problems. The following analogy may be invoked to underscore this point. At the beginning of flights on commercial airlines, attendants note that in the event of a decompression of the aircraft, an oxygen mask will descend from the overhead. If passengers are traveling with a small child or another dependent, they are advised nonetheless to get their own mask adjusted first before attempting to be of help. The therapist may consequently admonish a depressed patient, "Get your own oxygen mask adjusted first! What are you going to do to begin accomplishing this during the week? Consider this a decompression, an emergency, and what are you going to do to look after yourself so that you can look after your family?" Thus, the need for self-care is *reframed* as looking after the family and therefore presented in a more compelling manner. "What turns out to be changed as a result of reframing is the meaning attributed to the situation, and therefore its consequences, but not its concrete facts" (Watzlawick et al. 1974, p. 95).

Sometimes therapists can avoid constructing therapeutic tasks in terms of success and failure by framing them as *assessments*, preliminary to any effort to bring about change. For example, a therapist may encourage depressed patients to test whether social activities are as unsatisfying as anticipated or whether tiring themselves with exercise feels different from the fatigue they experience before it. They may also be encouraged to explore which demands and obligations make them feel better when they are tackled, which leave them feeling worse, and which will create problems later if ignored. Some of these assessments are deliberately left cryptic or openended. Thus, depressed patients may be asked to notice, in retrospect, when in the course of a week they have been free for a time from their ruminations and self-derogation. They should then later attempt more of the same activity and see if the same effect can be obtained.

The therapist must decide how to deal with observable signs of progress as they occur. In many instances, they invite another assignment, building in stepwise fashion upon what has already occurred. If that can be done without undue risk of failure, then that is the preferable course of action. Therapists, however, should be sensitive about the sometimes paradoxical drawbacks and pitfalls of improvement. It is important that small changes not become burdensome. In other words, they should not carry with them the demand that progress be maintained with new, more threatening initiatives. Change should not invalidate the depressed person's distress or his or her continued dissatisfaction with the status quo. Because most personal change involves a balance of positive and negative elements, it makes good sense to caution depressed persons that *there are drawbacks and even dangers to improvement.* Some persons request help but put the onus of change on the therapist. In arguing for the dangers of improvement, the therapist puts the burden back on the patient to demonstrate his or her willingness to make an effort.

Jamming interventions may be useful to reduce patients' sense of being under family members' critical gaze or of their otherwise being responsible to them. In the presence of the family members, the therapist may ask patients to hide progress from them and persist in pessimistic statements no matter how they feel. Thus, a depressed housewife had been badgered by her husband about seeking employment at a time when job opportunities were limited. The therapist encouraged her to do what she thought she could do, but regardless, she should leave moistened tissues and empty candy wrappers around the couch every night before he returned home. If asked about her progress, she should say no more than that she had spent the day feeling sorry for herself, despite whatever she had done. What she actually accomplished would thus be her concern alone for now.

Depressed persons are frequently avoidant and indecisive. They can find ample evidence that they are irresponsible and incompetent. Yet such an unsuccessful style of coping is often maintained by high standards and by a definition of the task at hand that makes any accomplishment seem insufficient and any effort seem futile. The therapist may utilize opportunities to reframe such apparent irresponsibility as the result of a willingness to accept too much responsibility. A suicidal woman complained that she deserved to die because she had been irresponsible and had disappointed her husband, children, and employer. The therapist could comment that suicide was the only exit she knew from the Superwoman role, and might say

> Other people would probably accept their limitations, or make excuses for themselves, but you do not allow yourself that, and so depression and attempting suicide is your way out. Being depressed at least slows you down. Yet, the problem with depression is that it sometimes lifts when you need it the most and you are again burdened with the sense that you can and should be able to do everything.

The therapist requested that the woman provide an antisuicide contract, but that she also take a brief leave from her stressful job. She protested that to do so would be irresponsible. "Superwoman would see it that way," the therapist agreed. "However, dead people make bad employees." Finally, a request was made that she develop a plan for how she would restrain herself for more than the week if her depression did not hold. Except for minimal efforts to deal with the children, she was to let problems be. By the end of the session, the woman expressed genuine relief. The therapist ended the session with, "And I'm not going to tell you to have a good week. That would be a set up. You would only have to work harder to keep yourself down."

This reframing technique is an intervention aimed at a positive framing of the patient's involvement in his or her predicaments. Its goal is to structure the patient's coping tasks and allow for progress in small steps. This intervention and technique serves to restrain someone from trying too hard when resources are depleted or situations are overwhelming. The rationale for such an intervention is that depressed persons are often able to infuse their feelings of sadness with feelings of badness and incompetence. They ultimately maintain their dysphoria by taking on too much, failing, or becoming avoidant of trying, and thus validating their negative view of themselves. Furthermore, they are often more likely to discover and utilize their resources if they are restrained from attempting too much rather than prodded to take on what they may see as overwhelming.

Working with Spouses

In working with spouses, it is important to not side with the spouse in an effort to prod the depressed person into action. Also, caution must be taken to not ignore spouses' clear statements that there is nothing wrong with their marriages except their partners' depression, if that is their position.

Just as it is important to acknowledge to depressed persons that it is understandable that they are depressed, so too should the therapist work to grasp and acknowledge whatever frustrations, sacrifices, and disappointments may color the spouses' reactions to their depressed partners and the prospect of their participation in therapy. The therapist should recognize how, in attempting to cope with the depressed partner, the spouse may have stifled complaints, faced what was seen as unjustified hostility and criticism, and made numerous, unappreciated concessions. The therapist should look for opportunities to connote these efforts positively, in terms of the spouse's absorption in efforts to help the depressed partner. He should further address how difficult it is to remain supportive in such circumstances. When possible, the therapist should link the occurrence of miscarried helping efforts to the positive intentions from which they spring. The basic theme is that people would not get trapped into such destructive interactions if they were not so committed to making a difference.

Sometimes the contribution of spouses to the predicament of their depressed partners is that they have remained aloof, indifferent, or unavailable. If so, the key is to increase their involvement in specific supportive efforts, even while helping them to avoid personalizing the depressed person's distress.

Usually, however, the issue is that the spouse is overinvolved in efforts to get the depressed person to feel better and act less dysfunctionally. There may have been a progression from initial efforts to be comforting and supportive, to advice and disputation of the depressed person's negative views, and then to coercion and characterological criticism (Coyne 1988). In the process, any sense of what is beneficial to either the spouse or the depressed person may be lost. In such situations, the therapist may pursue a course of *strategic disengagement*. As an experiment, the spouse is encouraged to limit efforts to be helpful to small gestures that do not allow an immediate acknowledgment. For example, the spouse might leave a note or small present or do a chore in the morning, knowing that the depressed person will not see this until later. Generally speaking, it is easier for spouses to remain humane and supportive when their responsibilities are limited and defined in terms of discrete small tasks, and when they are not anticipating immediate results for what they do. What often happens is helping becomes miscarried or deteriorates when someone cares too much or tries too hard to obtain an outcome that is not immediately within his control. The fundamental strategy is to connote positively the spouse's efforts and then encourage a deescalation and a refocus on what the spouse can do to take care of him- or herself. For example, the therapist might say:

> While I can appreciate what you are trying to do, it seems like the more you try, the worse it gets. Maybe it is just a matter of timing. . . . I am concerned that you'll wear yourself out and not be available when your partner needs you most. What can you do to take care of yourself, maybe allow yourself some rest and relaxation before plunging back into the struggle?

The therapist might even suggest that for the benefit of the depressed person, the spouse do something special for him- or herself on a schedule, whether or not he or she feels such efforts are needed.

Living with a depressed person can prove burdensome and frustrating, and spouses may find that any existing difficulties with irritability and anger control are uncovered and exacerbated. If they agree this has been so, they may be asked to contract with the therapist to avoid engaging in specific behaviors, such as cursing or yelling. This task is framed as a matter of personal development and even a challenge, and the patient's behavior is to be considered irrelevant. Thus, spouses are given heightened responsibility for their own behavior and are implicitly being asked not to fall back on the depressed person's provocation as an excuse for their own lapses.

Working with the Couple

Interventions with a couple build on what has transpired with the individual partners. Before asking that the two work together as a couple, the therapist is careful to acknowledge the problems in the relationship and to warn that many of the things they have attempted to do for each other will either backfire, go unrecognized, or be misunderstood. Only later will they be able to appreciate the helpfulness of what each is about to do now. The therapist suggests proceeding slowly and cautiously. He frames the immediate future as a time of change, one aspect of which is that the couple may need to tolerate what they do not want to be an enduring feature of the relationship.

When there are inhibitions in communicating problems, the therapist may need to be directive and encourage the couple to speak directly and not attempt to read the other's mind or guess how the other really feels. They may be specifically asked to make at least three unreasonable requests of each other before the next session in order to give the partner an opportunity to say emphatically, "No!" without feeling guilty.

With more overtly conflictual couples, the therapist may adopt the strategy of having them stage recurring arguments with more of a sense of theater or play. For example, with a couple in which the husband has taken to reacting harshly to any pessimistic or negative statement from his wife, the therapist first reviews with the husband how women might be different in that they benefit from simply having an opportunity to vent. Furthermore, men might make it difficult for women by taking responsibility to refute or resolve their complaints. It is further suggested that hearing oneself speak is different than silently thinking the same idea. Perhaps the wife needs to hear her own complaints without being distracted by his well-meant but unending efforts to help. The couple is then asked to stage situations in which she complains but he resists his urge to intervene.

One very important intervention is one in which the therapist looks for opportunities to express that the couple should appreciate their achievement. This is implied by the patients' situation not being worse than it is, and it identifies dignity and achievement in their efforts while highlighting their strengths or resourcefulness. This changes the focus to more positive behavior rather than focusing on the patients' shortcomings. The therapist may ask the partners individually how they have been able to make it as long as they have, despite their problems. If a comment about love or commitment is heard, the suggestion is made to find a way to better use this resource. If, however, the depressed patient expresses long-standing hostility toward the partner, the therapist then comments that this may represent a real loyalty. This paradoxically implies that the hostility is the partner's investment in what the partner feels or does, and that remaining hostile, at least for now, may be a way of keeping enough distance to reduce the hurt. This represents a positive reframing of the couple's feelings and behaviors.

Working with the Whole Family

Interventions with the family build upon what is being accomplished with the various family members. Oftentimes, the family is convened only briefly at the end of a session that has been divided among the parents and children. Full sessions with the whole family are likely only later in therapy. The therapist may use the presence of the whole family to give positive reframings of recent events in the family. He may note, for instance, when someone made a positive overture to other family members, felt rebuffed, and reacted angrily before anyone else could grasp what was occurring. The therapist might then also make the more general comment that for now it is the kind of family in which good things do not always reach their destination. The therapist should also listen for instances in which it is reported that one or more family members showed distress or pain without becoming angry, and when witnessing family members were able not to get angry or overinvolved. Similarly, the therapist should highlight when family members were successful in resolving misunderstandings or bad feelings about each other. Identifying such an occurrence, the therapist should label it as a sign of progress and praise everybody who took part.

Conjoint family meetings are also an opportunity to negotiate *quid pro quo* agreements that were developed in separate meetings with family members. Apologies may be exchanged and agreements announced. Such meetings may also allow the parents to present themselves as a united front and make joint announcements about rules, chores, and discipline. When possible, it is helpful for such meetings to end on a positive note and perhaps with the family committing themselves to some shared special activity. The therapist should be cautious about overestimating their ability to cooperate or their interest in spending time together, however.

Special Interventions

Focusing on Parenting

Depression interferes with effective parenting, and children of a depressed parent are at considerable risk for disturbance and behavioral problems themselves. Yet we should be cautious about blaming the depressed persons for what are more direct results of the withdrawal of the nondepressed parent, or of family stress, marital conflict, and preexisting family problems. Much of the risk to the children of depressed parents is eliminated in families in which the marital conflict is contained and the nondepressed parent is actively involved in disciplining and remains accessible to the children (Downey and Coyne 1990)

One important goal is to *decrease hostile-critical exchanges about disciplining the children*, both between the parents and with the children. It is much easier to get parents to renounce the use of criticism and name-calling than it is to get them to honor the agreement. More lasting change can come about only when rules are explicit, with set, passionless procedures for enforcing them. It may be useful to concentrate on one particular area of concern, such as homework, chores, or conflict between the children, and, at first, aim for only partial implementation of a plan. This may be all that can be reasonably achieved, and to insist on more would set the family up for failure.

The therapist may assist the parents in renegotiating responsibilities for enforcement of rules. Thus, by agreement, the nondepressed parent may temporarily take over responsibility for seeing that homework is completed and chores are done. Also, explicit *tagteam* arrangements may be implemented, by which one parent can pass responsibilities over to the other in an orderly and prearranged fashion. Nondepressed parents may also be asked to make explicit their intolerance of abusive and disrespectful behavior directed by the children toward the depressed parent.

Although these issues and interventions may seem common to any family in which there are parenting problems, the particular complications posed by the families of depressed persons should be noted. Efforts to work with such a family must take into account the effects of depression on one parent's functioning and of the likely withdrawal of the other parent; the limitations of the parents as a team; and the problems posed by children who have learned to exploit the family's difficulties. Furthermore, what is also different is the emotional reactivity of both the family as a whole and of particular family members. One person's distress becomes everybody's, sadness and hurt feelings become fused with hostility, and no one can expect much tolerance or understanding. Indeed, it is an indication of progress when either a parent or child can have a bad day without it leading to uproar in the family.

Focus on the Children

Therapists should make a point of granting children and, particularly, adolescents time to meet with them without the parents present. They often have specific concerns and a unique perspective on the family that would be lost if the parents were present. They may also appreciate time simply to ventilate their thoughts and feelings and get acknowledgment for what they have endured. Like spouses, children of a depressed parent need an understanding of why they cannot take responsibility for someone else's mood disturbance, even if they have the capacity to aggravate the situation. They may have been more aware of the depressed parent's irritability and anger than their sadness, and they may have personalized their withdrawal and lack of enthusiasm for the family. The offspring of depressed parents may need to obtain acknowledgment of how difficult life in their family has been for them.

The hostility between depressed persons and their children may be even more intense than that between depressed persons and their spouses (Weissman and Paykel 1974). Some will seek a deescalation of their conflict with their parents and will readily participate in a negotiation of a short truce or assumption of self-responsibility for specific tasks. Given the opportunity, children may even accept the task of orchestrating a special day for their depressed parent, such as a rescheduled Mother's Day. Some may make specific requests for a more positive involvement with their parents. It may be possible to assist the child in articulating a need for the nondepressed parent to get reinvolved in the family and thereby provide an initial reconnection for that parent that is less threatening than if the focus were on the attenuated marital relationship.

On the other hand, some adolescents may have settled into a pattern of oppositional behavior and may be unwilling to relinquish the freedom from rules or supervision that their family's problems have allowed them. *Defiance-based interventions* may, therefore, be in order. With this intervention, an uncooperative early adolescent was enjoined to break rules and be grounded so that his younger brother could discover that his parents were serious about enforcement without having to be grounded himself. When the adolescent refused, he was admonished that someone had to take on this difficult job and that he could do his brother a service.

The Depressed Child and the Game of Childhood Depression

Children of a depressed parent are six times more likely to be clinically depressed than other children (Downey and Coyne 1990). Yet their distress may go unrecognized in such a family. Also, depression usually occurs along with other problems, such as school refusal and angry and defiant behavior that proves distracting. Detection and diagnosis may require systematic interviewing of both the child and the parents.

Depressed children can be a handful. They can make nonsense out of the best-conceived parenting strategies, and by their misbehavior draw the parents into conflict with the school. They deny the influence and satisfactions for which parents and teachers strive so hard, and precipitate anger-control problems in adults usually characterized by self-restraint. They can leave their parents shocked and hating themselves for the strong reactions they elicit. A lot of initial work with parents of depressed children focuses on their vacillation between being enraged at them and incapacitated by guilt and remorse.

A labeling of a child's depression can be a way for parents to begin to appreciate that neither they nor their child can immediately snap the child out of a bad mood, although what the parents do makes a crucial difference in the long run. Labeling can cut down the outright cruelty that occurs and can also be useful to educate parents about an interactional pattern in which they may unwittingly be participating: the *game of childhood depression*. This term is used to explain why depressed children may seem to go out of their way to be defiant, throw tantrums for the most trivial of reasons, and struggle to get others upset with them.

Parents may feel that they love and accept their depressed children even if the children are exceptionally difficult. Although the children may succeed in getting parents to lose their temper and say hurtful things (from the parents' perspective), this regrettable behavior does not convey their true feelings. Depressed children, however, become convinced that others view them as negatively as they view themselves. The depressed children's perspective is that their parents are terribly disappointed in them and even hateful. When the children succeed in getting parents visibly upset, the children may be relieved that the parents are finally expressing their true feelings. It was the parents' niceness that was not genuine. The children may take some satisfaction in having exposed the parents, and once the parents are angry, the children may get even angrier for having been misled by the parents' nice behavior. The depressed children's game is thus to expose the negativity and hate that they believe is all around them. Bewildered parents may be shocked at their own feelings and behavior that depressed children are able to elicit. Yet they may ignore their own responsibility because they feel that depressed children are bringing it upon themselves. From the parents' perspective, the children are *creating* the parents' hostile behavior. Yet, from the children's point of view, they are merely *exposing* the parents' true feelings.

On the basis of this formulation, the parents may be encouraged to concentrate on not being drawn into the pattern. Their task is to work to preserve a calm but firm demeanor in dealing with the child's provocations, and this will be less difficult if they are clear about rules, but tolerant, and prepared to intervene before they get upset. They can state their position that they do not hate the child, but they are to avoid getting in prolonged arguments that are likely to escalate to a level of hostility that only confirms the child's negative view of the parents' attitude.

The therapist should offer the depressed child time alone and be patient and persistent when rebuffed. While some eagerly seek to talk with the therapist privately, others will not want the burden of sustaining a full session, and some will feign disinterest but wish to sit in with other family members, particularly siblings. Thus, a severely depressed preadolescent boy protested that he was only there to listen but stuck a note on the therapist's back stating "I like you" at the end of a session in which the family had been assisted in planning a weekend trip to a space museum.

As they become more comfortable, depressed children may accept help in identifying and articulating their feelings. Progress is being made when they are able to report expressing feelings, being criticized, or rejected, without first having a temper tantrum or sulking. The therapist should not underestimate their contribution to the emotional dysregulation of the family or their potential as a point of influence.

Psychodynamic Family Therapy

The psychodynamic family therapy shares the perspective of system-orientated family therapists who put great emphasis on the role of feedback within the family unit, which maintains a person in his or her depressed position. However, in contrast to systems theorists, the psychodynamic family therapist believes that the feedback for the maintenance of depressive interactions can also come from the past experiences. These experiences are thought to have imprinted a certain type of internal configuration and reality on the depressed person and other family members. This intrapsychic configuration generally results in the depressed person's selection of a marital partner who would be willing or potentially interested in participating in a depressive interactional pattern. The depressive interactional model is characterized by the expectation of frustration, disappointment, resentment, and distance within an intimate relationship in contrast to seeking satisfaction, pleasure, and intimacy, which hopefully is the goal of a nondepressive relationship. Being disappointed, neglected, or abused in early life results in the formation of a corresponding internal (intrapsychic) fantasy system. The depressed person enters a relationship with a depression-prone person with the mutual expectation for a vicious cycle of disappointment and provocation. The interaction is then marked by one of heightened irritability, which is mislabeled as *sensitivity*, provocativeness followed by mutual withdrawal. Thus, the psychodynamic therapist has been one of the strongest adherents to the concept of assortative mating from the early days of family therapy. The other important concepts utilized by psychodynamic family therapists include *shared unconscious conflict and fantasy systems* and *shared unconscious defenses*. The shared unconscious conflict and fantasy system is based on the expectation of neglect, disappointment, and abuse. The *shared unconscious defenses* refer to the collective efforts of the family members to conceal their pathological or pathogenic preoccupations. One common defense is a consistent pattern of blaming and counterblaming followed by *negative escalation* geared toward wasting the family's time and energy and thus concealing their wholehearted commitment to lack of enjoyment in life.

The psychodynamic family therapists are interested only in the part of the family history that is *dynamically alive* and repeats itself in the everyday interactions of the couple. Learning about the history of the family in the form of *living family history* (Ackerman 1958) is helpful to sensitize the therapist to the nature of the rigidities and peculiarities of family interactions. Three types of interactions are generally common in depressed patients based on conflictual and traumatic past experiences: conflict around *loss*, *sexual and physical abuse*, and emotional neglect and abandonment.

History of Loss

It is a common observation that the families suffering from a wide range of dysfunctions, particularly depression, have suffered a high level of loss in the early stages of family development. The impact of loss on the development of the family and its younger members is complex and multifaceted. The outcome of the loss includes (a) the generation of a pessimistic and hopeless attitude toward life (lack of coherence), (b) feelings of helplessness and the inability to alter their circumstances (lack of agency), (c) intense feelings of rage, and (d) interferences with the ego development due to the absence of lost family members who can serve as models for ego development and sources of emotional nurturance necessary to achieve this goal. Therefore, the psychodynamic family therapists pay particular attention to the role of the *unresolved early losses* and *their influence on the future life course* of the affected individual. The early losses are particularly pathogenic if they result in decompensation and pathological reactions in the remaining senior family members. The conflicts around loss tend to force a person to choose a partner with a tendency to be frustrating and rejecting and influence their common children in the same direction, too. An extension of the psychodynamic theory is the *intergenerational family theory*, which places particular emphasis on the repetition of similar phenomena in multiple generations. For example, a woman can treat her daughter as a representative of her mother who has died in her early life. The daughter can comply with the mother's expectations through the mechanism of *projective identification* by rejecting the mother. The same mechanism can be repeated in two or more generations, unless the appropriate circumstances result in its alleviation and correction. The intergenerational family theory can easily explain clinical phenomena such as multiple suicides or depressions in several generations of a family.

A significant contribution to the family therapy of depression is the work of Paul and Grosser (1985). Paul has described the long-standing distortions in object relationships following early unmourned losses in families. In a method designated as *correctional* or *operational mourning*, Paul explores assertively the losses in the patient's early life. Establishing himself as a model of empathic responsiveness, he helps the family member to grieve his or her early unmourned loss. Other family members identifying with Paul's approach make themselves available and assist the depressed person further in the mourning process. Paul's dramatic case histories demonstrate the power of his interventions and the liberating effect of the correction of the patient's current relational distortions.

The Role of Sexual and Physical Abuse

Recent literature draws very strong connections between the role of early sexual and physical abuse of patients, particularly women, and subsequent development of depression. Depression in women may be more correlated with the sexual abuse in their early childhood rather than with the breakup of their intimate relationships. Unfortunately, in many cases early sexual abuse by a parent and the loss of a parental figure by either divorce, separation, or rejection can occur together in the early developmental stages of a child's life. This can have compounding effects on the young child or adolescent. Sexual and physical abuse are particularly devastating if the other parent (or parents in cases of sexual abuse by a person other than a parent) does not side with the child and accuses her or him of lying about the abuse or complicity in the situation. The work of Main and colleagues (Main 1983, Main and Goldwyn 1984, Main et al. 1985) particularly explicates the differential outcome of physical abuse of the children in cases in which one parent is clearly against the abusing parent or participates in a collusive fashion through silence with the abusive parent.

One of the most devastating impacts of the sexual or physical abuse is the alteration of the child's internal image into someone who is "bad" or a "whore." This negative internal image makes the abused person particularly prone to place her- or himself in a situation in which she or he is victimized psychologically or physically by a spouse or, subsequently, by her or his children. A helpful clinical clue emerges when the person states in the session that she or he is being victimized, particularly by her or his child. Searching for association to past experiences of victimization may reveal dramatic, forgotten memories. For example, in a family session, a mother was constantly complaining of victimization by her 6-year-old son. The questioning by the therapist about the history of victimization met with an honest denial by the mother. Later on in the same session, she recalled that she was running naked in a room at the age of 5 with her older brother chasing her with the door closed. She was screaming, "We are going to get stuck" while running, and her mother and her sisters from behind the door were pleading with her brother not to do anything to her. She then recognized that the only explanation for the situation was that her brother was trying to put his penis into her genitals, and she was terrified that they would get stuck to each other in that position. This early victimization experience was making her particularly prone to repeatedly placing herself in disadvantageous positions with her husband and her child. She was victimized physically and emotionally by her young child who was acting like a tyrant with severe temper tantrums. The recovery of the memory was a significant step in assisting her to abandon her position as a victim and assert herself with more of a feeling of agency and effectiveness in different situations.

Emotional Neglect and Abandonment

Emotional neglect can result in the expectation of unpleasurable interactions with other people. At times, the impact of deprivation may be so severe that even the fantasy life of the person is significantly compromised and impoverished, and the person expects little gratification in real life, fantasies, or even dreams. There are usually years of lost opportunities in terms of lack of enjoyment, impoverished passionate life, or celibacy before families of such persons consult a therapist. At times, they may have failed many years of individual or family treatment based on their low level of expectation. The previous therapists may have felt totally defeated by such couples and have resorted to sarcastic or shame-producing interventions. The family, on their part, is full of complaints about the previous therapists, particularly in the form of lack of warmth, ungivingness, limited verbal exchanges, and so forth.

It is essential for the therapist to be able to unearth the emotional devastation pervading the life of the family in the present and in the past in order to produce adequate therapeutic leverage. In less seriously disturbed cases, a type of transference, improvement, or "cure" can happen when a couple, energized by the therapist's position as a parental figure, becomes engaged in producing pleasurable and successful interactions and activities. The additional benefit of positive reward and reinforcement of enjoyable activities can then enhance the motivation of the family members toward getting more out of life. The concept of healthy *entitlement* (Boszormenyi-Nagy and Spark 1973) is a helpful one with which to assist the family with the recognition that in early childhood they have not received much warmth, affection, nurturance, guidance, and input into their development due to the limitation of their parental circumstance and family crises. However, they have taken the impact of their early experiences as if they were not worthy or entitled to pleasure and success in their lives and have been depriving themselves in their contemporary life. Furthermore, they continue to deprive their children in subtle ways, as if they are trying to prove their parents right and implicitly accept the worthlessness of themselves and their children. The concept of pathological indebtedness and loyalty to the families of origin, proposed by Boszormenyi-Nagy and Spark (1973), has particular application here.

SUICIDE AS A SOLUTION

Family theorists have explored a variety of relational configurations in the family that attempts to solve the family conflict by extruding a particular member by promoting suicidal behavior. The exclusion of a particular family member in the form of a suicide attempt or successful suicide occurs at the time of actual crises, when the defensive mechanisms of the family can no longer maintain the family equilibrium without violating its integrity. Therefore, the suicidal behavior can be viewed as an attempt on the part of the family to maintain and manage its long-term relational conflicts by finding a solution in the form of extruding a family member as a scapegoat. Obviously, like all primarily defensive solutions, the suicidal behavior fails to remedy the long-standing conflicts, and the family continues with its chronic dysfunctions and imbalances, further burdened by the loss of a member and the subsequent guilt feelings.

The relational aspect of suicidal behavior can be manifested by the examination of the total communicational patterns in the family. Several studies have demonstrated that suicidal utterances are frequently supplemented by the expression of death wishes toward the suicidal patient on the part of other family members. This demonstrates the shared and collective aspects of suicidal decisions in the family, which are made through family consensus. The suicidal patient then complies dutifully with the destiny assigned him by the family. This framework makes common statements on the part of other family members such as "I would gladly open the window for you if you wish to jump out" more comprehensible.

The focus of family therapeutic intervention for depression and suicidal behavior in the adolescent is to bring to light the self-perpetuating dysfunctional patterns in the family. Such dysfunctional patterns fail to address the dissatisfactions in the family members effectively and attempt to maintain the status quo. The manifest sources of dissatisfaction are generally centered around the relationship of the adolescent with one or both of his parents. However, the exploration of the parent–child conflicts usually results in the unmasking of the covert collusion between the suicidal adolescent and one of the parents as a way of controlling the hidden marital conflicts or the disagreements between the parents and their families of origin. In order for treatment to succeed, it is essential that the conflicts between the senior members of the family be exposed in order to relieve the adolescent from the role of balancing the familial dysfunctions. This goal can be achieved more readily by supporting the parents to explore the roots of the dissatisfactions in the family rather than by confronting them aggressively, which can result in further resistance and defensiveness in the family system. If the treatment is progressing well, the parents will exhibit a willingness to work together in exploring covert dissatisfactions within the family and attempt at correcting them. The exploration of the marital dissatisfaction is followed generally by a move toward healthier *marital realignment*. The marital dissatisfaction in a suicidal family is frequently related to the long-standing interference by the families of origin with the functioning of the parents. It is essential that the parents form an alliance against the intrusion by the members of their families of origin and maintain their authority over their family of procreation.

Considering the suicidal behavior as the end result of the long-standing dysfunctional relationships in the family unit, the family as a whole should be given an active role in the control and management of the suicidal behavior. The need for the protection of the suicidal behavior is generally externalized when the hospital undertakes the responsibility for the management of the suicidal patient. The assumption of responsibility for the suicidal patient on the part of the hospital staff generally perpetuates the self-destructive behavior. It places the health professionals in the untenable position of picking up the pieces while the family continues to perpetuate the problem. However, the placement of the responsibility for the management of suicidal behavior on the family forces family members to negotiate solutions agreeable to everyone involved. In this way, the bargaining position of everyone in the family is enhanced while the unhealthy use of power, victimization, and intimidation by a faction of the family is minimized.

In families with multiple suicidal members, the intergenerational aspects of psychopathology assume an inordinate degree of importance. In such families, we find severe curtailment of the functional ability of the parents due to their insufficient differentiation from their families of origin. This configuration interferes with the parents' assuming a mature marital and parental position in their family of procreation. The parents' overall functioning may be so seriously impaired that they may not be able to provide the therapist with a minimum amount of clues or commentary on the nature of the family relationships. In such situations, intergenerational family therapy with the grandparents attending the sessions may be essential. It is generally more beneficial to include the parents of the mother and the father in separate sessions to avoid the unproductive bickering between the in-laws. The ultimate goal of treatment should be the enhancement of differentiation in the family of procreation to the point that they can function autonomously without constant reliance on their extended families.

SUMMARY

The families of depressed persons have considerable heterogeneity, and they are often beset by a daunting array of difficulties. The therapist should be careful not to replicate the family members' tendencies to personalize the pervasive dysfunction, or to be distracted by the family's more intractable problems from the small changes that are within reach. This is common particularly in the face of setbacks. It is important to keep a clear, flexible, set of goals in mind and not lose sight of why the family is willing to participate in therapy and what would allow them to get on with their lives without the need for the therapist. The suffering in such families is intense and usually more evenly distributed than it first appears. There is an almost contagious quality to their distress and despair. Working with such families often takes some real indelicacy. At times, the therapist may have to ask that family members override their sad feelings and even their empathy and enforce rules and hold to our agreements so as to make the family safer for more tender feelings. As we tell depressed mothers again and again, "If you are not feeling guilty about holding the line, you are not doing the right thing. On the other hand, if you are not looking after yourself, indulging yourself even, you are not going to be of any use to anybody."

REFERENCES

Ackerman, N. (1958). *The Psychodynamics of Family Life.* New York: Basic Books.

Boszormenyi-Nagy, I., and Spark, G. (1973). *Invisible Loyalties.* New York: Harper & Row.

Brown, G. W., and Harris, T. (1978). *Social Origins of Depression: A Study of Psychiatric Disorder in Women.* New York: The Free Press.

Coyne, J. C. (1988). Strategic therapy. In *Family Intervention in Affective Illness,* ed. G. Haas, I. Glick, and J. Clarkin. New York: Guilford.

Coyne, J. C., Downey, G., and Boergers, J. (in press). Depression in families: a systems perspective. In *Developmental Approaches to the Affective Disorders: Rochester Symposium on Developmental Psychopathology,* vol. 4, ed. D. Cicchetti and S. L. Toth. Rochester NY: University of Rochester.

Coyne, J., Kessler, R., and Tal, M. (1987). Living with a depressed person. *Journal of Consulting and Clinical Psychology* 55:347–352.

Downey, G., and Coyne, J. C. (1990). Children of depressed parents: an integrative review. *Psychological Bulletin* 108: 50–75.

Haley, J. (1973). *Uncommon Therapy.* New York: W. W. Norton.

Hinchcliffe, M., Hopper, D., and Roberts, F. J. (1978). *The Melancholy Marriage.* New York: Wiley.

Kahn, J., Coyne, J. C., and Margolin, G. (1985). Depression and marital conflict: the social construction of despair. *Journal of Social and Personal Relationships* 2:447–462.

Keitner, G., and Miller, I. (1990). Major depression and family functioning. *American Journal of Psychiatry* 147:1128–1137.

Main, M. (1983). Exploration, play and cognitive functioning related to infant–mother attachment. *Infant Behavior and Development* 6:167–174.

Main, M., and Goldwyn, R. (1984). Predicting rejection of her infant from mother's representation of her own experience: implications for the abused-abusing intergenerational cycle. *Child Abuse and Neglect* 8:203–217.

Main, M., Kaplan, N., and Cassidy, J. (1985). Security of attachment: in infancy, childhood, and adulthood. In *Growing Points in Attachment Theory and Research,* ed. I. Bretherton and E. Waters.

Main, M., and Weston, D. (1982). Avoidance of the attachment figure in infancy: descriptions and interpretations. In *The Face of Attachment in Human Behavior,* ed. C. P. Parkes and J. Stevenson-Hinde. New York: Basic Books.

Paul, N., and Grosser, G. (1985). Operational mourning and its role in conjoint family therapy. *Community Mental Health Journal* 1:339–345.

Sullivan, H. S. (1956). *Clinical Studies in Psychiatry*. New York: W. W. Norton.

Watzlawick, P. (1978). *The Language of Change: Elements of Therapeutic Communication*. New York: Basic Books.

Watzlawick, P., and Coyne, J. (1980). Depression following stroke: brief, problem-focused treatment. *Family Process* 19:13–18.

Watzlawick, P., Weakland, J., and Fisch, R. (1974). *Change: Principles of Problem Formulation and Problem Resolution*. New York: W. W. Norton.

Weissman, and Paykel (1974). *The Depressed Woman: A Study of Social Relationships*. Chicago, IL: University of Chicago Press.

10: PSYCHODYNAMIC MANAGEMENT OF DEPRESSED AND SUICIDAL CHILDREN AND ADOLESCENTS

Richard A. Gardner, M.D.

INTRODUCTION

I am in full agreement with those who claim that "for every crooked thought there must be a crooked molecule." There must be a neurological basis for all symptoms. There are some, however, who claim that this dictum makes the differentiation between the psychogenic and organic an anachronism, a residuum of medieval thinking. They would consider such differentiations to be in the category of questions like how many angels can dance on the head of a pin. Although I believe that it is true that there must be a neurological basis for all thoughts and feelings — because one must have a nerve cell to have a thought or a feeling — I do not believe that it necessarily follows that the differentiation between psychogenic and organic symptoms is irrelevant in modern times. Such differentiation concerns itself with the crucial question of *how* the molecule got "crooked." This is important because the more we know about the pathogenesis of a disorder, the better the likelihood we will be able to do something about it.

In addition, the differentiation has important therapeutic implications. If one believes that the molecule got crooked because of environmental (especially family) influences, then one is more likely to recommend psychotherapy, milieu therapy, family therapy, and other therapeutic approaches that involve personality changes in the patient and his or her associates. In contrast, if one believes that the etiology is metabolic, genetic, biological, and so forth, then one is more likely to have little faith in the therapeutic efficacy of environmental changes and more conviction that some drug (presently or in the future) will straighten out the molecule. This may very well be the case. This does not, however, negate the aforementioned arguments. Knowledge is power, and the more we know about the etiology of a disorder, the better we will be able to prevent and treat it. In addition, most of those who use medication in psychiatry will agree that they do not provide complete cures, that whatever straightening of the molecules such drugs can achieve, they still remain somewhat twisted. Accordingly, at this present state of our knowledge (or, more accurately, ignorance), we do well to utilize all therapeutic modalities, both biological and environmental.

A common way of dividing depressive symptomatology is into the *endogenous* and *exogenous*. Endogenous depression refers to depressive symptomatology that arises from within. Generally, genetic predispositions are considered to be present, but internal psychological factors are also operative. Exogenous depressions are generally considered to be the result of external stresses. Psychiatrists tend to be divided with regard to the relative importance of these two factors. In the 1940s and 1950s, primarily under the influence of psychoanalysis, depression was generally viewed as arising from internal psychological conflicts. The genetic predisposition was considered to be minimal, if not entirely absent. External factors were also considered to be important. In recent years, with the increasing popularity of the purely biological explanation, many psychiatrists view depression as resulting from genetic, metabolic, and biochemical abnormalities and do not pay much attention to the internal psychological factors and/or the external stresses. I consider the present shift toward the biological explanation to be unfortunate. I believe that there may be some genetic predisposition to depression, but it is small. I believe that the primary causes of depression in most (but not necessarily all) people relate to external stresses and internal psychological factors. The discussion here is based on this assumption.

I recognize that on this subject I am in the minority among my colleagues in the field of psychiatry. I have given serious consideration to new developments in the field that rely heavily on the theory of primary biological etiology, but I still hold that the weight of the evidence supports the position that adolescent depressions of the kind discussed in this chapter are best understood as manifestations of internal psychological and environmental processes. I am not referring to manic-depressive psychosis, in which the evidence for a biological genetic predisposition is strong. I am referring to the much more common types of depression seen in adolescence.

ENVIRONMENTAL FACTORS CONDUCIVE TO THE DEVELOPMENT OF DEPRESSION

With regard to the exogenous factors, it behooves the examiner to look carefully into the family and other environmental factors that may be contributing to the youngster's depression. I have described in detail (1992a) an evaluation that can serve this purpose well. Not to conduct such an exhaustive evaluation is likely to compromise the treatment because the examiner will be deprived of learning about the environmental factors that are likely to have contributed to the depression. And this is one of my strongest criticisms of biologically oriented psychiatrists. They generally do not delve deeply enough into the details of their patients' backgrounds. Committed to the notion that depression is primarily, if not entirely, biologically derived, they can justify their failure to conduct such an investigation. Subscribing to the biological theory also enables them to provide what appears to be a relatively quick and easily administered form of treatment, namely, medication. As I discuss later, antidepressants may be of symptomatic value in the treatment of the vast majority of depressions. But this is not inconsistent with my belief that environmental and psychological factors are the paramount etiological factors. Palliation is not the same as cure.

Accordingly, the examiner must try to ascertain what environmental factors have contributed to the depression. The evaluator does well to appreciate that depression is likely to emerge in many different types of dysfunctional families. Perhaps the youngster has been exposed to ongoing marital conflicts, especially those that culminate in separation and/or divorce. Exposure to and/or embroilment in custody litigation is an even greater environmental trauma because the youngster cannot but feel like a rope in a tug of war. The loyalty conflicts engendered by such litigation are enormous, and the likelihood that the youngster will become depressed when so embroiled is extremely high. In many such situations, meaningful therapy is impossible, so enormous are the environmental factors that are contributing to the depression. In these cases, I often refuse to treat, and offer to help resolve the custody dispute (either as a mediator or through court channels). It is only after the custody dispute has been resolved that I am in a position to decide whether therapy is still warranted. I have discussed in detail (1986) the ways in which custody litigation can contribute to a wide variety of psychopathological reactions including depression and suicide. Following divorce and remarriage, the stresses of adjusting to a new stepfamily, especially if there are numerous stepsiblings with whom the youngster has difficult relationships, may also contribute to depression. Perhaps the youngster suffers with a learning disability and thereby experiences inordinate academic stresses that can lead to depression (Gardner 1987). Some youngsters are likely to become depressed in their dealings with members of the opposite sex. The dating period can be extremely anxiety provoking, its gratifications notwithstanding. Rejections in this realm are a common source of depression (and even suicide) among adolescents. For older adolescents, unemployment may be a contributing factor.

Many youngsters become depressed over the socioeconomic conditions in which they have grown up. Patients used as subjects in studies of depression in childhood and adolescence often come from inner-city ghettos. It is easy to find depressed children in this environment. Many adolescents growing up in such areas use drugs as their antidepressant. Most of the studies on the effects of antidepressant medications on children use patients from these deprived areas. It is rare for such studies to derive their patients from affluent suburbs.

The youngster who does poorly in sports (possibly related to genetic and/or biological weaknesses) may become depressed in an environment that is highly sports-oriented. A youngster of average intelligence who grows up in a home with a sibling who is an academic "superstar" may also become depressed. The youngster who cannot live up to his or her parents' inordinately high academic standards is also likely to become depressed. My primary point is that the examiner should investigate every possible environmental factor that may produce depression and do whatever can be done to alter these factors. And such changes are most predictably accomplished when the therapist works with both the youngster and the parents.

INTERNAL PSYCHOLOGICAL FACTORS CONDUCIVE TO THE DEVELOPMENT OF DEPRESSION

Anger Inhibition

In addition to the exogenous factors, complex internal psychological mechanisms are also often operative in bringing about depression. One factor that may contribute to depression is inhibition in the expression of anger. The person's anger becomes turned inward and directed toward him- or herself. The inhibition of such rage is likely to produce depressed feelings. An ongoing state of frustration and its associated inner churnings of suppressed anger fuel the depressive affect. The failure to assert oneself and express pent-up hostility feeds into and intensifies depressed feelings. Furthermore, individuals who are inhibited in the expression of anger may develop self-flagellatory symptomatology. They constantly castigate themselves with comments such as "I'm stupid to have done that," "What a wretch I am," and "What a fool I've been." The person may justify such self-recrimination by dwelling on past indiscretions that may have long since been forgotten by others. These are trivial and do not warrant the degree of self-denigration that the individual exhibits. Errors and minor indiscretions become exaggerated into heinous crimes. When self-flagellatory symptoms are present, one can generally assume that such patients are fearful of and/or guilty over directly expressing anger to others, upon whom they may be quite dependent. They therefore direct their anger toward themselves, a safer target.

When working therapeutically with such patients, it is important to help them become less inhibited in the expression of their anger. They must be helped to assert themselves and direct their anger toward the source of provocation before it builds up internally and turns into suppressed rage and fury. The therapist must be ever alert to situations in which the patient suppressed self-assertion and resentment rather than deal more effectively and overtly with irritants. And the therapist must serve as a model for such self-assertion when the situation warrants it. Such patients may have grown up in families where the parents were similarly inhibited. The parents may have boasted that they have been married many years and never had a fight. In such a marriage, it is likely that one or both of the parents have anger inhibition problems. Many such inhibited youngsters may have been exposed to harsh disciplinary and punitive measures in the context of which they may have been told, "Nice boys and girls never say such things to their parents. They never even *think* such things."

Guilt

A further contributing factor to depression is guilt. By guilt I refer to the feeling of low self-worth experienced following thoughts, feelings, and acts that the individual has learned are unacceptable to significant figures in his or her environment. In essence, the guilty person is saying: "How terrible a person I am for what I have thought, felt, or done." Feelings of low self-worth attendant to guilt are likely to contribute to depressive affect and symptomatology. Guilt fuels the dysphoric mood and can deepen a depression. In addition, the self-flagellatory factors often operative in guilt often complement those produced by rage turned inward. Accordingly, the examiner does well to investigate factors that may be guilt evoking. As mentioned, many children are often taught to feel guilty about the expression of hostility toward a parent: "How can you do this to your mother?" and "What a terrible thing to say to your father." The examiner does well to look into things that the youngster might be doing that may engender guilty feelings. If the youngster has a healthy conscience, then performing acts such as cheating, lying, and stealing may be associated with guilt. In such cases, the guilt is appropriate, but it may still contribute to depression. In such circumstances, the therapist does well to make comments along these lines: "As long as you keep doing those things that you and I know are wrong, you are going to feel guilty and you will behave in a way that will contribute to the perpetuation of your depression."

Hendin (1991) points out that in Vietnam veterans, the guilt over the killing of civilians, as well as the guilt about surviving when close friends had not, often contributed to depression. The former cause of guilt may very well be appropriate, but the latter is generally viewed as inappropriate, even though it is extremely common. But both forms contribute to depression. However, there are youngsters who suffer with inappropriate or exaggerated guilt, such as guilt over sexual feelings, masturbation, or sexual activities at an age-appropriate level. Such an individual may be preoccupied with feelings of sinfulness. It is difficult to speak about sin without speaking about religion, and it is in this realm that the therapist may find himself dealing with a touchy subject. This problem notwithstanding, the therapist does well to try to reduce the feelings of sinfulness. Such patients should be helped to appreciate that most other people of the same religious persuasion do not take the rules so literally and are not overwhelmed with guilt over occasional transgressions. Parental input and that of a clergyman can sometimes be useful for such patients.

When working with patients who have excessive guilt, it is important for the examiner to appreciate that most patients have too little guilt, rather than too much guilt.

We are living very much in a psychopathic society. There are some therapists who work on the principle that the therapist should always try to reduce guilt and that increasing guilt cannot but be antitherapeutic. This is absurd. Most people need *more* guilt than *less* guilt. Accordingly, there are many situations in which the therapist must do everything possible to *increase* guilt in order to help turn the youngster from a psychopathic personality into a civilized human being, sensitive to the feelings of others.

But this is an aside. My main point is that youngsters with an inordinate degree of guilt are prone to become depressed, and anything that the examiner can do to reduce guilt will thereby contribute to the alleviation of depression.

Failure to Achieve Certain Aspirations

People who are prone to become depressed are often those with three sets of aspirations that must be maintained if they are to feel worthy. When these goals are not maintained, they tend to react with depressed feelings. The three goals are (1) the wish to be loved and respected; (2) the wish to be strong, superior, and secure; and (3) the wish to be good and loving rather than hateful and destructive. Some youngsters who are depressed have inordinate needs to be loved and respected. In response to some privations in this area, they may have exaggerated needs for compensatory respect and affection. These inordinate needs and demands may result in chronic feelings of dissatisfaction. It is the job of the therapist to help such youngsters develop more realistic goals with regard to the degree of love and respect they can reasonably hope to obtain from other human beings. Unfortunately, if they are swept up in the romantic love myth—which often promises enormous love and infinite respect—then their frustrations and disillusionment in this area are likely to be formidable. I have discussed in detail (1988, 1991, 1992b) what I consider to be the psychodynamic factors operative in romantic love. An understanding of these factors places the therapist in a better position to help adolescents understand this phenomenon and deal more realistically with its pathological elements.

With regard to the second set of aspirations—to be strong, superior, and secure—boys especially may experience frustration. In the macho world in which they grow up, any signs of weakness or even normal degrees of insecurity may not be tolerable. Inordinate aspirations in this realm are likely to result in the kinds of frustrations and disappointments that contribute to depression. The therapist must help such youngsters gain a more realistic view of what their potentials are and recognize that many who are seemingly stable in this respect are often presenting a facade. Such a youngster has to be helped to appreciate that even those who have exhibited genuine accomplishments still have feelings of insecurity.

With regard to the third realm—the wish to be good and loving rather than hateful and destructive—such youngsters may have the idea that there are all-loving people who do not harbor any hateful feelings at all toward anyone. They have to be helped to appreciate that all human relationships are ambivalent and that even the most loving person harbors deep-seated, hostile, and even hateful feelings. If the therapist is successful in convincing the youngster of the validity of this view, then aspirations may be lowered and this contributing element in depression reduced.

Dependency Problems

Individuals who easily become depressed are often quite dependent. Not being able to function adequately at age-appropriate levels, they easily slide back into more infantile levels where they gratify their dependent needs. Of course, such individuals require the presence of caretakers who will indulge their dependency demands. Such youngsters are likely to regress to infantile states of helplessness in stressful situations when they do not feel they have the capacity to cope. At such times, depressed patients become clinging and demand support and protection from those around them. It behooves the therapist to help such youngsters deal more adequately with the stresses of life, to learn more about how to cope with reality, and thereby to deal better with stresses. Also, they have to work with the caretaking individuals who might be indulging the dependency gratifications and thereby perpetuating the depression. Sometimes, this is more easily said than done, in that the caretakers may rationalize their indulgence to significant degrees. They may view the examiner who requests that they pull back and not provide such indulgences as being cruel and insensitive.

Reactions to Loss

Individuals who are depression prone are more likely to react in an exaggerated fashion to significant loss than those who do not become depressed. Sometimes the loss is realistic, such as the loss of a parent, sibling, or loved one. Sometimes the loss is symbolic, in that the individual considers the loss to be greater than it really is. A good example of this would be the loss of a boyfriend or girlfriend—someone who, in reality, could be replaced much more easily than the youngster can possibly imagine. Youngsters who are in the latter category should be helped to appreciate that an important factor in the romantic love phenomenon is the projection onto the loved person of one's own aspirations about what an individual should be. Often, it is useful to provide such youngsters with the traditional advice provided by parents after rejection by a boyfriend or girlfriend: "There's other fish in the sea," "I'm sure in a few days you'll be feeling much better," and "Why don't you try doing some fun things to take your mind off her (or him)." In situations in which the loss is more permanent, such as death and divorce, the youngster has to be helped to cope more adequately with these losses (Gardner 1983).

Teicher (1979) considers that an important loss that may contribute to the depression of an adolescent is the loss of the prepubertal family, which cannot be idealized during the adolescent period if the youngster is to move on along the track to adult independence. In retrospect, that family may be romanticized, and its loss in adolescence may contribute to depression. Most healthy adolescents transfer their loving and dependent feelings from their family onto peers of both sexes and form strong ties with peer substitutes. If such peer-substitute relationships have not developed, then the loss becomes more acute. This is one of the factors operative in teen suicides after the breakup of a romantic relationship. Accordingly, therapists do well to investigate in detail the particular losses that were operative in the patient's depression and to do everything possible to rectify these.

Because reaction to loss is such an important factor in depression and suicide, it is crucial that the therapist not be involved in a situation in which the patient is inappropriately rejected by him or her. There is no question that many depressed patients have killed themselves because of rejection by a therapist, the only person in their lives who they felt had any concern for them. I am not recommending that therapists treat depressed patients in any special way, especially in the direction of overindulgence. I am only emphasizing the importance of the therapist's being a caring human being who treats the patients with dignity and sympathy.

Depression and the Fight/Flight Reaction

The fight/flight reactions are of survival value. When confronted with a danger, organisms at all levels either fight or flee. This is an essential mechanism for survival. Some individuals are more likely to fight when confronted with a danger, and others are more likely to flee. It is probable that both genetic and environmental factors contribute to the pattern that will be selected. The healthy individual is capable of making a judicious decision regarding which mechanism to bring into operation when confronted with a threat. I view many depression-prone individuals as people who are fearful of invoking either of these survival mechanisms; that is, they are too frightened to fight because they do not view themselves as having effective weapons, and they fear flight because they do not consider themselves capable of surviving independently. They need protectors at their side — not only to protect them from the threats of others but to provide for them because they do not feel themselves capable of providing for themselves. They become immobile and paralyzed in a neutral position. They neither fight nor flee. In their immobility, they protect themselves from the untoward consequences they anticipate if they were to surge forward and fight the threat. In addition, their immobilization and failure to flee ensure their being protected and taken care of by their protectors.

The "success" of the depressive maneuver requires the attendance of caretaking individuals who will provide the indulgence and protection the depressive person requests, demands, or elicits. Without such individuals, the reaction may not be utilized. Well-meaning figures in the depressed person's environment are often drawn into the game, not realizing that their indulgence is a disservice. They may consider themselves loving, sacrificial, giving, and devoted. Although some of those qualities are without doubt present, the caretakers often fail to appreciate that the same maneuvers are perpetuating the depressive symptomatology. Therapists who work with depressed adolescents do well to consider this important possible contribution to the youngster's depression. These young people have to be helped to assert themselves and fight more ardently when the situation warrants it and to develop greater independence so they will not become immobilized and have to rely on caretakers when exposed to external stresses and threats. And the caretaking individuals have to be helped similarly to reduce their indulgence.

Nuclear War

We frequently read in newspaper and magazine articles the theory that growing up in a nuclear age can cause young people to become unmotivated and depressed. The prospect of being annihilated in nuclear warfare is said to contribute to poor motivation, boredom, and the lack of commitment to life. And this theory has been invoked to explain teen suicide as well. Although there are certainly youngsters who concern themselves with the prospect of a nuclear holocaust, I have not seen such concern contribute to the formation of clinical symptoms—depression, suicide attempts, or any other symptoms. Most (but certainly not all) of the youngsters I have seen in my office are not concerned significantly with issues such as politics, wars, and the possibility of a nuclear holocaust. They are much more concerned with their schools, friends, and family. When symptoms develop, they are usually derived from problems in these three areas. When one considers the adolescent's delusions of invulnerability, concerns with nuclear wars become even more remote. In fact, I would go further and say that most adolescents would believe that if there were a nuclear war, they would be among the survivors. And this is true not only regarding exposure to the initial blast but on the remote level of suffering future consequences of radioactive fallout, burns, and so forth.

Further Comments Regarding Psychotherapy with Depressed Adolescents

Clearly, it is crucial for the therapist to understand as fully as possible which of the multiplicity of psychodynamic factors are operative in his or her patient. Without such a basic foundation of information, therapy is compromised significantly. Dream analysis may be particularly useful in this regard. Hendin (1991) considers dream analysis to be particularly useful for determining the degree of suicidal risk, in that the suicide scenario commonly reproduces scenarios found in dreams that preceded the suicide. The dream may involve the individual being buried, depicted as already being in the coffin, or in the throes of death. Sometimes the dream depicts the individual as already dead. I will comment more about such fantasies in my discussion of suicide. Furthermore, an analysis of waking fantasies, especially those that are repetitious, and the focus of obsessive preoccupation can also provide information about the psychodynamics of the individual's depression.

In addition, one does well to consider the communicative element in depression and, especially, suicide. Depressed people are making a statement to those around them about their professions of uselessness and the desire to remove themselves from others notwithstanding. An interpersonal process is still going on, such as the desire for reunion with a dead person, a desire to wreak vengeance on those who have treated one badly, and the desire to be reborn again into a world in which there are happier relationships.

The therapist must be alerted to countertransferential reactions that may contribute to anger at the patient, especially anger over the patient's inordinate demands. These reactions may be a derivative of the dependency problem of the patient and/or the need to gain control over caretaking individuals. Threats of suicide may also be a cause of frustration and anger in the therapist and produce desires to get rid of the patient. If these threats are handled properly, in the psychotherapeutic process as well as in the hospital (if hospitalization becomes necessary; see later discussion), then the therapist is less likely to react with feelings of anger. Hendin (1991) describes in detail some of the subtleties and complexities of the therapist–patient relationship of depressed patients, especially with regard to the suicidal element. He gives particular emphasis to the threat of suicide as a very powerful weapon against the therapist, especially a therapist who is narcissistic.

Therapists who strictly adhere to the confidentiality principle in that they do not divulge suicidal risks have contributed to the deaths of their patients. Although adolescents certainly need their autonomy and a relationship with someone who is not a member of the immediate family, and a confidential relationship with a therapist can certainly contribute to the attainment of these goals, the therapist should consider that strict adherence to the confidentiality principle may give the patient the opportunity he or she needs to commit suicide.

SUICIDE

Suicide is the second leading cause of death in the United States for individuals between the ages of 15 and 24. (Motor vehicle accidents are the most common cause of death of children in their teens.) When there is an adolescent death in association with a motor vehicle accident — and the teen driver was the only person in the car — one should think of the possibility of suicide. Garfinkel (1989) states that 10 percent of *single* motor vehicle accidents involving one person are suicides. Accordingly, there is some overlap of the figures. And the suicide rate in this age bracket has been increasing. In 1950, the rate was 4.5 per 100, 000. This progressively increased to the point where in 1980 it was 12.3 per 100, 000. During the 1980s, the rate leveled off, but it is still at approximately 12 per 100,000 (Simmons 1987a, World Almanac 1991).

Firearms are the main vehicle for adolescent suicide. According to Garfinkel (1989), firearms account for approximately 40–55 percent of completed suicide during the adolescent period. Rosenberg and colleagues (1991) state that "the odds that potentially suicidal adolescents will kill themselves go up 75-fold when a gun is kept in the home" (p. 3030). The Centers for Disease Control (1988) report that in the year 1988, 1, 372 adolescents between ages 13 and 19 intentionally killed themselves with firearms.

Hanging is the second most common method. Garfinkel (personal communication, 1992) did a careful study of hanging suicides among adolescents and concluded that one-third of such deaths may not have been bona fide suicides but in fact were the result of sexual asphyxiation. Specifically, these youngsters appeared to be masturbating with the belief that reduction of blood flow to the brain would enhance the intensity of their orgasms. They masturbated hanging from a noose under the delusion that they would "beat the odds" and achieve this allegedly more intense orgasm and still defy death. Obviously, some of these youngsters did not "beat the odds." This situation is an excellent example of the adolescent's "delusions of invulnerability" (Gardner 1988).

According to Garfinkel (1989), drugs are the third most common cause of adolescent suicide, accounting for approximately one-third of such suicides. Again, it is difficult to differentiate between inadvertent overdoses and overdoses related to conscious attempts to commit suicide.

Obviously, some depressed patients become suicidal. It is important for examiners to appreciate that just about all human beings have suicidal thoughts at times. Life predictably produces frustrations, disappointments, and feelings of impotence. Everyone, at times, gets depressed. Many people will have the feeling that their lives are not worth it. Although it is impossible to obtain normative data regarding the frequency of such thoughts, it is reasonable to speculate that there is a gradation from the normal level of such thoughts to the pathological frequency. If the examiner worked under the assumption that normal healthy people *never* have such thoughts, then a much higher percentage of patients would be considered suicidal. One wants to learn about the frequency of such thoughts and, of course, the content. Content, especially, will be useful in helping the examiner differentiate between bona fide and fabricated suicide attempts and preoccupations.

I wish to emphasize at this point the importance of the examiner's not conducting a suicide evaluation under conditions of time constraints. That the evaluation may be considered urgent does not mean that the patient need be rushed through it. It is extremely unlikely that the patient is going to try to commit suicide in the therapist's presence. Accordingly, a few hours devoted to the evaluation is reasonable to expect of both the therapist, the patient, and the family. Physicians working in emergency rooms may be compromised in their ability to do a proper suicide evaluation, as is a therapist working in a clinic setting where the examiner is required to devote only a specific amount of time to each patient. Evaluators working for HMOs that are concerned with the cost effectiveness of the services provided may also be compromised in their ability to conduct an adequate evaluation for suicide. People do not tell surgeons that they must operate within a particular time frame. All appreciate the fact that the surgeon may not know exactly what to do until the patient is opened. The same principle holds for the psychiatric evaluation and is especially valid when one is considering the possibility of suicide. Evaluators do well, therefore, to refuse to conduct such examinations unless they are given the freedom to spend as much time as they consider warranted.

Therapists who work with adolescents may be asked to make a decision regarding whether or not a youngster who threatens suicide should be hospitalized. This is an extremely important question, and the ability of the therapist to differentiate between bona fide and fabricated suicidal threats may determine whether a youngster lives or dies. Accordingly, in the sections that follow, I present what I consider to be important differentiating criteria between the two groups. I believe that these criteria will most often enable the therapist to make a decision regarding which category the patient is in; however, there may be occasions when the examiner is not certain. Under these circumstances, it is best to err on the side of caution and to hospitalize the patient.

Bona Fide Suicide Attempts

The Presence of Deep Depression

First, I will describe those manifestations that generally indicate serious depression. When these factors are present, they significantly increase the likelihood that the suicidal threat is genuine. One wants to ascertain whether the threat is made by a youngster who is exhibiting a broader picture of moderately severe to severe depression. One wants to get a good idea about the depth of the depressive affect (dysphoric mood). Because this is a subjective state, the evaluator does well to make a detailed inquiry regarding exactly what feelings patients have when they say they are depressed. Like all things in life, there is a continuum. Suicidal risk is enhanced when the depressive feelings are deepseated. In such situations, the patient feels that a dark, black cloud has descended upon his or her brain, a specter that not only robs the individual of any capacity for pleasure but also produces a chronic state of psychological pain. The patient feels like he or she is moving through life like a zombie, with absolutely no desire to do anything. The term *anergia* is often used to describe this state of extremely impaired motivation and the feeling that one cannot do anything. Another term used for this phenomenon is *psychomotor retardation*. A related phenomenon is *anhedonia*, the inability to experience any pleasure, from any source whatsoever, including sexual. Even praises and rewards seem to have absolutely no effect on the youngster's mood. Persistent boredom may also be part of this constellation. Many adolescents who want to kill themselves claim that they really do not wish to die, but that they want to end the psychological pain associated with depressive affect.

Other common manifestations of severe depression are severe self-flagellatory and self-deprecatory statements ("I'm no good," "I'm useless," "I deserve to die," "I'm loathsome, wretched, etc."). Related to these feelings of self-denigration is the patient's inability to say anything positive about him- or herself. As mentioned, inhibition in the expression of anger may contribute to such self-flagellatory statements. The evaluator should ask at least two or three times, at various parts of the interview, whether the patient can think about anything positive to say about him- or herself. Statements of hopelessness about the future are common. Beck and colleagues (1985) found high ratings on a measure of hopelessness to be highly correlated with suicidal behavior. Profound feelings of helplessness, desperation, and despair are also strong indicators of bona fide suicidal intent. Another manifestation of severe depression is withdrawal from socialization and loss of interest in friends. If the withdrawal has exceeded 6 months, the danger of suicide is significantly enhanced.

Motivation for school and work may become seriously impaired, and the resultant deterioration of performance causes even further depression. There may be a change in eating habits, especially loss of appetite but, on occasion, compulsive eating. Sleep patterns also change, sometimes in the direction of insomnia and other times in the direction of excessive sleeping. Psychosomatic symptoms may also be present, for example, stomachache, headache, and, especially, fatigue. The youngster may exhibit a neglect in personal appearance with little concern for bathing, brushing teeth, and grooming.

Patients who spontaneously and frequently speak about their belief that no one will miss them if they die may be a serious suicidal risk. The youngster may make such statements as "I won't be a problem for you any longer," "Nothing matters," and "It's no use." If the youngster shows evidence of having attempted to get his or her "affairs in order," given away favorite possessions, and speaks about how things will be in the home after he or she is gone, then a serious sign of true suicidal intent is manifesting itself. This is an extremely important area to investigate. The realities may be that many close friends and relatives would suffer great grief if the youngster were to commit suicide. If, however, the patient *believes* that none of these individuals cares, then the suicidal risk is enhanced formidably.

The Presence of Psychotic Symptoms

The presence of psychotic symptoms, such as hallucinations and delusions, increases the suicidal risk. An extremely dangerous form of hallucination is one in which voices are telling the patient to kill him- or herself, especially if the youngster believes that the voices are gods or God's delegates. Particularly dangerous are delusions in which the patient views the suicide as a method for joining dead relatives in the afterlife. Of course, if the therapist believes that one does indeed have the opportunity to join dead relatives in the afterlife, then this might not be considered a delusion. It is hoped, however, that the therapist will be of the persuasion that at the age of 16 it is somewhat early for such reconciliation, and that it would be better to allow natural forces to determine when this great day of rapprochement takes place. Patients with such a delusion may also hear voices that encourage or order suicide to hasten the journey into the afterlife. Or the psychotic youngster may respond to delusions of persecution from which the only escape is to commit suicide. Other psychotic youngsters may kill themselves because they have reached the end of their tolerance for suffering the grief associated with their psychoses. Feelings of disintegration, the tensions associated with delusions and hallucinations, the rejections resulting from their inability to relate meaningfully with others, and even rejections by close family members bring them to the point of no longer wishing to live. Furthermore, high levels of chronic tension, unassociated with psychosis, may also predispose youngsters to suicide. Hendin (1991) points out that this factor is receiving increasing attention in recent studies.

The Presence of Formidable Rage

Hendin (1991), in an excellent article on psychodynamic factors operative in suicide, considers youngsters with enormous rage to be of high suicidal risk. Such individuals are filled with overwhelming anger that may even be acted out homicidally. The suicide may be a form of control exercised by people who are torn apart by their rage and violence. The combination of homicide and suicide is well known. People who have killed others have a suicide rate hundreds of times greater than those who have not killed (Hendin 1986, Wolfgang 1958). Here we see a combination of rage directed outward and rage directed inward, of destruction of others and destruction of self. In short, the presence of violence and a state of ongoing rage is an indicator of high suicidal risk. Not surprisingly, the most common source of such rage is dysfunctional family life. Shafii and colleagues (1985) found that there was significantly more parental abuse and rejection by the families of suicidal youngsters than by a control group. Often the parents communicate to the child that they don't want him or her to be part of the family (Sabbath 1969). Whether the parents began to feel this way before the child's behavior evoked rejection, or whether the child's behavior per se evoked the rejection, the net result is that the child does not feel wanted in the family, and the suicide may very well reflect compliance with the parental requests. Some children leave the home under these circumstances. Others kill themselves.

The Role of Academic Difficulties

There is an increased suicidal risk for patients with a learning disability, because such youngsters typically exhibit very poor judgment. Even if the threat is a manipulative gesture the youngster's poor judgment may result in the gesture's becoming an actuality. Learning-disabled children suffer enormously from their deficits. School exposes them to a situation in which they are constantly humiliated by their learning impairments, and they may be scapegoated mercilessly by their normal classmates with such epithets as "Ment" and "Retard." Even though somewhat protected in special classes, they are still known by the general student population as being "E-D kids." They cannot compete in sports because of neurological weaknesses, and they do not have the social skills to maintain meaningful relationships with peers. Even their parents are chronically disappointed with them. Their siblings consider them a source of humiliation and often will not invite friends to the home because of the embarrassment they suffer over the atypical behavior of the learning-disabled sibling. Accordingly, the presence of a moderate or severe learning disability increases the suicidal risk.

Youngsters with extremely high academic standards derived from parental perfectionism may become suicidal when they do not live up to their and their parents' aspirations. Disappointingly low scores on important examinations (such as the SATs) or failure to gain admission to their first-choice college may result in suicidal attempts by such youngsters. Generally, the inordinately high standards are not simply self-imposed; most often inordinate pressures are being placed upon the youngster by parents who are obsessed with high grades and prestigious academic institutions. Impaired functioning in school over a long period, as well as impairments in socialization, increases the suicidal risk. The manipulators are more likely to be functioning adequately in these areas.

The Presence of a Dysfunctional Family

It is important for the therapist to get a good idea about the degree of stability versus instability that exists (and existed) in the adolescent's home. This cannot be done adequately without interviewing the parents, individually and jointly. Furthermore, family interviews can also be helpful in this regard. The more unhealthy and/or chaotic the youngster's home life, the greater the likelihood that the suicidal gesture is genuine. Children who have been exposed to ongoing physical, psychological, and sexual abuse are much more likely to kill themselves than those who come from homes that are reasonably stable (Shafii et al. 1985). Children from unstable homes are more likely to be runaways, and suicide is more likely to occur among runaways. Obviously, a suicide attempt made by a runaway, when away from home, is not as likely to be detected by potential rescuers and interveners. Even though the youngster may be living at home at the time of the attempt, a history of running away increases the suicidal risk. And if the parents supported the youngster's leaving the home, then the suicidal risk is also enhanced because of the parental rejection signified by such support. These are the youngsters who claim that no one will care if they evaporate from the face of the earth, and they may be right.

The Setting and the Nature of the Suicide Attempt

When attempting to differentiate between true and false suicide attempts, it is important to get details about the setting in which the suicidal gesture took place and the exact nature of the gesture. Youngsters who make suicidal gestures when alone are more likely to commit suicide than those who do so in situations when a parent, sibling, or friend is either in the next room or expected quite soon. In the latter situation, people are being set up to discover the gesture before anything serious occurs. The seriousness of the gesture can also provide useful information about the youngster's true intent. If the youngster takes only a few pills from a large number in a single bottle, then it is most unlikely that the suicidal gesture was genuine. Taking pills, even in large quantities, generally speaks for a lower level of seriousness because of the youngster's recognition of the possibility that he or she may be saved. Wrist slashing, especially when superficial, is rarely a manifestation of a bona fide suicide attempt. If the attempt involved the use of a gun, obviously the risk of bona fide suicide is enhanced significantly. As mentioned, shooting oneself with a weapon is the most common method of committing suicide among teenagers (Gardner 1988, Simmons 1987b). But even if the youngster has not threatened to use a gun, if a gun is in the home it should be removed immediately, as should any pills that might be used for suicidal purposes. And the kind of firearm doesn't matter—whether it be a handgun, a rifle, or a shotgun. All varieties of firearms have the same risk (Brent et al. 1991). Hanging, the second most common suicide method used by adolescents, should be taken very seriously, even hanging in the aforementioned sexual asphyxia category. As mentioned, although miscalculation may be the primary factor here, it is still extremely risky. Neck slashing is also a very serious sign, and it is not only indicative of a bona fide attempt but also strongly suggestive of the presence of psychosis. However, psychotics represent only a very small fraction of all those adolescents who successfully kill themselves. Similarly, jumping out of a window, jumping off a roof, or leaping from a high place is obviously genuine, and even those who put themselves in a position where they are ready to do so are likely to be serious. However, merely threatening hysterically to take such an action — without any evidence that the youngster is inclined to do so — generally speaks for manipulation.

The Role of Substance Abuse

It is also important to investigate into the history of substance abuse. The abuse of alcohol adds to the suicidal risk. Under its influence, the youngster is more likely to exhibit poor judgment and diminished self-control, factors that may turn a fabricated, manipulative suicidal gesture into an actual suicide. Beck and Steer (1989) found that alcoholics have a five times higher than average chance of completing suicide. A similar situation holds for those who abuse drugs. (Again, I am not referring to death by overdose but to the effect of drugs on judgment and cognition.) Schaffer and colleagues (1988) describe drug and alcohol abuse as strongly associated with suicide by firearms. Accordingly, the authors warn strongly that guns should be barred from households that include a drug abuser or an alcoholic. Although each one of these factors alone is dangerous, the two combined are extremely explosive.

The Presence of Criminal Behavior and Impulsivity

Youngsters involved in criminal behavior are at high risk for suicide. They may be living in dread of being prosecuted and even jailed for their criminal actions. Or they may live in dread of retaliation for the failure to fulfill obligations with their criminal cohorts. I once saw in counseling the parents of a youngster who had committed suicide. The boy, himself, had never been a patient of mine in that he refused to join in with the parents in any aspect of treatment. He had involved himself in both drugs and gambling and had accumulated significant debts. His criminal creditors were constantly harassing him. In order to mollify them, he would borrow more money and gamble more. Thus, he sank even deeper into debt. Finally, he killed himself. It was clear that an important contributing factor to his suicide was the desire to bring about a cessation of his torment. Youngsters who have had difficulties with the law are often impulsive. They think primarily of the moment and do not consider enough the future consequences of their behavior. The same impulsivity that may result in their involving themselves in criminal acts may result in their making suicide attempts. Elderly people, being generally less impulsive, are more likely to plan their suicides — often far in advance. In contrast, youngsters, who are more likely to be impulsive, are more likely to kill themselves impulsively. It is for this reason that a gun in the home of an impulsive adolescent is often a lethal combination. Accordingly, the examiner does well to investigate this area, with regard to not only criminal behavior but impulsivity in other areas as well.

Past History of Suicide Attempts

One should also investigate the past history of suicide attempts. One should get details about the situations in which they occurred and the exact nature of the gestures. The greater the number of such gestures, and the more serious each of them was, the greater the likelihood that the suicidal threat under consideration is serious. Beck and Steer (1989) found that 36 percent of successful suicides in the 413 men and women they studied had made previous suicide attempts. A past history of self-destructive behavior and accident proneness also increases the suicidal risk. Accordingly, the therapist should look for the presence of masochistic tendencies and/or excessive guilt, guilt which the individual might wish to assuage by self-destructive acts — the extreme form of which is suicide.

Family History of Suicide

It is also important to investigate into the family history of suicide. If the youngster's mother or father has indeed committed suicide, then the risk that the youngster will do so as well is significantly increased. This not only relates to the modeling element but also to the privation that the youngster must have suffered following the death of the parent. Garfinkel (1989) describes one family in Vermont in which there were twenty-one successful suicides over three generations. This, too, is an extremely important differentiating criterion between the bona fide and the fabricated suicide attempt.

The Role of Past and Present Losses

Often, the suicidal gesture occurs following a loss or a rejection. Accordingly, one should find out about previous reactions to loss or rejection, whether they were tolerated well or whether the youngster reacted severely to them. The more pathological and/or exaggerated the past reactions to loss or rejection, the greater the suicidal risk with regard to the present episode. For example, a youngster might make a suicidal gesture following rejection by a girl friend. If there has been a long-standing history of depression and exaggerated reactions to such rejections, then the likelihood that this rejection will be accompanied by a bona fide suicidal gesture is increased.

Suicide Contagion and the Youngster's Concept of the Afterlife

Another factor that must be considered is that of the suicide of other adolescents in the community. If the youngster's suicide attempt was made at a time when other adolescents had committed suicide, especially others in the same area, the likelihood is increased that the youngster's attempt was genuine. This is sometimes referred to as *cohort effect, copycat suicide,* or *suicide contagion.* Suicide attempts, especially adolescent suicide attempts, sometimes become epidemic. Adolescents are always concerned with what their peers are doing and reflexively tend to go along with the "in" patterns of behavior, their professions of independence notwithstanding. One good example of this is the prevalence of anorexia and bulimia among today's youth. Articles on the subject appear consistently in teen magazines. Every classroom and every college dorm have their share of girls who suffer with the disorder. Suicide attempts are no exception to the phenomenon of acquiring the psychiatric disorder that is currently in vogue. Garfinkel (1989) describes an epidemic in Washington, D.C., in which eleven classmates of an adolescent boy committed suicide after he was killed in an automobile accident. In 1988, in Bergenfield, New Jersey, four youngsters committed suicide by carbon monoxide poisoning in a garage. Soon thereafter, a policeman prevented the suicide of two other Bergenfield youngsters who went into the same garage in order to commit suicide.

One factor that has contributed to the spread of the teen suicide phenomenon is the sensationalistic reporting of these deaths in the newspapers. Publicizing suicides not only fuels suicide epidemics but even provides potential suicides with suggested methods for killing themselves (the aforementioned Bergenfield garage suicide being an excellent example). This presents society with a dilemma. On the one hand, we live in a country where we pride ourselves upon our freedom of the press; to suppress, in any way, the freedom of newspapers to report such suicides would be unconstitutional. On the other hand, there is no question that the attention that such suicides provide these youngsters plays a role in encouraging others to perform similar acts. The freedom to describe them in the media, then, contributes to the death of many youngsters every year. One solution to this dilemma is for newspapers to *voluntarily* restrict such reporting to inconspicuous sections of the newspaper rather than to the headlines. In this way, the freedom of the press is in no way compromised, and the sensationalistic contributing factor to adolescent suicide will be obviated.

One could ask the question: "Okay, so the youngster is encouraged to commit suicide by the notoriety that peers have 'enjoyed' by their suicides. But don't these kids realize that suicide is final and that they won't be around to read the newspapers?" It may come as a surprise to the reader, but they may not appreciate that they won't be around. One does best to view adolescents as having the bodies of adults but the brains of children. If one had the opportunity to question adolescents who kill themselves in situations in which suicide is epidemic in their communities, the vast majority would speak of some fantasy relating to their ability to appreciate and even enjoy notoriety after they have died. The fantasy involves people reading about their deaths in the newspapers, crying bitterly at their funerals, and flagellating themselves for the terrible ways in which they treated the youngster. Here we see the vengeance factor operative in a very dramatic way. The fantasy might include the youngster's then getting the love that is not provided in life. The fantasy might involve the youngster's being in heaven and living without the pain and the privations suffered on earth. Or the fantasy might include a degree of attention far beyond what the youngster ever enjoyed in life. And this is especially attractive to withdrawn, alienated youngsters who were ignored and/or rejected to a significant degree. Suddenly, they will be famous. The hitch, of course, is that they will not be there to enjoy their notoriety. But they somehow lose sight of this obvious fact or delude themselves into believing that it will not be that way. Some even have the fantasy that

Hollywood will make a film of their lives and this, of course, will result in their becoming famous. The fantasy that they will be there to enjoy their popularity is an extension of the adolescent's delusions of invulnerability. It is also a manifestation of their cognitive simplicity.

Accordingly, therapists should focus on this particular area when evaluating adolescents with suicide potential. If the youngster does indeed harbor such delusions, then the therapist should do everything to get the youngster to consider other options, options that do not include the existence of some kind of an observing spirit following death. Of course, no examiner can say with 100 percent certainty whether or not such an afterlife exists. The therapist should, however, be reasonable enough on the subject to consider the *possibility* that there is no such existence and to get the youngster to consider that possibility as well. But, as mentioned, even if the therapist and patient both have deep convictions about the existence of an afterlife, it is hoped that the therapist will at least take the position that the decision regarding *when* an individual should enter into that realm should not be left to an adolescent but to whatever higher forces may be involved.

Hendin (1991) provides an excellent description of other suicidal fantasies commonly seen in suicidal patients. Rebirth fantasies are commonly seen. The individual suffers inordinately from what is considered to be a miserable existence, and the hope is that following the suicide, the individual will return to life in a happier situation and in a happier state of mind. Reunion fantasies are also seen, especially after the death of a loved one. The fantasy here is that there will be a reunion with the departed person in the afterlife. Another fantasy is that of retaliatory abandonment. An individual who is rejected deals with the situation by entertaining fantasies of suicide, thereby rejecting the individual who originally rejected the patient. This places control into the hands of the rejected one. Another common fantasy relates to the failure to live up to one's own and/or one's family's standards. Commonly, these are inordinately high in suicidal patients. They find the failure to live up to these unrealistic standards intolerable, and they kill themselves in order to bring about a cessation of the feelings of low self-worth that result from the failure to attain these unreachable goals. Once again, the therapist should help the individual appreciate the illogicality of these standards.

Social and cultural factors

Another factor that should be taken into consideration when assessing the severity of the suicidal risk is the location in which the youngster lives. Most studies indicate that the rate of suicide is greater in rural areas than in the more populated urban areas. Somehow, areas with very low population density produce more suicides than those in more crowded areas. States like Nevada, Alaska, and Wyoming have suicide rates among the highest in the country. Perhaps this relates to the isolation of such regions and the boredom that individuals living there may suffer, the beauty of the area notwithstanding. Perhaps the high rate in these states is related to their high population of Native Americans, a group that has a high suicide rate. As well as social factors, the therapist should consider the cultural factors that may be operative. In the Native American population, there is a high rate of alcoholism, unemployment, inadequate education, and a prevailing sense of hopelessness. All of these factors contribute to the high suicide rate in this group. But this is just one example. The therapist should also consider the patient's socioeconomic and/or ethnic group and investigate the suicide rates of those groups. If the rate is high, then the likelihood of the patient's being suicidal is increased.

The Suicide Note

If the youngster has left a suicide note, it may be an important source of information about whether or not the attempt has been genuine. One should examine it carefully, read every word, and try to determine which criteria are present. I am referring to those criteria that support not only bona fide attempts but fabricated attempts as well. If the note describes in detail the individuals to whom the youngster's possessions should be given, this increases the likelihood that the attempt is genuine. A suicide note in the form of a last will and testament also suggests serious intent. The circumstances around which the note was left and read may also provide useful information. A note mailed just before the attempt — a note that could not possibly reach the parents until *after* the death of the youngster — is more likely to be related to a serious gesture. This is also the case for unmailed notes that are not likely to be found until after death. In contrast, notes that provide advance clues to a forthcoming suicide attempt suggest manipulation because they give the finders a warning as well as time to interrupt the act.

Fabricated Suicide Attempts

In fabricated suicide threats and gestures, there is often an obvious manipulative factor operating. As mentioned, such threats or gestures commonly occur in a situation in which others are present or when there is every good reason to believe that others will arrive on the scene quite soon after the gesture. The motive is to evoke guilt and to manipulate individuals into complying with certain demands. The nature of the gesture is also a telltale sign as to how serious it is. The most common fabricated gestures are wrist slashing and the ingestion of a small fraction of a bottle of pills — often pills that the youngster knows or suspects are nontoxic. In these situations, one investigates into the events that led up to the suicidal gesture. Most often one will learn that the youngster has been thwarted with regard to some demand, and the gesture is an obvious attempt to get the parents to change their minds or to feel guilty over the way they have deprived the patient.

Sometimes these gestures serve to get the parents to bring the child to a therapist. Generally, this occurs in situations in which the parents have refused to recognize that the youngster has problems, and the suicide attempt can thereby be viewed as a ticket of admission into treatment. According to Toolan (1974), manipulative suicidal gestures are much more common in adolescent girls than in boys. However, the sex ratio of successful attempts is the reverse, with boys successfully killing themselves much more frequently than girls. In the literature, the general figures in both of these categories are four to one, that is, four girls make attempts to every one boy who makes an attempt, but four boys are successful to every girl who is successful. Schaffer and colleagues (1988), in their large study of teenage suicide, found even higher figures, namely, that five out of six teenage successful suicides are boys. Accordingly, the examiner should keep these figures in mind when conducting an evaluation. In short, if the patient is a girl, it is more likely that the gesture is fabricated; if the patient is a boy, a risk exists that the attempt is genuine (Wensley 1987).

Finally, there are the default criteria for deciding that the therapist is dealing with a fabricated suicide attempt. Specifically, the fewer bona fide criteria present, the greater the likelihood that the attempt is fabricated, and, conversely, the greater the number of bona fide criteria satisfied, the greater the likelihood that the attempt lies in that category.

HOSPITALIZATION

Introduction

Therapists who carefully consider all of the factors presented above will be in a good position to make a decision regarding whether the suicidal threat is genuine. However, as mentioned, in cases in which the therapist is uncertain, it is best to err on the side of caution and to recommend hospitalization. If the therapist does indeed believe that the suicidal risk is present, then he or she should pursue one of the following courses. If the therapist believes that the risk is present but might be reduced by intensive psychotherapy (e.g., 3 to 5 times a week, with the youngster and family) — and if the family is willing to become involved in such intensive treatment — then the therapist might well embark upon such a program and try to do everything possible to avoid hospitalization. But what about situations in which the family refuses both the intensive treatment program and hospitalization? Such reactions are common because denial is frequently seen in the families of suicidal patients (Garfinkel 1989). In such cases, I generally interrupt the patient's treatment and send a certified letter to the patient's family indicating that I believe that the choice is either intensive outpatient treatment or inpatient therapy. If they refuse intensive outpatient treatment and refuse hospitalization, I then state to the family that I am discharging myself from the case and am no longer assuming any responsibility for what happens thereafter. I am sure to include in the letter the name(s) of the hospital(s) that I recommend they take the patient to and offer to provide recommendations for other therapists if they wish to choose the intensive outpatient treatment option with someone else.

Let us consider the situation in which the therapist believes that the suicidal threat is so strong that immediate hospitalization is warranted, and that the aforementioned intensive psychotherapy would be very risky. And let us also consider the situation in which the patient and family refuse to go along with the recommendation for immediate hospitalization but are very desirous of an intensive treatment program and recognize its cost and investment of time and energy. Under these circumstances, I would, again, write a letter in which I remove myself from the case and explain the reasons why. Again, I would strongly urge them to reconsider their decision. It is important for the reader to appreciate that such letters are written not simply because it is a practice of good psychiatry but also because, considering the risks of malpractice suits at this time, they are judicious.

Let us now consider the situation in which the family refuses hospitalization but offers the alternative of 24-hour vigils by the parents and other family members. Therapists who agree to this program should hand in their certificates. There is no justification for going along with such a reckless course. Even paid hospital attendants in an institutional setting are not consistently alert enough during their vigils to prevent hospitalized patients from committing suicide on occasion. How then can one expect family members to be so? To believe that family members are going to conduct all-night vigils in rotation with one another is foolhardy and absurd. It just won't happen. Perhaps they may last a day or two, or even three, but not much longer. They are bound to slip up, and they are bound to be duped by the patient who is determined to commit suicide. Accordingly, if there is indeed a bona fide suicidal risk, the patient is likely to commit suicide under these circumstances. I rarely use the words *always* and *never*. However, this is one situation in which the therapist should *never* be party to such an arrangement. Under these circumstances, the most judicious thing for the therapist to do is to remove him- or herself from the case with an associated letter of explanation. In it, of course, the therapist must advise the parents to seek hospitalization for the patient.

I have a very conservative position with regard to hospitalizing adolescent patients. There certainly are indications for hospitalizing a youngster in this age bracket, but the majority of adolescent patients who are currently hospitalized would not have been so had I been the one to make the decision. I generally view hospitalization to be warranted primarily for people who are homicidal or suicidal, or who are in very special situations (to be described later) in which it is only by separation from their families that there is any hope for alleviation of their difficulties. Most patients' problems have both intrapsychic and interpersonal contributory elements. The therapist must work in both areas, which usually involves individual work and close work with family members. Plucking the person out of the family context, putting the individual in the hospital, and then treating that person in isolation from the family in the hope that such treatment will help the individual reintegrate him- or herself into the family is often misguided. Doing everything possible to keep the patient in the family, the environment wherein the problems arose and wherein the problems are best worked through, is, in my opinion, the preferable approach.

The Medical Model

One factor that contributes to the ease with which many therapists hospitalize relates to the influence of the medical model on psychiatric practice. Although it is true that the hospital may very well be the optimum place for the treatment of many physical disorders, it does not necessarily follow that the hospital is also the best place for the treatment of many psychiatric disorders. The reflex hospitalization of the patient often reflects doctors' blind following of the medical model.

The Hospital Business

It is important for the reader to appreciate (if he or she doesn't already) that many hospitals are basically businesses, often run and owned by nonmedical people. This is the case not only for private hospitals but, more recently, even nonprofit and voluntary hospitals as well. Under these circumstances, an empty bed means loss of income. The criteria for hospitalization then become expanded— often to include any situation that might justify hospitalization, no matter how weak the justifications. Many fancy and well-appointed hospitals charge enormous amounts of money ($800–1000 a day) and are nothing more than hotels. They look good on paper with regard to the kind of staff that is providing treatment, but little meaningful therapy is given. In such facilities, one of the most important (if not the most important) determinants of how long a patient will stay will be how much money the individual has. All other criteria are of secondary importance in determining the length of hospitalization. When the person runs out of insurance coverage (inevitable with such prices), the staff is suddenly talking about discharge from the hospital. At that point, the patient is referred back to the referring physician, just as a specialist in a hospital might refer back a patient to a referring general practitioner. The notion of the importance of continuity of treatment and the all-important ongoing therapist–patient relationship are of little concern to those in the hospital business. When they say that the average patient stays 21 days in their hospital, they are implying that that was all the patients needed, and that they were significantly improved and even cured following their sojourn in the facility. What the 21-day average really means is that that was just about all most of their patients could possibly afford before being forcibly discharged.

It is also important for the reader to appreciate that psychiatry is also a business, and that a psychiatrist referring a patient for hospitalization may do so more for financial gain than therapeutic indications. Most psychiatrists follow traditional practice in their private offices and charge a specific fee for a 45- to 50-minute session. In 1992, the going rate for most psychiatrists was $100 to $150 per session. In a hospital, however, one makes rounds (again, following the medical model). A patient may be seen for only 5 or 10 minutes, and the psychiatrist may easily get away with charging not only standard fees but even more because insurance companies tend to pay more money for people who are in hospitals. Under these circumstances, earning $1, 000 in an hour is not uncommon. And when patients complain about this, they are told that their disgruntlement is just another manifestation of their psychopathology, and that if they were healthier they wouldn't be complaining so much.

The Teaching Hospital

Another factor that influences the decision regarding hospitalization relates to the situation in teaching hospitals, those closely affiliated with medical schools. These hospitals have an obligation to provide patients for medical students, interns, and residents. In addition, most teaching hospitals train psychologists, psychiatric social workers, and sometimes nurse practitioners, pastoral counselors, and others who want to become therapists. It would seriously compromise the reputation of such an institution if it did not have a good supply of patients for all these students and their teachers. Once again, the criteria for hospitalization become loosened in order to provide such teaching material.

Situations in which Hospitalization Is Warranted for Depressed Adolescents

Certainly, when there is a bona fide suicidal risk, hospitalization is warranted. The hospital must be one in which the personnel are specifically trained to deal with suicidal patients, and the setting must be one in which the utmost care is taken to deprive the potentially suicidal patient of the opportunity to kill him- or herself. One cannot be too stringent on this matter. Even with the most skilled care, and even with significant dedication on the part of hospital personnel, patients successfully commit suicide in such settings.

There are other factors that should be considered when deciding whether or not a depressed adolescent needs hospitalization. The suicidal risk may or may not be present, but these other factors argue strongly for the judiciousness of hospitalization for such patients. For example, the patient's home life may be so chaotic and the family so incapable of working through their problems that the only way to prevent further deterioration of the youngster is to remove him or her from the home. Under these circumstances, the hospital may be viewed as a way station to placement elsewhere. These are situations in which the family has proven itself to be unworkable regarding any kind of therapeutic intervention. Such crisis intervention is certainly indicated. However, even then, day hospitals will sometimes serve (Westman 1979). Under these circumstances, the hospitals may provide a structure that does not exist in the home. The environment is far more predictable than the chaotic one of the home. And these factors are generally salutary.

Teicher (1979) considers one of the benefits of hospitalization to be the availability of other people, on an ongoing basis, who may serve to compensate for the interpersonal losses that may have played a role in the depression. He states: "The 'mothering' atmosphere of the ward [preferable to a private room for a young person], plus the support of the other patients, offers a caring, protective, and safe milieu" (p. 693). One may have difficulty discharging these patients from the hospital. They tend to cling to the staff and to other patients. Hospitalization for such youngsters has both its advantages and disadvantages. One hopes that the advantages of substitute relationships will outweigh the disadvantages of the exaggerated dependency that may be engendered in the hospital setting.

It is important for therapists to appreciate that even under these circumstances, there are certain elements in the hospital program that are antitherapeutic. I have already mentioned the lack of continuity of treatment and the lack of appreciation of an ongoing therapist–relationship as the cornerstone of effective psychotherapy. Another drawback is that the youngster is being placed in an environment with other disturbed adolescents, who may be suffering with moderately severe to severe psychiatric disorders. Whatever benefit may be derived from the healthy therapeutic milieu of the administration and caretaking personnel, there is no question that exposure to other sick adolescents has many antitherapeutic elements. Certainly, one of the aims of treatment is to help the adolescent relate better to peers. But with peers who are severely disturbed, more unhealthy than healthy behavior may be learned. It is common for parents, when visiting such facilities, to comment that their youngster will be placed with a lot of "crazy kids." Traditionally, such parents are reassured that there is nothing antitherapeutic or dangerous about such placement, and that their concerns are unwarranted. At best, this is naive; at worst, the reassurance is duplicitous. It is often not believed by the reassurer, but he or she doesn't want to lose a good customer.

Furthermore, it is important to appreciate that hospitalized patients may be affected detrimentally not only by their fellow patients but by the caretaking individuals as well. The view that these people represent paragons of mental health is simple-minded. Although there are certainly many humane and dedicated individuals who devote themselves to the care of the mentally ill, there are others who do not fall into this category. Some of the sickest people gravitate toward jobs in psychiatric hospitals. Many are borderline and some even psychotic. Many are sadistic, psychopathic, or just plain lazy and uninterested. Accordingly, therapists should take this factor into consideration before recommending hospitalization.

I recognize that some readers may think that I have a somewhat jaundiced view of the value of hospitalization for adolescent patients. It is a view derived primarily from the "outside." What I have seen of the "inside" comes from my residency days as well as my 30 years' experience as an attending psychiatrist at a large New York City hospital. Furthermore, over the years I have seen many patients in my private practice who have been placed in a wide variety of hospitals, both public and private. In addition, I have lectured at both private and public hospitals in twenty-five to thirty states over the last twenty five years. At the hospital with which I am affiliated in New York City (The New York State Psychiatric Institute at the Columbia Presbyterian Medical Center), I have supervised residents who have patients admitted to the inpatient service. My experience has been that the younger the patient, the less the likelihood I would have recommended hospitalization. This is certainly the case for many, if not most, of the patients on the children's inpatient service. With regard to adolescents, the same principle holds: the younger adolescents, generally, are less likely to require hospitalization than some of the older ones. And the older ones have generally been youngsters with flagrant psychotic episodes, who probably do require hospitalization because of the danger to themselves and others if they are not placed in a protected setting. The reader who is interested in further discussion of hospitalization of adolescent patients should refer to articles by Rinsley (1974), Stone (1979), and Zinn (1979).

REFERENCES

Beck, A. T., and Steer, R. A. (1989). Clinical predictors of eventual suicide: a five-to-ten-year prospective study of suicide attempters. *Journal of Affective Disorders* 17:203–209.

Beck, A. T., Steer, R. A., Kovacs, M., and Garrison, G. (1985). Hopelessness and eventual suicide: a 10-year prospective study of patients hospitalized with suicidal ideation. *American Journal of Psychiatry* 142:559–563.

Brent, D. A., Perper, J. A., Allman, C. J., et al. (1991). The presence and accessibility of firearms in the homes of adolescent suicides: case-control study. *Journal of the American Medical Association* 266:2989–2995.

Centers for Disease Control (1988). *Compressed Mortality Files.* Hyattsville, MD: Centers for Disease Control, National Center for Health Statistics.

Gardner, R. A. (1983). *The Boys and Girls Book about One-Parent Families.* Cresskill, NJ: Creative Therapeutics.

——— (1986). *Child Custody Litigation: A Guide for Parents and Mental Health Professionals.* Cresskill, NJ: Creative Therapeutics.

——— (1987). *Hyperactivity, the So-Called Attention Deficit Disorder, and the*

Group of MBD Syndromes. Cresskill, NJ: Creative Therapeutics.

———— (1988). *Psychotherapy with Adolescents.* Cresskill, NJ: Creative Therapeutics.

———— (1991). *The Parents Book about Divorce.* 2nd ed. Cresskill, NJ: Creative Therapeutics.

———— (1992a). *Psychotherapeutic Techniques of Richard A. Gardner.* Rev. ed. Cresskill, NJ: Creative Therapeutics.

———— (1992b). *Self-Esteem Problems of Children: Psychodynamics and Psychotherapy.* Cresskill, NJ: Creative Therapeutics.

Garfinkel, B. (1989). Adolescent suicide. *Psychiatry Letter of the Fair Oaks Hospital* 7(1):1-6.

Hendin, H. (1986). Suicide: review of new directions in research. *Hospital Community Psychiatry* 37:148-154.

———— (1991). Psychodynamics of suicide, with particular reference to the young. *American Journal of Psychiatry* 148:1150-1158.

Rinsley, D. B. (1974). Residential treatment of adolescents. In *American Handbook of Psychiatry: Vol. 2*, ed. G. Caplan, pp. 353-366. New York: Basic Books.

Rosenberg, M. L. (1991). Guns and adolescent suicides. *Journal of the American Medical Association* 266(21):3030.

Sabbath, J. C. (1969). The suicidal adolescent: the expendable child. *Journal of the American Academy of Child Psychiatry* 8:272-289.

Schaffer, D., Garland, A., Gould, M., et al. (1988). Preventing teenage suicide: critical review. *American Journal of Child and Adolescent Psychiatry* 27:675-687.

Shafii, M., Carrigan, S., Whittinghill, J. R., and Derrick, A. (1985). Psychological autopsy of completed suicide in children and adolescents. *American Journal of Psychiatry* 142:1061-1064.

Simmons, K. (1987a). Adolescent suicide: second leading death cause. *Journal of the American Medical Association* 257 (24):3329-3330.

———— (1987b). Task force to make recommendations for adolescents in terms of suicidal risk. *Journal of the American Medical Association* 257 (24):3330-3332.

Stone, L. A. (1979). Residential treatment. In *Basic Handbook of Child Psychiatry: Vol. 3*, ed. S. I. Harrison, pp. 231-262. New York: Basic Books.

Teicher, J. D. (1979). Suicide and suicide attempts. In *Basic Handbook of Child Psychiatry: Vol. 2*, ed. J. D. Noshpitz, pp. 685-697. New York: Basic Books.

Toolan, J. M. (1974). Depression and suicide. In *American Handbook of Psychiatry: Vol. 2*, ed. G. Caplan, pp. 294-306. New York: Basic Books.

Wensley, S. (1987). Portrait of adolescent suicide. *P & S (Columbia University, College of Physicians & Surgeons)* 7(2):14-17.

Westman, J. C. (1979). Psychiatric day treatment. In *Basic Handbook of Child Psychiatry: Vol. 3*, ed. S. I. Harrison, pp. 288–299. New York: Basic Books.

Wolfgang, M. (1958). An analysis of homicide-suicide. *Journal of Clinical and Experimental Psychopathology 19.* 208–218.

World Almanac (1991). *The World Almanac and Book of Facts.* New York: World Almanac (Pharos Books, A Scripps Howard Company).

Zinn, D. (1979). Hospital treatment of the adolescent. In *Basic Handbook of Child Psychiatry: Vol. 3*, ed. S. I. Harrison, pp. 263–288. New York: Basic Books.

11: PSYCHODYNAMIC PSYCHOTHERAPY WITH DEPRESSED CHILDREN AND ADOLESCENTS

Jules Bemporad, M.D.
G. Pirooz Sholevar, M.D.
Linda Schwoeri, M.A., M.F.T.

INTRODUCTION

This chapter describes depression and depressive symptomatology in children and adolescents within a framework of the child's developmental process. In espousing a developmental perspective, one sees depression as the result of cognitive, affective, and physical changes in the child and in his or her ability to experience and express the feelings attached to the state of depression. Therefore, the symptoms, causes, and treatment of depression vary according to the age of the child. All forms of mood disorder can be found in children and adolescents, but the forms increase in frequency and severity as the child reaches adolescence. Depression-like states in childhood depend on the level of cognitive and social developments in the child. However, all ages have in common the general, more contemporary view that depression is a "fundamental human experience that automatically arises subsequent to significant losses or frustrations in everyday life" (Bemporad 1988, p. 26).

Because of the many physical and emotional changes children experience within each stage of growth, the symptoms of depression in childhood must be considered within a developmental framework in addition to the overt symptomatology described in *DSM-III-R*.

The child's cognitive abilities, the dynamics of his or her personality, and its defensive structure must be evaluated in relation to age, developmental level, and the family's level of functioning or pathology. These factors are relevant especially if there is a history of family depression, frequent separations, losses (real or threatened), or rejections that might precipitate a depressive episode.

THEORETICAL CONCEPTS

The contemporary psychoanalytic view of depression incorporates the classical concepts expressed by drive theory, ego psychology, object relations theory, and self psychology. The fundamental concept in the genesis of depression is *narcissistic vulnerability* to disappointment, frustration, and deprivations. This vulnerability is based on the depression-prone person's excessive dependence on external sources rather than on internal ones to maintain self-esteem. The excessive need for gratification is exhibited by the assumption of a passive position by the depressed person for nurturance from others, rather than reliance on his or her own actions. Simultaneously, the depressed person becomes prone to excessive anger and rage toward others who fail to provide gratification or to help the person achieve his or her aspirations and expectations.

Although the reliance on others to feel worthy about oneself may be considered pathological in adults, in children this dependency may be considered a normal situation resulting from the human animal being born in a state of relative immaturity and requiring a high degree of parental care for adequate development. Therefore, many of the depressive reactions of childhood may be understood as justifiable if considered from a developmental perspective.

Depression is viewed as a fundamental ego state and as the emotion associated with helplessness in meeting one's aspirations and ego ideals (Bibring 1953). It is equated with a major reduction in one's sense of well-being regardless of the cause. Sandler and Joffee (1965) explain the loss of the object as significant, because it coincides with the loss of the source of gratification for one's state of well-being supplied by the lost object. The state of well-being defined by Sandler and Joffee originates in the child's satisfactory and optimal relationship with his primary caregiver, mainly the mother. This state is characterized by an internal representation of the mother as a need-gratifying person whose presence is associated with the feeling of well-being, enjoyment, relaxation, hopefulness, and optimism. An unsatisfactory mother–child relationship results in a feeling of deprivation. The infant's experience of the mother as frustrating and depriving results in the infant's feeling joyless, tense, hopeless, and unable to evoke positive responses from the object and, by extension, from the external world of reality. This state of loss of the feeling of well-being is equated with depression.

Jacobson (1953, 1964, 1971a) has delineated the internal structural components correlated with the states of well-being and depression. The fundamental internal structure is *self-representation* as the crucial agency that is formed within the context of the mother-child relationship and correlates with the subsequent sense of identity and affective disposition. In cases of an optimal parent–child relationship generated within the context of loving parenting, the schema matures and develops over time, and the child's self-image is cathected with libido, resulting in a positive sense of self and optimism regarding others. An unstable and poorly delineated self-image cathected with a relatively high proportion of ambivalent and aggressive energy, together with a highly frustrating and depriving mother–child relationship, results in low self-esteem. Low self-esteem and poor self-image are characterized by an unstable view of one's self in different situations, an aggressive cathexis of the self-presentation, feelings of helplessness, and the inability to have an impact on the environment. This lack of agency describes feeling unable to evoke positive nurturance and love from the object, feeling hopeless about the present, and fearing the lack of emotional coherence in the future. In essence, what has been lost is the affective state of well-being associated with one's relationship with the object (Sandler and Joffe 1965).

Kohut's theory of self psychology (Kohut 1971) has particular relevance to the phenomenon of depression, particularly the types of depression correlated with the experiences of deficits in early developmental stages. Kohut proposes that the self can be seriously damaged or destroyed as a result of unempathic or absent parenting. The disturbances of self can be exhibited by depression due to the absence of satisfactory selfobject relationships and selfobject experiences. Deprivation of the empathic, joyful responses of selfobject figures can result in what Kohut has called *empty depression*. It is manifested by a depletion of self-esteem and lack of vitality in contrast to *guilty depression*, which is predominantly manifested by persistent self-rejection and self-blame.

The Role of Ego Regression

The role of ego regression has received insufficient emphasis in psychoanalytic literature. Fenichel (1945) has commented on ego regression resulting in the loss of boundaries between self and object representations in the depressive states. There is a regressive identification with the lost love object. The loss of selfobject boundaries can explain the feelings of self-reproach and guilt following rejection and frustration by the object, rather than externally directed aggression and assertiveness. Fenichel's (1945) formulation of ego regression does not place sufficient emphasis on massive ego regression in severely depressed persons. In such cases, the ego regression exhibits itself by withdrawal from the primary objects, withdrawal from the external world and external sources of gratification, loss of enjoyment in activities, and to some degree the loss of ego capacities and social skills necessary for engagement with other people and activities. The impairment of ego functions has been best described in the cognitive area but also includes impairment of concentration, attention, observation, initiative, and memory. The passive posture of the depressed person who is open only to passive gratifications from external offerings is probably related to ego regression and has been previously described as evidence of oral fixation.

The early object relationship experienced in the mother–child dyad is the fundamental source of gratification and nurturance and is the crucial first step in wooing the child to turn toward the outside world. If the early mother–child relationship is based on a relatively high level of frustration, it would make the person's relationship with the external world tenuous, leaving him vulnerable to withdrawal in the face of frustration, failure, and deprivation. The tenuous nature of this relationship with the external world is manifested in common symptoms of overt and covert depression such as *anergia* (lack of initiative), tendency to *social isolation* (withdrawal from objects), and *anhedonia* (lack of enjoyment in activities). The phenomenon of ego regression has therapeutic ramifications. It limits the impact of treatment because of the patient's partial withdrawal and low engagement with the therapist. It may require specific and active therapeutic interventions to reestablish the relationship with the external world.

In summary, the contemporary psychoanalytic theories of depression emphasize the role of childhood antecedents of depression in terms of actual absence or death of a parent early in life or, more likely, negative experiences related to the loss, such as inadequate substitute or lack of involvement with the replacement. Childhood exposure to abuse, neglect, or family discord and living with a depressed parent, particularly in early childhood, are etiologically significant. Depression is viewed as analogous to a sense of loss of some aspect of self through the loss of selfobject relationships or the selfobject experiences related to it. Therefore, the loss can be the result of the loss of a person, an achievement, or some valued experience on which the individual has relied to support his sense of self.

IMPLICATIONS OF EARLY SELFOBJECT EXPERIENCES

The contemporary psychoanalytic theories of depression pay significant attention to contemporary adult antecedents as well as the current social stressors in the person's life. Among the major adult antecedents of depression may be the selection of a neurotic object who is also depressed, depression prone, socially isolated, or burdened with characterological problems or substance abuse. Depression-prone adults through assortative mating may choose partners who are depressed or exhibit severe personality disorders and enter marital relationships characterized by chronic marital discord and lack of intimacy. This can frequently result in separation, divorce, or in chronically unhappy unions. These marriages are characterized by lack of meaningful communication, unclarity of marital roles, absence of problem solving, and a high level of dissatisfaction. Therefore, the contemporary view of depression emphasizes the continuation of disturbances in object relationships in adult life by continuation of relationships patterned after unsatisfactory and frustrating experiences in early parent–child relationships. The absent or distorted family image and the internalization of the unsatisfactory parental marriage (Sonne 1991) are part of the distorted internal image of the child.

The intrapsychic deficits and conflicts in depression-prone

persons may also result in the reestablishment of subsequent relationships that are devoid of intimacy. The lack of intimacy with the object is an additional source of vulnerability to depression due to the lack of narcissistic nurturance and the need for constant narcissistic gratification and reassurance that the depressive requires to feel whole.

The contemporary psychoanalytic views of depression are consistent with the view of Sullivan (1953), who has emphasized the importance of the interpersonal milieu of the patient in the genesis of depression, and more recent empirical studies on attachment bonds (Bowlby 1969, 1977, Rutter 1972); the relationship between external stressful life events and depression (Klerman et al. 1984, Paykel et al. 1969); and the role of intimacy (Brown and Harris 1978). It is consistent with the views of Rochlin (1959), who has emphasized the role of injury to one's narcissism. When narcissism is threatened, the person feels humiliated and his self-esteem is injured. Rochlin emphasizes the appearance of aggression as a secondary defensive function in order to restore the self-esteem and assert one's value. He assigns a secondary place to the role of inwardly turned aggression which was emphasized in the early stages of the psychoanalytic movement (Abraham 1927, Freud 1923, 1957).

Depression is currently viewed as the result of a lack or inadequate internalization of narcissistic supplies that foster and maintain a positive self-regard despite the unavoidable losses and frustration of everyday life. The depression-prone individual may be further hampered by the development of a tendency toward self-blame, an inhibition over discovering alternative activities that could bring a sense of worth, and difficulties in relationships that often result in a poor choice of marital partners.

DEVELOPMENTAL PERSPECTIVE ON DEPRESSION

Infancy

Depressive behavior is observed mainly in infants who are separated from their mothers. After a period of angry protest, the infants show unhappiness, withdrawal, and apathy. It is debatable whether this is an example of true depression or mourning, or a reaction to the deprivation of the stimulation supplied by the mother figure. Infants do appear distressed by the separation from their mothers and after some time do withdraw into a sort of detached state described by Bowlby (1969). However, the distress appears to be in response to the needed security and warmth of the mother. The infant is capable of a type of suffering and may be in pain, but the relationship between this phenomenon and the later pain of depression in adults may be questioned due to the immaturity of the infant. This view as well as Bowlby's is more sanguine than that of Spitz (1946), who described a malignant state of depression in infants that included symptoms of weight loss, insomnia, lack of response to people, and a faraway gaze when separated from and not reunited with their mothers. Based on a developmental perspective, dysphoric moods would be considered more transient and responsive to improvements in the infant's and toddler's stimulation and environmental situation.

Early Childhood

Prior to school age, children show depressive symptoms directly in response to the environmental deprivation of love or the gratifying approval of parents. Depression in this group is exceedingly rare, again due to the cognitive immaturity of the children, which may protect them from true mood disorders. Also, at this young age, verbalization needed for the expression of feelings is still relatively primitive, and the child tends to translate affect into action and to substitute love objects. The child also has not yet developed a harsh conscience, which may contribute to the depressive process. The younger child is most reactive to situational stresses and immediate effects of the loss of significant others who provide him or her with nurturance, mirroring, and security. Therefore, a change to a more nurturing environment at this age may be of great therapeutic benefit by allowing the child to experience a needed sense of being appreciated and to be understood for his or her abilities or talents as well as deficiencies. This environmental change can help alleviate many of the frustrations and foster a sense of emotional well-being.

When frustration and losses arise, the child may become inhibited, clinging, frightened, sad, and unwarrantedly serious. Still lacking proficiency in verbal skills, he or she may be unable to identify or describe the feelings through language but may convey the situation via doll play. Activity still becomes a way of compensating for disappointments and losses, and the child quite readily notices rewards as well as punishments arising in the environment at home or at play.

Early Latency (Ages 5–6)

Symptoms begin to change somewhat at this age. They appear as sadness, withdrawal, and unsustained crying, but they are still directly related to the frustrating, depriving situation at hand. Children at this age are becoming more social and interactive with peers. Their social and cognitive skills are developing. They are aware of their subjective experience but may not as yet know that they can control their affect cognitively. They are unable to reason that instead of being sad, they can attempt to exert some control by not thinking about what makes them sad. They also do not know that others have different perspectives, making it difficult to understand the intentions of others. During this age, the children often confuse fantasy with reality in thoughts and perceptions of self. Unable to maintain a constant or accurate estimation of self, they often give up when disappointed, and this in time can lead to feelings of hopelessness and helplessness. However, they are more able to enjoy peer-oriented activities such as kindergarten and are more reactive to the positive action of nonfamilial adults such as teachers. The child is still primarily sensitive to what the parents expect of him or her, is still dependent on positive, gratifying parental responses, and is therefore quite vulnerable to the signs of parental disapproval. Unaware of his or her own abilities and limits, the child may instinctively inhibit any actions that might lessen that needed parental approval and can easily assume responsibility and guilt for events not within his or her control. This is particularly so in abusive situations. Fortunately, this is a resilient age, and children can and do learn to actively attend to more positive situations that distract them from whatever might be causing unhappiness.

Treatment Considerations

Younger children manifest depressive responses following the loss of love of a parent or the significant others who provided nurturing, mirroring, and security. Treatment, therefore, should attempt to foster such self-psychological functions as twinship and idealizing of the child's selfobject needs. Treatment addresses these through the following:

1. Play should be used as a communication tool as well as a tool for creative expression. The therapist should appreciate the child's efforts and help him or her decrease some inhibitory tendencies by encouraging involvement through fantasy play.

2. Work should be with the caretakers and centered on providing understanding of the child's developmental needs. Family therapy is often necessary to assess and confront the family's unrealistic and harsh expectations and demands on the child.

3. The child should be moved to a more nurturing environment if the caretaker is not responsive to making changes.

4. The therapeutic relationship should be aimed at gratifying the child's emerging needs for self-esteem and approval because it offers the child a selfobject through which his or her talents, abilities, and personality can be acknowledged and utilized to build a positive sense of self.

Older Latency (Ages 9–12)

Children at this age present with typical adultlike symptoms of depression and with low self-esteem that now appear to be self-generated. Their dysphoria has both cognitive and affective components. At this age, the child is more capable of making deductions about his or her circumstances and is better equipped to express them. Depending on the parental standards, the children may have internalized unrealistic modes of evaluating themselves as well as others. The dysphoria is no longer an immediate reflection of their environment; it is now generated from within the child and is demonstrated in his or her developing self-esteem. The children have *cognitive distortions* in regard to their abilities. They believe they are repulsive and deficient and will never be loved unless they succeed in all things. Their developing conscience exaggerates their sense of guilt and responsibility; therefore, they feel that they cannot meet parental expectations unless they are perfect. However, they are still not capable of higher level abstract thinking and, therefore, are unable to project themselves into the future, limiting their awareness of circumstances to the here and now.

The child in this stage is focused on competitiveness, perfectionism, and ambition. It is a time when acceptance and performance in extrafamilial activities are becoming very important to one's self-regard. The pubescent child starts to depend less on the home environment and more on peers and school for praise and acceptance. However, the child still fears being unable to meet the parental ideals and in the face of this failure, fears threats to the still valued parental relationship. These children are now much more aware of themselves in relation to their group. They do a lot of sizing up, and one distinction of this time is that they feel they cannot attain the internalized parental ideal both outside and inside the family. They may become depressed and perceive themselves as personal failures. Depression at this age has both an affective quality and a more cognitive evaluative quality to it. It is no longer in direct response to stimulants in the environment; the child has within himself personal sources of dissatisfaction resulting from internalized standards that are often unrealistic or unattainable.

Treatment Considerations

Treatment should involve shared activities such as games, mutual storytelling with interpretations, and conversation that provides a type of restructuring of the child's self-evaluation (Bemporad 1982).

Adolescence

The depression in the adolescent appears as a type of dysphoria marked by cognitive distortions and rapid shifts in mood in response to even minor life events. Prior to adolescence, children are not able to project themselves into the future. However, in adolescence there is an obsession with time. The adolescent is now able to connect his present experience to what might happen in the future. However, he does not yet have the ability to take the adult perspective in order to modulate this new cognitive ability. Therefore, an adolescent may believe that being stood up on a date means he or she will never be capable of having a relationship or that flunking one test indicates continued academic failure. This lack of moderation in predicting one's future may account for the urgency and sense of helplessness seen in adolescence.

Also in adolescence, a new social role is required as one moves more and more outside the family. The adolescent's budding new sense of self-worth requires that others accept and acknowledge his or her ideas as valuable. There is an increased vulnerability to depression created by a seemingly inordinate need for external nurturance and affirmation to secure an acceptable sense of self-esteem. Bibring (1953) defines self-esteem in terms of a tension between narcissistic needs and desires and the ego's awareness of its ability to accomplish. As they try to create a satisfactory sense of self outside the family orbit and in a new social setting, adolescents have difficulty regulating self-worth, and this subjects them to labile, depressed moods. The symptoms appear as extreme fluctuations of mood following mild or trivial frustrations as well as gratifications. Put-downs, criticisms, and threats to the already injured sense of self are reacted to with pain, hurt, and intense humiliation. Understandably, the adolescents may not have developed appropriate and gratifying compensatory mechanisms for their losses, rejections, or shortcomings. Some may not have had the needed loving selfobjects in the past, and as a result they appear labile, confused, and vulnerable to episodes of depression.

The adolescent struggles more so now because he can make judgments about his abilities and liabilities and may no longer be using the childhood defenses of denial or distraction to mediate these situations. Adolescence "is the time when childhood fantasies along with childhood toys are discarded with an inescapable feeling of loss and resignation" (Bemporad 1988, p. 27). Adolescents are not prepared to face the tasks at hand, especially in the area of sexual development and the feelings and fears of intimacy related to sexuality. Competitiveness, the feeling of inadequacy, shame, rejection, and disappointment inherent in adultlike activities intensify their already threatened sense of self-worth. To the adolescent, even minor events take on great significance, as witnessed by the desperation and urgency with which these events are often met.

Adolescents also fear the freedom that is attached to separating and individuating from their family. Many view freedom as an ordeal in which exist powerful temptations and guilt as well as responsibility to loved ones. In a family context, the problems of adolescence appear in relation to ambivalence over independence versus dependence. The adolescent struggles to convince others that he or she is no longer a child yet behaves in a manner that continually challenges the parent's ability to support the adolescent's desire to be seen and treated as a mature person.

Treatment considerations

The psychodynamic treatment of depressed adolescents aims at allowing them to develop the skills necessary to meet the tasks of this developmental phase, or to correct those internalized prohibitions or ambitions that lead to maladaptive ways of seeing the self. The therapist acts more as a mentor than an analyst, becoming a more realistic parent.

Suicide

The subject of suicidality should be examined according to the developmental level of the child or adolescent. The child's concept of death changes over time. Prior to age 5, death is seen as a temporary and reversible state, as if the individual is still alive but asleep. Between the ages of 5 and 9, the child begins to appreciate and fear death as a state in which there is a permanent separation from the loved ones. According to Cytryn and McKnew (1979), prior to age 14, suicide attempts are considered actions of impulsive, angry children with low frustration tolerance who are living in chaotic, multiproblem homes. After puberty suicide becomes an attempt to alter a living situation that is intolerable or becomes a means of punishing someone. Suicidal gestures and behavior in adolescence, especially after age 14, are therefore more of a risk because of the cognitive, affective, and social development at that stage.

TYPES OF DEPRESSION

Efforts to arrive at typologies of childhood depression remain in debate and create problems for the clinician. Cytryn and McKnew (1979), however, have proposed a classification that differentiates between a depressive, affectual response and depressive illness. They classify three types of depression:

1. *Acute depressive reaction* is usually the result of some clearly identifiable cause, such as a severe trauma created by the loss of a loved one, or the loss of nurturance by someone who had provided care in the past. Children suffering from this type exhibit clear symptoms of depression for a short time but recover quickly because they have a good premorbid history of personal and family adjust-

ment. It might be difficult to differentiate these children from those who exhibit a grief or mourning reaction in response to loss.

2. *Chronic depressive reaction* is characterized by the presence of depressed mood and behavior with no history of a precipitating event. Children with this type of depression do not adjust well to situations and present with a syndrome of persistent sad affect, sleep and eating disorders, and suicidal thoughts and threats. At least one parent may have a recurring depression.

3. *Masked depressive reaction* is presented with no overt depressive symptomatology, but there is an underlying depression manifested in sad affect and depressive themes in fantasy, drawing, and conversation. It is characterized by hyperactivity, aggressive behavior, psychosomatic illness, or delinquency. The child's acting out usually covers the underlying depression while defending the child against despair.

Bemporad (1982) discusses two types of depression related to the developmental period of adolescence:

1. *Anaclitic depression* is described as a type of depression in which the youngster is unable to cope with the psychosocial developmental tasks of adolescent life because of prior developmental failures. Panic, anxiety, somatic complaints, and a sense of being overwhelmed are some of the symptoms exhibited. Adolescents with this type continue to require the support of parental figures to help them function adequately and to make adjustments to their peer environment.

2. In *introjective depression*, the child is able to separate from his family and is developmentally ready for adolescence. However, the child experiences unrealistic self-expectations that interfere with the tasks of this developmental period.

TYPES OF DEPRESSION: A NEW MODEL

Karasu (1991) has provided a comprehensive psychodynamic model for a sensitive integration of multiple psychoanalytic views of depression. His model integrates the diverse points of view offered by multiple developmental metatheorists and describes the diverse maturational level of the patients. Karasu has described clinical signs and symptoms of each type of depression as well as some guidelines for therapeutic interventions. He has proposed four basic prototypes of depression: dyadic deficit depression (DDD), dyadic conflict depression (DCD), triadic deficit depression (TDD), and triadic conflict depression (TCD). Each type of depression is etiologically correlated with the unresolved conflicts or deficits based on different types of parent–child relationships; furthermore, each type of depression is related to the specific psychosexual phase of the child's development, intrapsychic maturation, and possible psychopathology.

Dyadic Deficit Depression (DDD)

Psychodynamic and Clinical Manifestations

DDD is the product of disturbances in the early mother–child relationship with a psychologically absent, unloving, unpredictably available, or insecurely bonded mother. The symptoms of patients include feelings of helplessness, with a pleading quality, clinging dependency, anxiety, dread of sense of self, self-blame, loneliness, hypochondriasis, and a yearning for affection. Weight gain, over-sleeping, sexual difficulties in the form of impotence or disturbances of arousal are common in adults. Patients are vulnerable to experiences of deprivation and disappointment from childhood to adulthood. They tend to perpetuate their sense of helplessness and unworthiness by undermining their relationships at school or work, or in social situations. They suppress their aggressive feelings because they fear abandonment and, likewise, negate their abilities and function below their capacity.

Therapeutic Techniques

Treatment should include the provision of a reliable, active, nurturing, and empathic relationship between the therapist and the child. The establishment of an empathic relationship with the patient can help generate a cohesive and positive self-representation that mitigates against hurt and injury. The patient's attention should be drawn to the limitations of the mother without generating a litany against her. This reorganization of internal feeling helps the patient refrain from self-blame for the past or present failures of the parental figure (Karasu 1992). Engaging these patients requires special intervention techniques. The patient should be helped to acquire skills to relate to others in the external world. The secondary gains from depression in terms of receiving attention in response to helplessness and the primary gains in terms of maintenance of unworthy and self-defeating internal objects should be interpreted.

Patients tend to experience the therapist as a depriving parent and arouse guilt in him. This is a phenomenon that should be interpreted early and repeatedly in treatment.

Dyadic Conflict Depression (DCD)

Psychodynamic and Clinical Manifestations

DCD represents a conflict over being controlled and made dependent versus being independent. The internal conflicts generally originate in the separation-individuation phase of development and are related to the struggle over autonomy and the establishment of a cohesive sense of self. Once the patient discovers that he or she lacks control over objects, he or she struggles to gain such control. As a result of this struggle, the patient constructs an internal view of the objects as intrusive, demanding, controlling, and conditionally accepting or loving. This may result in the establishment of an unrealistic ego ideal and expectation of self based on the fantasy that by being conscientious and perfect one would evoke acceptance and love from the external object. As a result, such people end up with an unachievable ego ideal. The struggle to control others, in an effort to prevent being controlled, makes these patients particularly vulnerable to feelings of failure and shame. As adults, such patients frequently reject the wish to have children in order to feel in control and clean. They are also prone to directing their aggression outward as a preventative measure against depression. At the time of real or fantasied loss and failure, their aggression may be temporarily directed toward themselves. Control issues surface clinically as bulimia, anorexia, substance abuse, or promiscuity.

Therapeutic Techniques

Treatment requires that the therapist tolerate hostility from the patient without retaliating. The patient blames the therapist for many shortcomings in order to achieve dignity and self-respect based on the patient's unrealistic perspective on life. The fear of engulfment and being controlled by the therapist is a prominent underlying dynamic. Strong attempts to defeat self and the therapist in order to maintain self-definition and independence are prominent. This results in escalating negative transference feelings in which the therapist is experienced, incorrectly, as being disapproving.

Triadic Deficit Depression (TDD)

Psychodynamic and Clinical Manifestations

TDD is related to the psychological absence of the father, who may be viewed as abusive or at least insensitive. The negative view toward the father is extended into the lack of belief in authority or socially accepted ideals. Such patients follow commands more out of fear of retaliation than from an internalized feeling of guilt. Therefore, their goals are primarily centered around attainment of external gains in life. Their relationships are vacillating and unstable. In cases where a good-enough dyadic relationship with the mother has been achieved, both male and female patients may form a highly dependent relationship with females.

The fathers of such patients frequently lack respect for themselves and devalue their wives. Therefore, the male or female children in such families grow up with devalued self-image based on identification with the paternal attitude of devaluing women as love objects. In cases of high dependence upon females, the loss of an exclusive dependency relationship, a business failure, or a physical illness may bring about depression.

Clinical features of TDD patients include complaints that have the quality of phallic frustration. The patients tend to be sexually and financially exploitative of others, emphasize productivity, and maneuver others to gain ground, self-esteem, and power. They tend to marry "up," as if making a business deal, and to establish a semblance of respectability while neglecting their family and children.

Therapeutic Techniques

Treatment is ultimately directed toward reorganization and repair of the internal images of a discredited father and devalued mother. The therapist is called upon to remain uncompromising in his or her values in order to gain the credibility needed for internal reorganization to occur.

The patient's low expectations and discrediting of the therapist are based on distorted internal images and need to be interpreted early. Other measures include helping the patients to give up their excessive reliance on external props for self-esteem, countering the panic that life would be totally empty without such external props, and learning new modes of deriving pleasure and meaning in a real relationship by attaining an altruistic commitment to it. The pseudo-intimate and manipulative modes of relating need to be interpreted. Keep in mind and counter the high likelihood of the patient's premature dropping out of treatment after attainment of limited favorable changes.

Triadic Conflict Depression (TCD)

Psychodynamic and Clinical Manifestations

Clinical manifestations of TCD arise from conflict proper and inhibition over sexuality and aggression, which are repressed and remain unconscious. The conflicts are primarily phallic in nature. They arise over sexual desires and aggression based on an unrealistic assignment in early childhood of value to parents and children relative to each other. Therefore, the children develop conflict over competition and rivalry, which results in either aggression or inhibition of initiative. Sexual inadequacy and submission or excessive aggressiveness is prevalent.

The clinical symptoms are precipitated by phallic losses, failure of aspirations, and superego transgressions that result in feelings of castration, inferiority, and ineffectiveness. Superego transgressions are defended against by undoing and consequently self-punishing behavior. The fear of success, loss of self-respect, and anxiety regarding entitlement, deservedness, and meaningfulness are also common. Patients may enter treatment when things are going well, which may promote depression, survivor's guilt, guilt due to success, and self-directed aggression. Dictates from the superego make patients excessively responsible toward their families and children.

Therapeutic Techniques

Treatment should focus on superego distortions rooted in early life foundations. Classical transference and resistance interpretation serve as the mutative factors in treatment. The reconstruction of sources of conflict in the early relationship of the patient and his or her parents as manifested in intense transference reaction (transference neurosis) is necessary.

EGO REGRESSION IN DEPRESSION

The manifestations of ego regression in depression can be pervasive. In addition to the affective dimension, the ego regression may manifest itself in disturbances in the patient's behavior, sensations, imagery, cognition, interpersonal and social relationships, and neuropsychological–biochemical substrates (Lazarus 1992). The different aspects of ego regression may result in social withdrawal, anhedonia, and anergia.

Therapeutic Techniques

In addition to the establishment of a therapeutic relationship with the patient, empathically based diagnosis, reconstruction of the patient's early life experiences, and specific behavioral and psychosocial interventions can be quite helpful or necessary to address the patient's ego regression and restore his or her functioning. Such measures have been broadly described by cognitive psychotherapy (Beck 1967, 1991) and to some degree by multimodal therapy (Lazarus 1992). The cognitive therapist addresses the cognitive distortions of the patient, particularly in the form of the *depressive triad* representing a negative view of self, negative and hostile view of the object, and pessimistic and negative view of the world and the future.

Behavioral interventions by the therapist address the patient's withdrawal from gratifying behavior and overinvolvement in meaningless drudgery. Lazarus (1992) suggests establishing a catalogue of rewarding activities and constructing a checklist of pleasant event schedules. The aim is to establish numerous behaviors, sensations, images, ideas, people, and places that have been historically rewarding to the patient. This may include very simple, ordinary, everyday activities that are potentially reinforcing events.

Affective interventions consider anger and rage as occurring secondary to depression and frustration. The display of sympathy and attempts to cheer up the patient tend to aggravate the depressive reaction and therefore should be avoided. More effective is the establishment of standard anxiety reduction methods such as relaxation. A behavioral technique such as the use of calming self-statements may be helpful. The end product is the establishment of a repertoire of self-assertive and uninhibited responses that tend to reduce depression.

In order to reduce the impact of depression on sensation, exercise is prescribed. Interventions in the imagery dimension can be helpful to conjure up vivid images and to recall past successes. Such methods can be used effectively in treatment sessions and can result in the stimulation of fantasies as an intermediate step to activities.

In the cognitive dimension, Ellis (1962, 1989) has proposed methods of cognitive disputation that are geared toward the alteration of irrational self-thoughts, imperatives, and consequent standards that are impossibly high. Other cognitive distortions include dichotomous divisions, overgeneralizations, negative expectations, and selective abstractions. Many self-defeating ideas are encased in schemas that act as central organizing ideas and belief systems. These schemas undermine the patient's sense of self and others and result in the patient feeling unworthy of happiness.

Interpersonal interventions encourage the patient to participate in a significant network of other people and to respond in an adaptive way to their demands. The appropriate use of assertiveness instead of overly aggressive or overly submissive responses is necessary. Learning to say no, asking for favors from others, expressing positive feelings, and volunteering criticism and disapproval with style are social skills that help the patient handle interactions.

The recognition that moderate and severe depression, regardless of the precipitating psychological factors, can influence the neurochemical balance of the patient has recently gained significant importance. The low side-effect profile of new antidepressants makes their use particularly helpful. The patient should be encouraged to view the medication as a helpful agent in the overall endeavor to overcome depression and reestablish a satisfactory and gratifying life style rather than as a magic bullet that can eradicate depression by itself (Lazarus 1992). The medication is particularly effective in addressing the ego-regressive aspects of depression, increasing libido, and decreasing sleep disorders.

CASE HISTORIES

Carol: An Early Latency Child

Identifying Information

Carol, a 6-year-old girl, was referred for psychotherapy when she threatened to jump from a third-story window because her great-grandmother showed attention to a neighbor's child. Carol, a shy, sad-looking child, initially volunteered little information. Her reticence and inhibition decreased markedly as she got to know her therapist, and she eventually showed a deep need for and appreciation of the therapist's empathic understanding and warmth.

Background Information

Carol's mother was 16 years old when she delivered her. She is now in prison for prostitution and for selling heroin. Carol was given to her maternal grandmother, who was only 30 at the time Carol was born. The grandmother died shortly after Carol's birth, and Carol subsequently went to live with her 52-year-old great-grandmother. This arrangement was not successful because the great-grandmother became resentful about having to care for Carol and, when drunk, would physically and verbally abuse her.

At age 4, Carol tried repeatedly to run away to a neighbor's house, where she felt better cared for. Her suicide attempt at age 6 was admittedly her way to get her great-grandmother's attention.

Observations from Play

Carol's doll play involved a young girl named Hazel, who was occasionally beaten up and yelled at by her drunken doll mother. Although her play accurately reflected her real life situation, Carol could give no reasons for these events. The mother doll beat the Hazel doll, and Hazel felt sad. Neither Hazel nor the mother doll was perceived as unworthy or bad; these events simply occurred. Hazel tried to get the mother doll's love because it "made her feel better" and because the mother doll would then "buy her toys."

Treatment Process

After a few weeks, Carol became open and cheerful in the therapy sessions. Work with the great-grandmother centered on trying to create a better home environment for Carol. However, despite efforts to change the woman's attitude, it became clear that she had simply exhausted her capacity to be responsible for another child at this stage of her life. Carol continued to play out sequences of neglect, abuse, and loneliness as the caretaker's efforts diminished. She was then placed in a nurturing foster home, where she has done well, the initial dysphasia having disappeared. Carol continued her relationship with the therapist, who involved the foster parents in attempting to partially remedy the past deprivations of her life and guide her toward continued normal development.

Discussion

Carol's history is one of deprivation due to the very early loss of the maternal figure and the absence of satisfactory caretakers who could compensate for that loss. Subsequent caretakers were abusive and neglectful, adding to her loss of positive and rewarding relationships. This case is representative of the developmental period of early latency in that Carol was not able to be reflective of her situation and, instead, reacted directly to it by running away and later attempting suicide. She was not able to verbalize her feelings and could only create the atmosphere of abuse and deprivation through the play figures. She also was unable to hold the figures accountable, and no psychological motivation could be seen for the abusive, rejecting behavior beyond the drinking that was observable when the abuse occurred. Her dependent needs for acceptance and attention from parental figures were clear. The attempts to create a better environment eventually proved rewarding, and the child's ability to forge other relationships with nurturing figures indicated her ability to at least partially bounce back.

Carol's case can be considered a DDD type of depression, as described by Karasu.

Paul: An Adolescent

Identifying Information

Paul, an 18-year-old college dropout, was seen following a suicide attempt, in which he took a large number of assorted pills after a girlfriend decided to break off their relationship. He intended to die, but the mixture of pills was fortunately not lethal. When first seen, Paul could hardly carry on a conversation, was in extreme mental torment, and repeatedly stated that he wished he was dead. He appeared paralyzed by an overwhelming sense of pain and despair despite all his brilliance and mental ability. He broke down into tears upon the mention of his lost love, repeating that without his girlfriend, his world was empty and life was no longer worth living. He felt incomplete and deprived of any hope of happiness without her. He also could neither eat nor sleep, but rather paced his bedroom at night.

Background Information

Paul had always been shy and seclusive. He had difficulty separating from his mother, was afraid of peers, and exhibited erratic school performance despite having a superior intellect. He found it difficult to express his feelings and suffered severe stomach cramps in times of distress. His mother was plagued with migraine headaches, and his sister had developed an ulcer in childhood. Both Paul and his sister had superior intelligence, and the mother utilized this gift by insisting that they excel in academics.

In his early teens, Paul became truly depressed when he compared himself with other boys. He felt like an outsider around them and was unable to relate to most of them. He was painfully shy in social situations, often developing stomachaches at parties or dances. Instead of revealing his painful feelings to anyone, he tried to find solace in solitary hobbies and in muscle building. Despite attempts at compensation, he continued to see himself as unmanly and inadequate. He kept his room a mess and dressed in a shabby fashion in a futile attempt at rebellion against his mother. He had difficulty being with her but also felt that he needed her to direct his life and give him structure. Paul grew up very naive about crucial aspects of life. His sole responsibility was to make good grades; other tasks were discouraged.

When he entered an out-of-town college, Paul was totally bewildered and lacked experience caring for himself. He quit college to avoid failing in his first year. This caused him to feel disgraced becaused he had not succeeded in his strongest area, intellectual achievement. At the time of this self-devaluation, he met his girlfriend, Carrie. Carrie accepted him as he was and without conditions. She allowed him to feel worthwhile and deserving of love. She became the fulcrum of his existence and filled his thoughts so much that he could not attend to his studies. He dropped out of college again. After about a year of intense involvement, Carrie decided that she was too young to stay with him and broke off the relationship. Paul attempted suicide shortly thereafter.

Family Dynamics

Paul's mother had grown up with wealthy parents and was given much in terms of material comforts; however, she received little love and warmth. Her parents valued social standing, outward appearance, financial success, and upward mobility. She was a loving and giving mother as long as her children behaved in an overly polite, exemplary manner and made top grades. If either faltered, she became furious or subjected the children to long lectures. Paul's father also came from a prominent family but had chosen music as a career. He achieved moderate success as a musician but was unable to support his family in a manner comparable to his own or his wife's childhood experience. He was a more relaxed, fun-loving individual who lived for art and seemed satisfied with his accomplishments. He was, however, ashamed that he could not give more to his family, and this kept him in a secondary role in family matters. He and Paul rarely talked when together.

Paul's parents truly loved each other, but there was a constant undercurrent of resentment from Paul's mother and a sense of failure from Paul's father. Both parents hid their feelings from other people and continued to present themselves as if they were still very wealthy. Paul's mother developed a sense of inferiority over her limited financial state because she was snobbishly treated as a poor relation by her wealthier siblings. Her attempt at vindication was to force her children to succeed, thereby justifying her choice of Paul's father as a marital partner.

Treatment Process

It took a long time for Paul to think about life without Carrie. He had depended on her for his validation as important and worthwhile. The relationship helped him to fight off chronic depression and low self-esteem. He continued to dwell on his symptoms rather than discuss his angry feelings about Carrie's leaving him, his mother's treatment of him, and his therapist's not doing more to help him. When his facade of stoicism was later interpreted to him, it opened up discussion of his need to cover feelings of inferiority. He was as yet unable to see that he had used his relationship with Carrie to fulfill his narcissistic needs. However, he did begin to appreciate how his denial of hostile feelings of being overwhelmed by his mother, fear of hurting others, and his restriction of social contacts had predisposed him to becoming depressed. Paul's case fits with Karasu's DCD classification and exhibits conflict over dependency, unrealistic, ideal ego expectations, and the resultant feeling of shame.

CONCLUSION

Depression is a fundamental human experience subsequent to significant frustration and losses and can include the feeling of helplessness and dramatic reduction in self-esteem. The affective, cognitive, and physical changes experienced in such situations comprise the depressive disorder and the symptomatology, which varies in expression. The developmental stage and age of the child produce complex diagnostic configurations and may require specific therapeutic strategies and methodologies. This developmental perspective includes two major dimensions: (1) the achievement of a *triadic* versus a *diadic* stage of interpersonal development and (2) the role of a deficit or conflict that interferes with the developmental progression and functioning of the individual in each stage. These two dimensions can then provide clues to the selection of the more promising therapeutic and intervention strategies. The developmental paradigm described in this chapter can be applied to children, adolescents, and adults to enhance therapeutic effectiveness.

REFERENCES

Abraham, K. (1927). Notes on the psycho-analytic investigation and treatment of manic-depressive insanity and allied conditions. In *Selected Papers on Psychoanalysis*, trans. D. Bryan and A. Strachey, pp. 248–279. London: Hogarth, 1911.

Beck, A. T. (1967). *Depression: Clinical, Experimental and Clinical Aspects*. New York: Harper & Row.

—— (1991). Cognitive therapy: a 30-year retrospective. *American Psychologist* 46:368–375.

Bemporad, J. (1982). Management of childhood depression developmental consideration. *Journal of Psychosomatic Medicine* 23(1):272–279.

—— (1988). Psychodynamic treatment of depressed adolescents. *Journal of Clinical Psychiatry* 49(9):26–31.

Bibring, E. (1953). The mechanism of depression. In *Affective Disorders*, ed. P. Greenacre, pp. 13–48. New York: International Universities Press.

Bowlby, J. (1969). *Attachment and Loss, II: Separation*. New York: Basic Books.

—— (1977). The making and breaking of affectional bonds, II. Some principles of psychotherapy. *British Journal of Psychiatry* 130:401–431.

Brown G., and Harris T. (1978) *Social Origins of Depression: A Study of Psychiatric Disorder in Women*. London: Tavistock.

Cytryn, L., & McKnew, D. (1979). Affective disorder. In *Basic Handbook of Child Psychiatry*, ed. J. Noshpitz. New York: Basic Books.

Ellis, A. (1962). *Reason and Emotion in Psychotherapy*. New York: Lyle Stewart.

—— (1989). Rational-emotive therapy. In *Current Psychotherapies* ed. R. J. Corsimi and D. Wedding, pp. 197–240. Itasca, IL: Peacock.

Fenichel, O. (1945). *The Psychoanalytic Theory of Neurosis*. New York: W. W. Norton.

Freud, S. (1923). The ego and the id. *Standard Edition* 19:66.

_____ (1957). Mourning and melancholia. *Standard Edition* 14:237–260.

Jacobson, E. (1953). Contributions to the metapsychology of cyclothymic depression. In *Affective Disorders*, ed. P. Greenacre. New York: International Universities Press.

_____ (1964). *The Self and the Object World*. New York: International Universities Press.

_____ (1971a). *Depression*. New York: International Universities Press.

_____ (1971b). *Depression: Comparative Studies of Normal, Neurotic and Psychotic Conditions*. Madison, CT: International Universities Press.

_____ (1973). The depressive personality. *International Journal of Psychiatry* 11:218–221.

Karasu, B. (1991). The worst of times, the best of times: psychotherapy in the 1990s. *Journal of Psychotherapy Practice and Research* 1:2–15.

_____ (1992). Developmentalist metatheory of depression and psychotherapy. *American Journal of Psychotherapy* 46(1) January.

Klerman, G., Weissman, M., Rounsaville, B., and Chevron, E. (1984). *Interpersonal Psychotherapy of Depression*. New York: Basic Books.

Kohut, H. (1971). *The Analysis of the Self*. New York: International Universities Press.

Lazarus, A. (1992). The multimodal approach to the treatment of minor depression. *American Journal of Psychotherapy*, 46(1):549–554.

McKnew, D., Cytryn, L., Etron, A., et al. (1979). Offspring of patients with affective disorders. *British Journal of Psychiatry* 134:148–152.

Paykel, E. S., Myers, J. K., Dienelt, M. N., et al. (1969). Life events and depression: a controlled study. *Archives of General Psychiatry* 21:753–760.

Rochlin, G. (1959). The loss complex. *Journal of the American Psychoanalytic Association* 7:299–316.

Rutter, M. (1972). *Maternal Deprivation Reassessed*. London: Penguin.

Sandler, J., and Joffee, W. G. (1965). Notes on childhood depression. *International Journal of Psycho-Analysis* 46:88–96.

Sonne, J. (1991). Triadic transferences of pathological family image. *Contemporary Family Therapy* 13(3):219–229.

Spitz, R. A. (1946). Anaclitic depression: an inquiry into the genesis of psychiatric conditions in early childhood, II. *Psychoanalytic Study of the Child* 2:312–342. New York: International Universities Press.

Sullivan, H. S. (1953). *The Interpersonal Theory of Psychiatry*. New York: W. W. Norton.

12: CURRENT PSYCHOPHARMACOLOGIC TREATMENT RESEARCH OF DEPRESSED CHILDREN AND ADOLESCENTS

John O. Viesselman, M.D.
Elizabeth B. Weller, M.D.
Ronald A. Weller, M.D.
Shahnour Yaylayan, M.D.

OVERVIEW

This chapter is a clinical review of the psychopharmacologic treatment of child and adolescent depression. To utilize psychotropic agents effectively in depressed children and adolescents, depression should be accurately diagnosed according to standardized criteria. Also, an awareness of the specific symptoms of depression targeted for treatment is important. In treating children, a working knowledge of the pharmacokinetics of psychotropic agents in this age group is important because they can differ significantly from those in adults. Side effects of the medications should be known. When medications are prescribed, the importance of medical follow-up must be understood. Finally, the evidence for the effectiveness of antidepressant medications in child and adolescent depression should be considered. Data from both controlled and uncontrolled studies will be summarized, and caveats regarding the pharmacologic treatment of children and adolescents will be considered.

DIAGNOSIS OF DEPRESSION

The occurrence of depression in children historically has been recognized but had tended to be defined more as a symptom than a syndrome or a disorder until recently (Cantwell 1983). Bipolar disorder was not felt to exist in children and often was misdiagnosed in adolescents (Carlson and Strober 1978). However, many reports now support the existence of both unipolar and bipolar affective disorders in children (Carlson and Cantwell 1980, Weller and Weller 1984). Not only do children and adolescents have both bipolar and unipolar affective disorders, but these disorders can be diagnosed using the same criteria as for adults with some minor modifications that take into account a child's developmental level.

A diagnosis can be more accurate and, thus, more helpful if standardized diagnostic criteria are regularly used by clinicians experienced or trained in their use. Several structured diagnostic interviews are available, and clinicians unfamiliar with criteria-based diagnosis can improve their diagnostic skills by becoming familiar with their use. The Diagnostic Interview for Children and Adolescents (DICA) (Herjanic and Campbell 1977), the Diagnostic Interview Schedule for Children (DISC) (Costello et al. 1984), and the K-SADS, based upon the Schedule for Affective Disorders and Schizophrenia for Children (K-SADS) (Puig-Antich and Chambers 1978) are a few of the interviews that can be used. These interviews have been used to establish the diagnosis in many of the antidepressant drug studies in children and adolescents. Diagnoses made by structured interview have better reliability and face validity than diagnoses made by unstructured clinical interview (Cantwell and Baker 1989, Gutterman et al. 1987). Both children and their parents need to be interviewed to obtain diagnostic information because the reports of symptoms by children differ from those reported by their parents (Kovacs 1978). By utilizing multiple informants, more information can be obtained.

The criteria for diagnosing mood disorders in children and adults are basically the same in the *DSM-III-R (Diagnostic and Statistical Manual of the American Psychiatric Association, Third Edition, Revised* (American Psychiatric Association 1987). However, certain difficulties may arise in using adult criteria to diagnose children. For example, melancholia is difficult to diagnose in children because their current depression is usually their first episode, and they are not old enough to have a personality disturbance or to have previous somatic treatment such as antidepressant medication. Having had previous episodes, a good previous response to tricyclics, and no personality disturbance prior to the first major depressive episode are three of the nine criteria for melancholia. Thus, for a child to meet *DSM-III-R* criteria for melancholia, he or she would typically have to meet five of the remaining six criteria, which in effect makes the criteria much more restrictive for children than adults.

Children with depression also have frequent somatic complaints, conduct symptoms, antisocial behavior, alcohol and drug use, aggressive outbursts, agitation, and mood-congruent hallucinations associated with affective episodes. In adolescents, psychiatric symptoms of bipolar disorder may be so florid as to suggest schizophrenia. The distinction between primary affective disorders and primary conduct, drug, alcohol, schizophrenic, or somatic disorders can often be clarified by determining the onset of symptoms. For example, if symptoms of conduct disorder are severe and predate the onset of the affective disorder, then a diagnosis of a secondary mood disorder and a primary conduct disorder is more likely than a diagnosis of a primary mood disorder (Carlson and Cantwell 1980).

Seasonal affective disorder (depression with seasonal pattern) may also be difficult to diagnose in children. For example, children with school problems may do fine during the summer and begin to manifest behavioral and affective symptoms when school starts in the fall. Since fall is the usual onset specified for seasonal affective disorder, it can be difficult to determine if affective symptoms occurring at this time are truly seasonal or are being precipitated by the stresses associated with starting school. Finally, children may lose a parent by death or have their family disrupted by divorce and present with depressive symptomatology that actually represents a state of bereavement (Weller and Weller 1990).

The types of depression described in *DSM-III-R* are listed in Table 12–1. Almost all have in common the presence of a *major depressive episode*, which is defined by *DSM-III-R* criteria as the presence of five or more of the following signs and symptoms for 2 weeks or more: (1) depressed mood; (2) loss of interest or pleasure; (3) significant weight loss or weight gain; (4) insomnia or hypersomnia; (5) psychomotor agitation or retardation; (6) loss of energy

TABLE 12-1

TYPES OF DEPRESSION ACCORDING TO *DSM-III-R*

Major depressive disorder, single episode or recurrent
Major depressive disorder, melancholic type
Major depressive disorder, with seasonal pattern
Major depressive disorder, with psychotic features
Dysthymia
Depressive disorder, not otherwise specified
Bipolar disorder, depressed
Cyclothymia
Adjustment disorder with depressed mood
Organic mood disorder
Uncomplicated bereavement

or fatigue; (7) feelings of worthlessness or excessive or inappropriate guilt; (8) decreased concentration; and (9) recurrent thoughts of death, suicide, or a suicide attempt or plan for committing suicide. Many of the studies reviewed in this chapter used these or very similar criteria to diagnose a depressive episode in children and adolescents.

EPIDEMIOLOGY

The incidence and prevalence of childhood and adolescent depression vary according to age, the sample selected, and the criteria and instruments used to diagnose depression. In preschoolers, the prevalence was about 0.3 percent (Kashani and Sherman 1988), and in prepubertal children the prevalence was about 1.8 percent. In 14- to 16-year-olds, the prevalence was 4.7 percent, which is close to adult levels (Robins and Regier 1991).

The prevalence of depression is much higher in clinically derived samples. In pediatric inpatients, the rate is about 7 percent, and in pediatric neurologic inpatients about 40 percent. In psychiatric inpatients, the rate varies from 13 to 59 percent, depending on the study. In psychiatric outpatients, it is about 28 percent (Kashani and Sherman 1988), and in an educational diagnostic clinic, it was about 53 percent (Weinberg et al. 1973).

NEUROENDOCRINE FINDINGS

Neuroendocrine research in child psychiatry is in its infancy. Some of the preliminary neuroendocrine findings in children are similar to those found in adults; however, the findings are few and varied. Weller and Weller (1988) have reviewed these findings in some detail. In general, about 20 percent of children are hypersecretors of cortisol. Forty to seventy percent of children do not suppress cortisol after being given dexamethasone. These findings are inconsistent because of the varied methodology employed in the studies, so the authors could not draw any general conclusions. However, the preponderance of evidence suggests that neuroendocrine findings similar to those seen in adult depression are present in some subset of depressed children and adolescents.

PSYCHOPHARMACOLOGIC TREATMENT

Historically, psychopharmacology in psychiatry has focused on symptoms. Symptoms can be dichotomized into target symptoms and side effects. Each symptom category requires baseline assessment and follow-up. Target symptoms may be clinically defined during the initial diagnostic work-up and then followed during treatment for improvement. However, studies to evaluate efficacy of a psychotherapeutic agent require a more systematic approach. Rating scales for assessing severity of depression, such as the Children's Depression Rating Scale (CDRS) (Poznanski et al. 1985), the Child Depression Inventory (CDI) (Kovacs and Beck 1977), the Bellevue Index of Depression (BID) (Petti 1978), and the Children's Depression Scale (CDS) (Lang and Tisher 1978), have been used to evaluate treatment response. The CDI and CDS are self-rating scales, and the CDRS and BID are administered by clinicians. The CDRS is similar to the Hamilton rating scale (HAM-D) (Hamilton 1960), and the CDI is similar to the Beck Depression Inventory (BDI) (Beck et al. 1961), and has been the most widely used depression rating scale. These instruments allow the researcher to be more thorough and systematic about assessing target symptoms and follow-up.

Side-effect symptom checklists also allow the same thoroughness in assessing the occurrence of adverse medication effects (Asberg et al. 1970, Gittelman-Klein and Klein 1973). Baseline assessments of side effects and target symptoms should be made prior to initiating treatment because symptoms may often be mistakenly ascribed to medication after it is started. Clinically, baseline data can be used to facilitate discussion with the patient as to whether the effect is due to the medication or merely attribution.

MEDICAL ASPECTS

After depression has been diagnosed and target symptoms and side effects have been assessed, the patient's medical status should be determined prior to initiating drug treatment. The initial medical work-up should include baseline ECG; measurement of height, weight, and vital signs; and blood tests. Blood tests should include CBC and differential, liver function tests, electrolytes, creatinine and BUN, and thyroid function tests.

The baseline ECG is necessary because at high blood levels, the antidepressants and their metabolites affect cardiac conduction (Preskorn et al. 1983). Without a baseline ECG, the clinician would not know if a finding of conduction defects was due to the antidepressants or was a preexisting condition. Also, because the blood level of antidepressants and their active metabolites is extremely variable in children and adolescents (Preskorn et al. 1989), blood level determinations of antidepressants and their metabolites are necessary to determine if children and adolescents are at risk for cardiac conduction effects and as a clinical guide for when to get repeated ECGs during treatment.

Preskorn and colleagues (1983) described an ECG study of sixteen children undergoing treatment with imipramine (IMI). Their ECGs were read by cardiologists blind to their treatment status and to their IMI and desmethylimipramine (DMI) blood levels. The PR and QT intervals were measured. Patients with plasma levels above 350 ng/ml had prolongation of the PR interval great enough to meet criteria for first-degree heart block. Children were then divided into two groups, one with total IMI plus DMI plasma levels less than 225 ng/ml and the other with levels greater than 225 ng/ml. Intracardiac conduction was slower and more impaired in those with plasma levels greater than 225 ng/ml. The high plasma level group also had higher diastolic blood pressures and heart rates. These findings emphasize the need for a baseline ECG and vital signs and antidepressant plasma levels.

Such levels are important because cardiac side effects are related to plasma levels and not mg/kg dosages. Preskorn and colleagues (1989) administered fixed 75-mg dosages of IMI to sixty-eight children. They found a 22-fold variability in IMI plus DMI levels, a 12-fold variability in IMI levels, and a 72-fold variability in DMI levels. The range of IMI plus DMI levels was from 25 to 553 ng/ml, of IMI from 20 to 236 ng/ml, and of DMI from 6 to 435 ng/ml. Thus, at a single fixed dose of IMI, a patient could either be subtherapeutic or toxic. Table 12–2 summarizes these results (adapted from Preskorn et al. 1989).

Children and adolescents require different dosages of medication to achieve the same plasma levels as in adults because of age-related differences in pharmacokinetics (Jatlow 1987). This is due to differences in the total volume of distribution of drugs, in the percent of body fat per total body weight, and in the rates of hepatic metabolism.

Volume of distribution is a significant factor in determining the levels for drugs, such as lithium, which are primarily distributed in body water. Volume of distribution is less of a factor for antidepressants because most antidepressants are lipophilic and their distribution is more affected by differences in body fat. Body fat changes with growth and development and varies according to gender. For example, a normal-weight 9-year-old girl will have a lower percentage of body fat than a normal-weight 16-year-old girl. However, a 9-year-old boy may have a greater percentage of body fat than a 16-year-old boy. Differences in volume of distribution due to body fat are probably no more than about 5 or 10 percent and by themselves do not explain the considerable variation in plasma levels.

Children and adolescents generally require much higher dosages to achieve the same plasma levels observed in adults. This is most likely due to their increased rate of hepatic metabolism. The rate of hepatic metabolism in prepubertal children is twice that of adults and even greater in children less than 5 years of age. The rate of metabolism decreases to adult levels around the age of 15 (Moriselli 1977). Some variability may also be accounted for by children who are rapid and slow metabolizers. However, the relationship between rapid and slow metabolizers and plasma levels of antidepressants in children has not yet been elucidated.

Some of the most notable adverse side effects of tricyclic antidepressants are due to their anticholinergic properties. These side effects are the same as those seen in adult patients: dry mouth, blurred vision, constipation, delayed micturition, and urinary retention. At higher tricyclic blood levels, cognitive changes and EEG changes can occur. These are reversible with a decrease in dose (Preskorn et al. 1983).

TABLE 12-2

IMI AND DMI PLASMA CONCENTRATION VARIABILITY[a]

Study	N	Age range	Diagnosis	Daily dosage	IMI variability	DMI variability	IMI + DMI variability
Rapoport et al. (1980)	40	7–12	Enuresis	Fixed 75 mg	NA	NA	15
Potter et al. (1982)	32	7–13	Enuresis	Fixed 75 mg	5.5	26	NA
Weller et al. (1982)	11	7–12	MDD	Fixed 75 mg	2.2	7	6
Puig-Antich et al. (1987)	30	9.6 ± 1.5	MDD	3–5 mg/kg	16	37	27
Preskorn et al. (1988)	68	6–14	Mixed[b]	Fixed 75 mg	12	72	22

[a]Adapted from Preskorn et al (1988). VAR (variability) = highest value/lowest value.
[b]Mixed = enuresis and MDD.
NA = not available.

Based on these findings, children should be started on low doses of tricyclics. After pharmacologic steady state has been achieved, their plasma levels should be measured. Steady state occurs after being on the same dose of medication for approximately 5 days (Weller et al. 1982). Plasma levels should be drawn 8 to 12 hours after the last dosage of medication. Steady state plasma levels should be repeated after each dosage adjustment until the combined IMI plus DMI levels are in the therapeutic range, which is greater than 125 ng/ml. Since ECG changes are primarily seen above 225 ng/ml, the ECG should be repeated as soon as the plasma levels are in the 125–225 ng/ml range and thereafter with each increase in dosage.

One of the major concerns about treating children and adolescents with antidepressants is that the cardiac conduction effects of the medication at higher doses might lead to cardiac failure and even death. Recently, Riddle and colleagues (1991) and Popper and Elliott (1990) discussed the occurrence of sudden death in children who had been taking tricyclic antidepressants. They presented information on three children who had died unexpectedly and speculated on the possible causes of the sudden deaths. They suggested that besides the cardiac effects of tricyclic antidepressants, other factors may have contributed to the deaths, such as a history of prior cardiac disorders, blood pressure and pulse changes, extreme physiologic stress, overheating, dehydration, tricyclic antidepressant–induced seizures, prior seizure disorders, interactions with over-the-counter medications or caffeinated drinks and foods, other unspecified drug interactions, and abrupt tricyclic antidepressant withdrawal. Because the information available on the three cases was limited, many of these possibilities were not addressed in the case reports.

The diagnostic characteristics and plasma levels of the tricyclics of the children who died are not clear. Two of the three children who died were being treated for attention deficit hyperactivity disorder and two of the three children had normal or low plasma levels of the tricyclic. Because the information available on these children was so limited, definite conclusions about the cause of the deaths could not be drawn. However, because the children were taking tricyclics, the possibility that they contributed to the deaths should be considered. A careful history and prescribing and cardiac monitoring should always be employed when using tricyclic antidepressants. The history should include information about the child's propensity for seizures, or a history of seizure disorder and any concurrent medication the child may be taking. The baseline ECG should be obtained before any medication is started, and medication should be prescribed at a low intial dosage and followed carefully.

EFFECTIVENESS OF PHARMACOLOGIC TREATMENT

Pharmacologic treatment of depression in adults is the paradigm for treating children and adolescents with medication. The effectiveness of treating adult depression with medication has been well established (Morris and Beck 1974). Depending on the adult population studied, 65 to 90 percent of adults with depression respond to antidepressants.

Ryan (1990) recently reviewed the use of antidepressants in children and adolescents. Because antidepressants that have a variety of ring structures are now available, he refers to them as *heterocyclic antidepressants*. The majority of the psychopharmacologic studies reviewed concern the tricyclic antidepressants. Some of the uncontrolled studies reviewed refer to the use of lithium and monoamine oxidase inhibitors. Controlled studies of psychopharmacologic treatment of depression in children and adolescents provide the best data on efficacy (Table 12-3). Because results differ for prepubertal children and adolescents, they are discussed separately. Later uncontrolled studies are reviewed (Table 12-4). Because these studies are not controlled, the evidence is less convincing. As can be seen, the results of the uncontrolled studies are more positive than those of the controlled studies. However, examining the uncontrolled studies provides some information in assessing the effectiveness of antidepressants in children and adolescents with depression.

CONTROLLED STUDIES IN CHILDREN

Only studies that used systematic diagnostic criteria to establish diagnosis, structured rating scales to assess improvement, and were published after 1976 were included. No further references to methodology will be made unless they are clinically relevant.

Puig-Antich and colleagues (1987) studied the effect of antidepressant medication in children with depression. They studied

TABLE 12-3

CONTROLLED STUDIES OF ANTIDEPRESSANT TREATMENT OF DEPRESSED CHILDREN & ADOLESCENTS

Author	Group	Criteria	Duration	Drug	Daily dosage	Drug response %	Placebo response %
Puig-Antich et al. (1987)	Child	RDC	5 weeks	IMI	3.25–5.0 mg/kg	9 of 16 (56)	5 of 22 (68)
Preskorn et al. (1987)	Child	DSM-III	6 weeks	IMI	25–150 mg	NA	NA
Geller et al. (1989)	Child	RDC	8 weeks	NT	27.5–115.0 mg	8 of 26 (30.8)	4 of 24 (16.7)
Geller et al. (1990)	Adol.	DSM-III	10 weeks	NT	67.3–121.3 mg	1 of 12 (8.3)	4 of 19 (21.1)
Kramer et al. (1981)	Adol.	Clinical	6 weeks	AMI	200 mg	8 of 10 (80)	6 of 10 (60)

NA = not available.

TABLE 12-4

Uncontrolled Studies of Drug Treatment in Depression

Author	Group	Criteria	Medication	Daily Dosage	N	Response (%)
Puig-Antich et al. (1979)	Child	RDC	IMI	50–145 mg	13	46
Preskorn et al. (1982)	Child	DSM-III	IMI	≤ 5 mg/kg	16	75
Petti et al. (1983)	Child	DSM-III	IMI	75–225 mg	21	67
Kashani et al. (1984)	Child	DSM-III	AMI	45–110 mg	9	67
Geller et al. (1986)	Child	RDC	NT	20–50 mg	22	64
Strober et al. (1990)	Adol.	RDC	IMI	150–300 mg	34	30
Ryan et al. (1986)	Adol.	RDC	IMI	1.7–5.2 mg/kg	34	44
Robbins et al. (1989)	Adol.	DSM-III	Tricyclics (TCAS)	NA	12	92
Ryan et al. (1988a)	Adol.	RDC	Li + TCAs	Li, 600–1500 mg	14	43
Ryan et al. (1988b)	Adol.	RDC	MAOIs	NA	23	62
Strober et al. (1992)	Adol.	RDC	Li + TCAs	Li, 0.66–1.19 mEq/L	24	42
Jain et al. (1992)	Adol.	DSM-III-R	Fluoxetine	20–80 mg	31	74

NA = not available.

thirty-eight prepubertal children who had major depressive disorder according to research diagnostic criteria (RDC) (Spitzer et al. 1978). The subjects were both inpatients and outpatients. The diagnosis was determined by two child psychiatrists who independently assessed the children. Depressed children were admitted to the study if they received a diagnosis of major depressive disorder by both psychiatrists and were excluded if they were medically ill or had other psychiatric disorders.

Of the thirty-eight subjects who were randomly assigned, sixteen were assigned to IMI and twenty-two were assigned to a placebo. After a 2-week drug-free period, they were started on either IMI or a placebo three times daily. IMI was started at a dose of 1.5 mg/kg/day and was gradually increased to 5 mg/kg/day. The dosage was maintained at this level from day 12 to day 35, which was the end of the study. The raters did not know the treatment condition or plasma levels. Children who were rated as only slightly or questionably depressed or anhedonic at the end of the study were considered responders.

The response rate for children on IMI was 56 percent, and the rate for children on the placebo was 68 percent. This was not a significant difference. The log (plasma IMI + DMI) significantly predicted clinical response ($p < .003$), and children who responded to active medication had higher plasma levels (mean 284 ± 225 ng/ml) than children who did not respond (145 ± 80 ng/ml). The authors concluded that because of the high placebo response rate (68 percent), they were unable to detect any effect of the active medication. They recommended that in future studies, all the children have a placebo washout phase several times a week to eliminate placebo responders prior to starting active medication. They also suggested the medication dosage be based on plasma IMI plus DMI levels rather than on a fixed mg/kg basis.

This study failed to demonstrate a clinically significant difference in response between children who had been treated with IMI or treated for the same length of time with a placebo. Among the children in the active medication group, there was a tendency for the response to be related to plasma IMI plus DMI levels. However, what this means is uncertain, because active medication was no different than the placebo.

Preskorn and colleagues (1987) also studied the effect of IMI in depressed prepubertal children. Twenty-two prepubertal children aged 6 to 12 were studied. The children were inpatients at the time of the study. They met *DSM-III* criteria for major depressive disorder and had been depressed for at least 30 days. They were diagnosed using the DICA, and the severity of their depression was rated using several systematic clinical rating scales. The dexamethasone suppression test (DST) was done on all patients.

After a 1-week baseline evaluation period, children who had not improved were randomly assigned to either IMI or a placebo. This was a double-blind study. A psychiatrist who was not involved with the children's clinical treatment or evaluation adjusted the dosage of IMI after 2 weeks of treatment so the IMI plus DMI level was between 125 and 250 ng/ml. The children were treated for 6 weeks total and evaluated for response to medication (or placebo) at the end of both the third and the sixth week.

The children treated with IMI had a bigger decrease in their severity ratings than those treated with the placebo. For example, at the end of the sixth week of treatment, the severity ratings of the children treated with IMI showed a 43 percent improvement over baseline compared with only a 35 percent improvement for children treated with placebo. When those children who were nonsuppressors on the DST were considered separately, 51 percent of the children treated with IMI improved, compared with only a 32 percent improvement for children treated with the placebo. These differences were statistically significant.

This study shows that the severity of symptoms improves more with active antidepressant medication than with a placebo. They did not mention the percentage of children who "responded" to medication, but they did mention the magnitude of symptom reduction. Children who were taking IMI were rated as less severely depressed (more improved) than children who took a placebo after treatment. IMI-treated children who were DST nonsuppressors had a more marked decrease in their symptoms than the corresponding placebo-treated children. This is the only controlled study that demonstrates a difference from a placebo. It may be that children who are DST nonsuppressors are more severely ill than DST suppressors and have a more biological depression, which is more likely to respond to antidepressants.

Geller and colleagues (1989), in another double-blind study, evaluated the effectiveness of nortriptyline (NT) versus a placebo. In this study, they made sure that the children were treated with adequate therapeutic dosages of medication. They studied fifty depressed outpatient children aged 5 to 12 who remained depressed at the end of a 2-week placebo washout phase. The children had been depressed for at least 2 months. They met RDC or *DSM-III* criteria for major depression. They were assessed with rating scales and were classified as responders if their ratings indicated minimal or no depression at the time of evaluation.

The children were randomly assigned to a placebo ($n = 24$) or NT ($n = 26$) and treated for 10 weeks. Their plasma levels were adjusted to be within the 60–100 ng/ml range. There was no difference in response between NT-treated patients and those receiving placebo. In fact, the response rate in both groups was quite low. The rate of response in the NT group was 30.8 percent and in the placebo group was 16.7 percent. The authors speculated that the low response rate may have been related to the chronicity or severity of the depression. It also might be that adrenergic medication may not be as effective in children, or that the plasma level selected as therapeutic may have been too low.

This study failed to demonstrate any difference between NT and a placebo. The children had been clinically depressed for 2 months or more and remained depressed after an initial 2-week period of nonspecific placebo treatment. They were treated with therapeutic dosages of NT at blood levels believed to be therapeutic in children. The rate of response was very low for both the placebo and medication.

In summary, the controlled studies in prepubertal children failed to demonstrate any difference between a placebo and active antidepressant medication treatment. The only positive finding for medication is that it does seem to reduce the severity of depressive symptoms more than a placebo. Thus, from the controlled studies it would appear that children treated with antidepressants are more symptomatically improved than placebo-treated children, but there is no difference in the percentage of children who respond to antidepressants or a placebo.

CONTROLLED STUDIES IN ADOLESCENTS

In adolescents, the situation is similar. Geller and colleagues (1990) studied the effectiveness of NT in depressed adolescents. Fifty-two depressed adolescent outpatients between the ages of 12 to 17 were studied. The authors diagnosed major depressive disorder according to *DSM-III* criteria. After a 2-week placebo washout period, the adolescents were randomly assigned to a placebo (n = 19) or NT (n = 12). All were followed for an additional 8 weeks.

Plasma levels of NT were then adjusted to be within the therapeutic range, 60–100 ng/ml. Outcome was assessed using rating scales. The adolescents were classified as responders if their ratings indicated minimal or no depression at the time of assessment.

The response rate was similar in the NT and placebo groups. Correlations of severity with plasma levels suggested that the adolescents with higher plasma levels did worse than those with lower levels. Overall, 8.3 percent of the NT group and 21.4 percent of the placebo group responded. This response rate was even lower than in Geller and colleagues' (1986) similar study of prepubertal children.

This study failed to demonstrate any difference between NT and a placebo in adolescents. It is similar to the results in prepubertal children. The response rate was even lower than in prepubertal children, and there was a suggestion that higher levels of medication were associated with a poorer response.

The only other double-blind placebo-controlled study of antidepressant treatment of adolescents was done by Kramer and Feiguine (1981). This was a study that was done earlier than the more recent studies by Geller and colleagues (1990). Their diagnoses were less precise and their follow-up assessments were less systematic than the later studies. However, because they were evaluating the effectiveness of an antidepressant other than IMI (amitriptyline), this study deserves mention.

They compared amitriptyline (AMI) with a placebo in twenty adolescents with depression. They used a structured interview to diagnose depression, but they also used the Minnesota Multiphasic Personality Inventory (MMPI) to verify the diagnosis. Because the MMPI is a cross-sectional instrument, all that is apparent is that the adolescents were depressed at the time they took the test. However, since precipitants, duration, and severity are not addressed by the MMPI, it is not clear how depressed the children actually were or how long they had been depressed. In this study, the depression criteria resembled those of Feighner and colleagues (1972), which are similar to *DSM-III* criteria.

The adolescents were randomly assigned to a placebo or AMI

and treated for 6 weeks. A placebo washout phase and plasma level monitoring were not used. Overall, 80 percent responded to AMI and 60 percent responded to the placebo. These findings demonstrate that children who are depressed have a high placebo response rate.

This study showed a nonsignificant difference between AMI and placebo. The percentage of children who responded to either was high. This study does not demonstrate that the clinical response to AMI is any different than the response to the placebo.

Both controlled studies of antidepressant treatment of depressed adolescents do not demonstrate any significant difference between antidepressant treatment and a placebo. This does not mean that antidepressants do not help, but it does mean that it has not yet been demonstrated. It also means that more controlled studies need to be done to answer this question, because in practice, antidepressants are frequently prescribed to children and adolescents who are depressed. The scientific evidence to support this clinical practice at the current time is lacking.

UNCONTROLLED STUDIES IN CHILDREN

Uncontrolled studies of antidepressant treatment in children and adolescents are included here because they may give us some clinical indication about which antidepressants may eventually prove to be helpful. Since antidepressants are currently being used clinically, it is useful to look at the uncontrolled studies to gain some understanding of which clinical variables may be relevant when prescribing (see Table 12-4).

Limitations of uncontrolled studies include lack of blindness, small sample size, lack of controls, failure to monitor blood levels, and outdated diagnostic criteria. In general, response rates are higher in uncontrolled studies. Controlled studies are done to eliminate biases that can result from the limitations mentioned above. Thus, the following uncontrolled studies in children and adolescents should be interpreted with this in mind.

Puig-Antich and colleagues (1979) studied the response of depressed children to IMI. The patients were thirteen prepubertal children ages 6 to 12. They were interested in determining if any clinical predictors of response could be determined. Major depression was diagnosed according to RDC (which are the same as

DSM-III criteria). Subjects had two diagnostic interviews scheduled 2 weeks apart. To be included in this study, they had to meet criteria for depression both times. Eleven were outpatients and two were inpatients. They were treated with IMI for 5 weeks, and plasma levels of IMI were obtained. The dosage range of IMI was from 50 to 145 mg/day. The children were considered responders if they were rated as not depressed or minimally depressed at the time of reassessment.

The overall response rate was 46 percent. Responders had a higher mean plasma IMI plus DMI level (231 ng/ml) than nonresponders (128 ng/ml). There was a positive correlation between plasma level and therapeutic response. The greatest response occurred in the patients with plasma levels greater than 200 ng/ml. Based on this, the authors suggested that a plasma IMI plus DMI level of greater than 146 ng/ml separated responders from nonresponders. Thus, in this study it appeared that there was a positive relationship between plasma level of medication and the clinical response of the child. Higher levels seemed to be associated with a better response.

Preskorn and colleagues (1982) also looked at the issue of predicting clinical response based on blood levels. They also used IMI to treat depressed children. They treated twenty prepubertal children ages 7 to 12. All met *DSM-III* criteria for major depression on the DICA. Rating scales were used to assess improvement, and plasma IMI levels were done. All the children were inpatients. IMI was used only in subjects who failed to improve after an initial 2-week period of inpatient counseling, observation, and assessment.

The children were treated with a fixed dosage of 75 mg of IMI for the first 3 weeks. After this period, if there was no response and adverse side effects were present, the dosage was decreased to 50 mg. If there was no response and no adverse side effects were present, the dosage was raised to a maximum of 5 mg/kg/day. The children were then treated for an additional 3 weeks with the adjusted dosage. The treating physician making the dose adjustments was blind to the plasma levels of IMI. This was to ensure that knowledge of the blood levels did not bias the physicians' clinical impressions.

Remission was defined as a score of 1 or 2 on the clinical global impression scale (CGI) and a score of 10 or less on the CDI or CDRS. Remission occurred in 92 percent of the children with plasma levels of IMI and DMI between 125 and 225 ng/ml. Only one of four children with plasma levels outside this range remitted. Of sixteen children completing the study, twelve were responders. Thus, the overall response rate was 75 percent. Antidepressant response was most strongly correlated with total IMI and DMI levels. This study found that children with higher blood levels of the medication seemed to respond better.

Petti and Conners (1983) looked at the clinical response to IMI in children who had depression associated with other conditions. The other *DSM-III* conditions included depressive neurosis, other reaction of childhood depression, unsocialized aggressive reaction with depression, overanxious reaction, and runaway reaction. They studied twenty-one inpatients aged 7 to 13. The presence of depression was determined by the BID. The children were treated with IMI up to 5 mg/kg/day or 200 mg/day, whichever was lower. The actual range of dosages was from 75 to 225 mg daily. The children's response was evaluated by a rating scale. Improvement in one or more behaviors on the scale was the criteria indicating a positive response. Accordingly, 67 percent of the children were responders. Plasma IMI levels were not done. This clinical study showed that IMI seemed to be effective in depression associated with other diagnoses.

Kashani and colleagues (1984) studied the effect of AMI in depressed children. They used a double-blind crossover design to assess the effect of either AMI or a placebo. The children were nine inpatients aged 9 to 12 who met *DSM-III* criteria for major depressive disorder. Children and parents were interviewed initially and reinterviewed at the end of each follow-up period using the BID. After a 3- to 4-week baseline period, patients were randomly assigned to either AMI or a placebo for 4 weeks and then crossed over to the alternative treatment for another 4 weeks. AMI was increased to a fixed dosage of 1.5 mg/kg/day after 3 days. The final dose of AMI ranged from 45 to 110 mg per day.

Of the children who improved, the children taking AMI had a much greater degree of improvement than the children taking the placebo. Plasma levels were not measured. This investigation indicated that while both medication- and placebo-treated children improved, the medication-treated children seemed to improve more.

Geller and colleagues (1986) attempted to determine if there was a therapeutic blood level of antidepressants in children treated with NT. They treated twenty-two outpatients 6 to 12 years of age with NT. Children met both RDC and *DSM-III* criteria for major depressive disorder. The CDRS rating scale was used for baseline and follow-up assessment of severity of depression. The patients were drug-free for 2 weeks and then started on NT. They were treated with a fixed dose of either 10 mg b.i.d. or 25 mg b.i.d. of NT based on their rate of drug metabolism. During the study, the raters were blind to the rate of metabolism and plasma levels.

In this study, 64 percent responded. The dosage and blood levels of the responders were significantly higher than those of the nonresponders. Higher levels and doses predicted greater improvement on the rating scale. Nine of the fourteen responders had plasma levels greater than 60 ng/ml. At the end of the study, seven of the eight nonresponders responded when their plasma levels were adjusted to be within the 60–100 ng/ml range. Based on this study, the authors suggested the therapeutic range of NT for children was 60–100 ng/ml. Although these findings were suggestive, this study indicated that when children were given enough medication, most of them seemed to respond.

The uncontrolled studies in children generally suggest that antidepressant medication is helpful in depression. The findings are much more optimistic than the findings in the controlled studies. As would be expected from uncontrolled studies, the rates of response were higher, and more correlations of blood levels with clinical response were found. These findings are probably in the direction expected by the clinical investigators and seem to demonstrate the reasons controlled studies are needed.

UNCONTROLLED STUDIES IN ADOLESCENTS

Uncontrolled studies usually form the clinical basis for more controlled research. They provide the clinicians and researchers with early suggestions about which therapies may hold promise and which may not. The uncontrolled studies in depressed adolescents basically addressed the same issues as the studies in prepubertal children. The initial studies attempted to determine if antidepressants were helpful and if therapeutic response could be predicted by clinical parameters similar to those in adults.

Ryan and colleagues (1986) evaluated how depressed adolescents respond to IMI and if blood levels were helpful in predicting response. The 34 adolescents aged 10 to 17 met RDC for major depression. They came from both inpatient and outpatient settings. They were treated for 6 weeks with IMI and plasma levels were measured. Response was defined as a significant increase in pleasure and interest as noted on the rating scale. Raters were blind to plasma levels. Overall, 44 percent of the adolescents were responders. There was no correlation between total plasma levels and response. Therefore, from this study adolescents seemed to respond to antidepressant treatment, but their response was not related to their plasma level of medication.

Strober and colleagues (1990) also studied the response of depressed adolescents to IMI. They used an approach similar to that of Ryan and colleagues (1986). They tried to determine if plasma levels could predict a therapeutic response to IMI. They treated thirty-four inpatient adolescents aged 13 to 18 who met RDC and *DSM-III* criteria for major depression. Their dosages averaged 222 mg/day for 6 weeks. The rate of response in this study was 30 percent. The plasma levels did *not* differentiate responders from nonresponders. They did not find that plasma levels could predict the response of adolescents to IMI. In addition, the number of adolescents who responded to medication was low.

Clinically, the adolescents in this study were very depressed and had failed to respond to the placebo. Therefore, they can be considered as more treatment resistant than the usual adolescent with depression. Just as they did not respond to the placebo, they also did not seem to respond to IMI. Although this study was an uncontrolled study, it was more scientifically rigorous, and the results were similar to the controlled studies.

Robbins, and colleagues (1989) evaluated the effectiveness of psychotherapy, milieu treatment, and antidepressants in adolescents with depression. They studied fifteen inpatient adolescents with major depression according to *DSM-III* criteria. They used the K-SADS for diagnosis and follow-up assessments. Response was defined as "slight" or "not at all" ratings for depression and anhedonia on the rating scale. The patients received 6 weeks of intensive psychosocial treatment followed by a trial of a variety of tricyclic antidepressants. All also were given a DST.

The patients were treated with a variety of antidepressants. The antidepressants used were DMI (10), IMI (2), AMI (2), and

NT (1). The patients were treated with dosages that produced plasma levels in the therapeutic ranges appropriate for adults. Twelve of the fifteen completed a trial of a antidepressant. Of the adolescents who completed the antidepressant trial, 92 percent were responders.

None of the DST nonsuppressors had responded to psychosocial treatment alone. One DST nonsuppressor responded to a combination of DMI and lithium carbonate. All seven of the patients who were DST nonsuppressors and completed the antidepressant trial responded to medication (six responded to antidepressants alone, and one responded to antidepressants and lithium). Five of twelve patients who were DST suppressors responded to medication also.

This study is of interest because all the adolescents had been treated with intense psychotherapy and psychosocial treatment for 6 weeks prior to treatment with medication. They had failed to respond. They therefore represent adolescents who are treatment resistant and who might be started on antidepressants after psychosocial treatment had failed. This is a common situation seen in clinical practice.

In an effort to increase the effectiveness of antidepressants, attempts have been made to augment their actions by treating patients concomitantly with augmenting medications such as lithium. This strategy has received only minimal study in children and adolescents.

Ryan and colleagues (1988a) studied the effect of augmenting tricyclic antidepressant treatment with lithium carbonate in fourteen adolescents. They had major depression according to RDC. Diagnoses were made using the K-SADS-P (Kiddie-SADS) based on the schedule for affective disorders and schizophrenia and the CGI was used to assess severity and improvement. The patients were three males and eleven females. They were from 14 to 19 years of age. They were treated with antidepressants for 1 to 9 months. About 80 percent had been treated at least 2 months before lithium carbonate augmentation was started. Outcome was assessed retrospectively by chart review using the CGI. A responder had a severity CGI rating of mild to borderline. An improved patient was described in the patient's record as "much to very much improved." Forty-three percent of the patients in this clinical chart review were much to very much improved, and 21 percent showed some improvement. The remainder (36 percent) did not respond. This study was descriptive and retrospective. It was done by chart review and was uncontrolled for the individual biases of the clinicians who were treating, and the results should be considered with these limitations in mind. These findings suggested lithium augmentation seems to be helpful after an adequate trial of tricyclics has failed.

Strober and colleagues (1992) also studied the effect of lithium augmentation on adolescents who had failed to respond to IMI. Their results were almost identical to Ryan and colleagues' (1988a) study. They studied the twenty-four adolescents who had failed to respond to IMI in their previously cited study (Strober et al. 1990), using the same methods. In addition, they added lithium carbonate in dosages sufficient to achieve levels in the 0.7–1.2 mEq/L range. The adolescents showed a 42 percent response rate to lithium augmentation. In addition, the response was cumulative with maximal response being observed after 3 weeks of lithium augmentation. According to this study, the clinician should stick to the lithium augmentation for at least 3 weeks before deciding that augmentation is not effective. Taken together, both Ryan and colleagues' (1988a) and Strober and colleagues' (1992) studies provide more convincing evidence that there exists a subpopulation of depressed adolescents who respond to the addition of lithium carbonate in therapeutic doses to their medication regimen.

One of the older uncontrolled studies of lithium suggested that it might be of benefit in children and adolescents with affective symptoms. Gram and Rafaelson (1972) studied thirteen male and five female adolescents diagnosed psychotic according to the World Health Organization (WHO) classification system. (This study was not included in Table 12–3 because that table is concerned with the antidepressant treatment of depression only. This study is mentioned here because it suggests an effect of lithium on depressed mood.) All of the children studied were in a special school and were followed by teacher and parent rating scales constructed for the study. The patients were treated using a double-blind placebo-controlled crossover randomized clinical trial. They were treated with either lithium sulfate or a placebo for 6 months and then crossed over to the alternative treatment for 6 months. Lithium levels were maintained in the 0.6–1.0 mEq/L range. Overall, nine of the eighteen patients responded positively to lithium and only one of eighteen to the placebo. Lithium showed the most noticeable effects on decreasing aggressiveness, decreasing hyperactivity, and improving mood. Although not specifically mentioned by the author, this suggests that lithium by itself may have an antidepressant effect in adolescents. This also might have been due to the presence of bipolar disorders among the so-named psychotic adolescents. This study was one of the early studies suggesting that lithium might be helpful in children and adolescents having affective symptoms.

In addition to lithium, monoamine oxidase inhibitors (MAOIs) and fluoxetine have been clinically studied in children and adolescents with depression. Ryan and colleagues (1988b) reviewed the charts of twenty-three adolescents who had been treated with MAOIs. All met criteria for major depression, definite or probable, by RDC using the K-SADS-P. Response to medication was determined by having one of the clinicians involved in the adolescent's care review the chart and rate global improvement on a 5-point scale (good, fair, slight, none, worse). Eighteen of the adolescents were on a tricyclic antidepressant and MAOI combination and four on MAOIs alone. Tranylcypromine and phenelzine were the MAOIs used. The rate of good improvement due to the tricyclic antidepressant and MAOI combinations was 62 percent. Another 13 percent had a fair response. Because most of these patients were treated with the MAOI and tricyclic antidepressant combination, it is not clear how much of the clinical response can be attributed to the MAOI alone.

Compliance with treatment can be a major problem with many adolescents. As a result, it was carefully assessed in this study. There were seven patients (30 percent) who were noncompliant with dietary restrictions. One patient made a suicide attempt, four patients were deliberately noncompliant (18 percent), and two patients (9 percent) were accidentally noncompliant. The 30 percent rate of noncompliance needs to be carefully considered before prescribing MAOIs to adolescents with refractory depressions.

Jain and colleagues (1992) studied the effect of fluoxetine in depressed children and adolescents. Their study was also a chart review study similar to the MAOI study mentioned above. They reviewed the charts of thirty-one hospitalized children and adolescents. One-third of the patients were in the prepubertal age range, and the remainder were adolescents. The children were not separated according to prepubertal or adolescent status, and the results were reported for the sample as a whole. This is unfortunate because preceding studies suggest that depressed prepubertal children may respond better than depressed adolescents. The children were diagnosed with major depression according to *DSM-III-R* criteria, and their response was assessed by the CGI rating scale. The dosage of fluoxetine ranged from 20 to 80 mg per day. The average dosage was not reported. Sixty-four percent of the patients received only 20 mg/day, 25 percent received 40 mg/day, 9 percent received 60 mg/day, and one patient (2 percent) received 80 mg/day.

Overall, 74 percent of the children and adolescents were judged to be responders, and 54 percent were judged to be much to very much improved. Thirty-nine percent of the children had an additional diagnosis such as attention deficit hyperactivity disorder, oppositional-defiant disorder, or conduct disorder. Thirty-five percent of the children received another medication, such as lithium or neuroleptics, concurrently. Because of the mixed characteristics of the sample and the presence of other effective medications, it is difficult to know if the therapeutic effects were related just to fluoxetine or to the combination. However, the authors point out that they observed no difference between those treated with fluoxetine alone and those with fluoxetine in combination with other medication. The most common reason for discontinuing fluoxetine was irritability or hypomaniclike symptoms. Although this study is uncontrolled, it does suggest that fluoxetine may be helpful in adolescents and children with depression.

The studies of Strober and colleagues (1990, 1992) and Ryan and colleagues (1986) deserve some additional comment. Although they were not randomized double-blind placebo-controlled studies, they were systematic and thorough. They studied well-defined populations of adolescents and were specific about their exclusion and inclusion criteria; had a placebo washout period; used structured interviews for diagnosis and follow-up; used accepted criteria for diagnosis; and used plasma levels to determine the correct dosage of IMI. Despite this, they still found relatively low response rates, rates consistent with the rigorous double-blind studies. The response rate was 30 percent for Strober's study and 44 percent for Ryan's study. However, in looking at Ryan's data, it appears as if eight of his subjects might have been prepubertal. If they were removed, the response rate for the remaining pubertal subjects would decrease to about 38 percent. This would be similar to Strober's findings. Thus, the response rate for antidepressants in children and adolescents with resistant depressions seems to be at best about 30 to 35 percent judging from both studies. So far, this has been found to not differ from the response rate to a placebo.

As is the case with prepubertal children, the uncontrolled studies show therapeutic optimism about the effectiveness of antidepressants in adolescents. The controlled studies that have been done have yet to justify that optimism. The uncontrolled studies, however, also indicate further studies that need to be done. Lithium, MAOIs, and augmentation strategies need to be studied more rigorously. These uncontrolled studies suggest that the indications for use of medication in adolescent depression may be forthcoming.

SUMMARY

In general, the more rigorous studies show low rates of response to antidepressants in children and adolescents suffering from depression. The available studies in children and adolescents do not demonstrate a significant advantage of active medication over placebo. The three double-blind placebo-controlled studies in prepubertal children did not demonstrate that the response rate to active medication differed significantly from the response rate to the placebo. The double-blind placebo-controlled studies in adolescents also indicated that the rate of response to antidepressants was no greater than to the placebo. The only controlled study supporting the effectiveness of antidepressants was the study by Preskorn and colleagues (1987), which showed IMI to be more effective than a placebo in reducing the severity of depressive symptoms. Also, the study by Kashani and colleagues (1984) suggests a similar finding for AMI, although that finding failed to reach statistical significance.

Although at the current time there is no evidence from controlled studies that there is any difference in the frequency of response to medication or a placebo, the degree of improvement in depressive symptoms may be greater in those children treated with antidepressants. Stated another way, children and adolescents who improve when treated with antidepressants show a greater degree of symptomatic improvement than children and adolescents who improve when treated with a placebo. The magnitude of improvement also seems to be greatest in children who are DST nonsuppressors. These findings are certainly preliminary and tentative. They need to be replicated by other well-designed experimental and clinical studies.

RECOMMENDATIONS

Given the current findings regarding the response of children and adolescents to antidepressant treatment, what should treatment be in children who meet criteria for depression? The psychopharmacologic treatment of children and adolescent depression should be undertaken cautiously. Patients and their parents need to be interviewed and a *DSM-III-R* diagnosis determined. The symptoms targeted for treatment need to be determined, and treatment should be based on these symptoms and the *DSM-III-R* diagnoses. According to current evidence, the patient should be treated and observed for 2 or more weeks without medication, unless the severity of depression precludes this approach. During this time, patients should receive psychotherapy and support. If they fail to respond to this initial approach and continue to be significantly depressed, they can be started on antidepressants. A DST should be done on inpatients; however, this is not always feasible in outpatients.

Although the literature indicates that the response rate to medication or a placebo is the same, it also indicates that the response rate to medication is higher than the response rate to a placebo in children who are DST nonsuppressors. The purpose of the DST is to help identify this subgroup of children and adolescents who are more likely to respond to antidepressants. For this reason, it is important to identify this group whenever possible.

Children and adolescents who do not respond to psychotherapy represent a population of children with treatment-resistant depressions. Antidepressants seem to ameliorate depressive symptoms in these children more than does a placebo. Although the response rates are low, children do respond, and a trial of medication is justifiable.

Once it is clinically decided to use antidepressants, low dosages should be started initially to avoid toxicity in slow metabolizers. The medication chosen should be one with which there is the most cumulative experience and which is approved for use in children (e.g., IMI). The dosage of medication should be based on blood levels whenever possible. Doses should be increased until within the therapeutic range based on the blood levels. Therapeutic ranges for IMI plus DMI are 125–225 ng/ml, and for NT 60–100 ng/ml. Patients should be treated for at least 6 to 10 weeks with plasma levels in the therapeutic range before switching to another medication.

An ECG should be done as part of the initial work-up. As previously mentioned, the ECG is a necessary part of the initial evaluation. At higher plasma levels of antidepressants children can develop conduction defects and cardiac irregularities. A baseline ECG will allow the clinician to determine if any abnormalities observed after the child has been on antidepressants are likely due to the medication or were previously present at the time of the initial work-up. If conduction defects are already present, then the clinician can also determine if the potential benefit of medication justifies the risk. Tricyclic antidepressants should not be started if the PR interval is $\geq$ 0.21 seconds or the QRS interval is $\geq$ 0.12 seconds. If after treating with antidepressants the heart rate exceeds 130 bpm, the blood pressure is > 130 mmHg systolic or 85 mmHg diastolic, the QRS interval is > 30 percent over baseline, or the PR interval is > 0.21 seconds, the clinician should seriously consider either decreasing or discontinuing the antidepressant. When the plasma levels are in the therapeutic range, a repeat ECG should be done. If the medication is to be increased further after therapeutic plasma levels are reached, then the ECG should be repeated with each additional increase.

Plasma levels of antidepressants should be obtained after the patient has achieved pharmacologic steady state. Steady state usually occurs after 5 to 7 days on the same medication dose for most antidepressants. Plasma levels should be drawn 8 to 12 hours after the last dose, so that the resultant level reflects the low average blood level rather than a peak level. The values quoted in this chapter are based on blood levels drawn as such.

The target symptoms and side effects need to be followed clinically and carefully and vital signs taken at each visit. When antidepressants are discontinued, they should be tapered rather than abruptly discontinued to prevent any possible withdrawal effects. Children and adolescents have been noted to experience a flu-like syndrome when antidepressants are abruptly discontinued. If a medication is to be used that is not currently approved by the FDA for use in children, the parent and child need to be informed. In any event, appropriate parental consent and assent of the child need to be obtained. By considering these principles and precautions, it is possible to effectively and safely treat children and adolescents with psychopharmacologic agents, such as antidepressants, when it is clinically indicated.

The studies of pharmacologic treatment of depression in children and adolescents are few, and controlled studies for newer antidepressants, MAOIs, and lithium augmentation have not been done. Lithium may be effective as an antidepressant alone or may be used to augment the response to antidepressants. MAOIs need to be used with caution because of compliance problems in children and adolescents; however, they may be helpful in treatment-resistant depressions and dysthymic disorders. The serotonergic medication fluoxetine may be effective in children and adolescents. However, there are no published controlled studies for the other serotonergic medications, clomipramine and sertraline.

The current state of psychopharmacologic treatment of depression in children and adolescents is in its toddlerhood. The available studies show a glimmer of promise for the effectiveness of medication. Multicenter studies need to be done. Newer medications need to be studied in randomized double-blind placebo-controlled clinical trials. Studies comparing the effectiveness of psychotherapy and medication need to be done. It is hoped that in the coming years, research and a scientific approach to treatment and outcome will reveal what works and what does not.

REFERENCES

American Psychiatric Association (1987). *Diagnostic and Statistical Manual of Mental Disorders.* 3rd ed. rev. Washington, DC: American Psychiatric Association.

Asberg, M., Crenhohn, B., Sjoquist, F., et al. (1970) Correlation of subjective side effects with plasma concentrations of nortriptyline. *British Medical Journal* 4:18–21.

Beck, A. T., Ward, C. H., Mendeson, M., et al. (1961) An inventory for measuring depression. *Archives of General Psychiatry* 4:562–571.

Cantwell, D. P., (1983). Depression in childhood: clinical picture and diagnostic criteria. In *Affective Disorders in Childhood and Adolescence*, ed.

D. P. Cantwell and G. A., Carlson, pp. 3-18. Jamaica, NY: Spectrum.

Cantwell, D. P., and Baker, L. (1989). Stability and natural history of *DSM-III* childhood diagnoses. *Journal of the American Academy of Child and Adolescent Psychiatry* 28:691-700.

Carlson, G. A, and Cantwell, D. P. (1980). A survey of depressive symptoms, syndrome and disorder in a child psychiatric population. *Journal of Child Psychology and Psychiatry* 21:19-25.

Carlson, G. A., and Strober, M. (1978). Affective disorders in adolescence: issues in misdiagnosis. *Journal of Clinical Psychiatry* 39:59-66.

Costello, A. J., Edelbrock, C., Dulcan, M. K., et al. (1984). Final report to NIMH on the Diagnostic Interview Schedule for Children. Unpublished manuscript.

Feighner, J. P., Robins, E., Guze, S. G., et al. (1972). Diagnostic criteria for use in psychiatric research. *Archives of General Psychiatry* 26:57-63.

Geller, B., Cooper, T. B., Chestnut, E. C., et al. (1986). Preliminary data on the relationship between nortriptyline plasma level and response in depressed children. *American Journal of Psychiatry* 143:1283-1286.

Geller, B., Cooper, T. B., Graham, D. L., et al. (1990). Double-blind placebo-controlled study of nortriptyline in depressed adolescents using a "fixed plasma level" design. *Psychopharmacology Bulletin* 26:85-90.

Geller, B., Cooper, T. B., McCombs, H. G., et al. (1989). Double-blind, placebo-controlled study of nortriptyline in depressed children using a "fixed plasma level" design. *Psychopharmacology Bulletin* 25:101-108.

Gittelman-Klein, R., and Klein, D.F. (1973). School phobia: diagnostic considerations in light of imipramine effects. *Journal of Nervous and Mental Disorders* 156:199-215.

Gram, L. F., and Rafaelson, O. J. (1972). Lithium treatment of psychotic children and adolescents. *Acta Psychiatrica Scandinavica* 48:253-260.

Gutterman, E. M. O'Brien, J. D., and Young, J.G. (1987). Structured diagnostic interviews for children and adolescents: current status and future directions. *Journal of the American Academy Child and Adolescent Psychiatry* 26:621-630.

Hamilton, M. (1960) A rating scale for depression. *Journal of Neurology, Neurosurgery and Psychiatry* 23:56-62.

Herjanic, B., and Campbell, W. (1977) Differentiating psychiatrically disturbed children on the basis of a structured interview. *Abnormal Child Psychology* 5:127-134.

Jain, U., Birmaher, B., Garcia, M., et al. (1992). Fluoxetine in children and adolescents with mood disorders: a chart review of efficacy and adverse effects. *Journal of Child and Adolescent Psychopharmacology* 2:259-263.

Jatlow, P. L. (1987). Psychiatric pharmacoscience of children and adolescents. In *The Progress in Psychiatry Series*, ed. C. Popper, pp. 29-44. Washington, DC: American Psychiatric Press.

Kashani, J. H., Shekirn, W. O, and Reid, J.C. (1984). Amitriptyline in children with major depressive disorders: a double-blind crossover pilot study. *Journal of the American Academy of Child Psychiatry* 23:348-351.

Kashani, J. H., and Sherman, D. D. (1988) Childhood depression: epidemiology, etiological models, and treatment implications. *Integrative Psychiatry* 6:1-21.

Kovacs, M. (1978) The interview schedule for children (ISC): interrater and parent–child agreement. Unpublished manuscript.

Kovacs, M., and Beck, A. T. (1977). An empirical clinical approach toward a definition of childhood depression. In *Depression in Childhood: Diagnosis, Treatment, and Conceptual Models*, ed. J. G. Schulterbrandt, pp. 1-25. New York: Raven.

Kramer, A. D., and Feiguine, B. A. (1981). Clinical effects of amitriptyline in adolescent depression. *Journal of the American Academy of Child and Adolescent Psychiatry* 20:636-644.

Lang, M., and Tisher, M. (1978). *Children's Depression Scale.* Victoria, Australia: Australian Council for Educational Research.

Lucas, A. R., Lockett, H. J, and Grimm, F. (1965). Amitriptyline in childhood depression. *Disorders of the Nervous System* 26:105-110.

Morris, J., and Beck, A. T. (1974). The efficacy of antidepressant drugs. *Archives of General Psychiatry* 30:667-674.

Moriselli, P. L. (1977) *Drug Disposition During Development.* New York: Spectrum.

Petti, T. A. (1978). Depression in hospitalized child psychiatry patients: approaches to measuring depression. *Journal of the American Academy of Child Psychiatry* 17:49-59.

Petti, T. A., and Conners, C. K. (1983). Changes in behavioral ratings of depressed children treated with imipramine. *Journal of the American Academy of Child Psychiatry* 22:355-360.

Popper, C. W., and Elliott, G. R. (1990). Sudden death and tricyclic antidepressants: clinical considerations for children. *Journal of Child and Adolescent Psychopharmacology* 1:125-132.

Potter, W. Z., Calil, H. M., Suffin, T. A., et al. (1982). Active metabolites of imipramine and desipramine in man. *Clinical Pharmacology and Therapeutics* 31:1146-1152.

Poznanski, E. O., Freeman, L. N., and Moklos, H. B. (1985). Children's depression rating scale, revised September, 1984. *Psychopharmacology Bulletin* 21:979-989.

Preskorn, S. H., Bupp, S. J., Weller, E. B., and Weller, R.A. (1989).

Plasma levels of imipramine and metabolites in 68 hospitalized children. *Journal of the American Academy of Child and Adolescent Psychiatry* 28(3):373–375.

Preskorn, S. H., Jerkovich, G. S., Hughes, C., et al. (1988). Depression in children: concentrative dependent CNS toxicity of tricyclic antidepressants. *Psychopharmacology Bulletin* 24:275–279.

Preskorn, S. H., Weller, E. B., Hughes, C. W., et al. (1987). Depression in prepubertal children: dexamethasone non-suppression predicts differential response to imipramine vs placebo. *Psychopharmacology Bulletin* 23:128–133.

Preskorn, S. H., Weller, E. B., and Weller, R. A. (1982). Depression in children: relationship between plasma imipramine levels and response. *Journal of Clinical Psychiatry* 43:450–453.

Preskorn, S. H., Weller, E. B., Weller, R. A., and Glotzbach, E. (1983). Plasma levels of imipramine and adverse effects in children. *American Journal of Psychiatry* 140:1332–1335.

Puig-Antich, J., and Chambers, W. (1978). *The Schedule for Affective Disorders and Schizophrenia for School-Age Children* (Kiddie-SADS). New York: New York State Psychiatric Institute.

Puig-Antich, J., Perel, J. M., Lupatkin, W., et al. (1987). Imipramine in prepubertal major depressive disorder. *Archives of General Psychiatry* 44:81–89.

Puig-Antich, J., Perel, J. M., and Lupatkin, W. et al. (1979). Plasma levels of imipramine (IMI) and desmethylimipramine (DMI) and clinical response in prepubertal major depressive disorder: a preliminary report. *Journal of the American Academy of Child Psychiatry* 18:616–627.

Rapoport, J. L., Mikkelsen, E. J., Zavadil, A., et al. (1980). Childhood enuresis. *Archives of General Psychiatry* 37:1146–1152.

Riddle, M. A., Nelson, J. C., Kleinman, C. S., et al. (1991) Sudden death in children receiving norpramin: a review of three reported cases and commentary. *Journal of the American Academy of Child and Adolescent Psychiatry* 30:104–108.

Robbins, D. R., Alessi, N. E., and Colfer, M. V. (1989) Treatment of adolescents with major depression: implications of the DST and melancholic clinical subtype. *Journal of Affective Disorders* 17:99–104.

Robins, E. L., and Regier, D. A. (1991). *Psychiatric Disorders in America.* New York: The Free Press.

Ryan, N. D. (1990). Heterocyclic antidepressants in children and adolescents. *Journal of Child and Adolescent Psychopharmacology* 1:21–31.

Ryan, N. D., Meyer, V., Dachille, S., et al. (1988a) Lithium antidepressant augmentation in TCA-refractory depression in adolescents. *Journal of the American Academy of Child and Adolescent Psychiatry* 27:371–376.

Ryan, N. D., Puig-Antich, J., Cooper, T., et al. (1986). Imipramine in adolescent major depression: plasma level and clinical response. *Acta Psychiatrica Scandinavica* 73:275–288.

Ryan, N. D., Puig-Antich, J., Rabinovich, H., et al. (1988b). Case study. MAOIs in adolescent major depression unresponsive to tricyclic antidepressants. *Journal of the American Academy of Child and Adolescent Psychiatry* 27:755–758.

Spitzer, R. L., Endicott, J., and Robins, E. (1978). Research diagnostic criteria: rationale and reliability. *Archives of General Psychiatry* 35:773–782.

Strober, M., Freeman, R., and Rigali, J. (1990). The pharmacotherapy of depressive illness in adolescence: I. An open-label trial of imipramine. *Psychopharmacology Bulletin* 26:80–84.

Strober, M., Freeman, R., Rigali, J., et al. (1992). The pharmacotherapy of depressive illness in adolescence: II. Effects of lithium augmentation in nonresponders to imipramine. *Journal of the American Academy of Child and Adolescent Psychiatry* 31:16–20.

Weinberg, W. A., Rutman, J., Sullivan, L., et al. (1973). Depression in children referred to an educational diagnostic center: diagnosis and treatment. *Journal of Pediatrics* 80:1065–1072.

Weller, E. B., and Weller, R. A. (1984). Current perspectives on major depressive disorders in children. Monograph Series. Washington, DC: American Psychiatric Press.

—— (1988). Neuroendocrine changes in affectively ill children and adolescents. *Neurologic Clinics* 6:41–53.

—— (1990). Grief in children and adolescents. In *Psychiatric Disorders in Children and Adolescents*, ed. B. D. Garfinkel, G. A. Carlson, and E. B. Weller, pp. 37–47. Philadelphia: Saunders.

Weller, E. B., Weller, R. A. Fristad, M. A., et al. (1988). Depressive symptoms in acutely bereaved children. 41st Annual Meeting of the American Psychiatric Association, Montreal, Canada, May 7–11.

Weller, E. B., Weller, R. A, Preskorn, S. H., and Glotzbach, R. (1982). Steady-state plasma imipramine levels in prepubertal depressed children. *American Journal of Psychiatry* 139:506–508.

13: PREVENTIVE INTERVENTION WITH CHILDREN OF DEPRESSED PARENTS

William Beardslee, M.D.
Linda Schwoeri, M.A., M.F.T.

INTRODUCTION

There is now extensive empirical evidence that growing up in a family with a parent who has an affective disorder presents a grave risk to children. This risk is intensified during the crisis years of adolescence. There has been increasing emphasis on the need for preventive interventions for such youngsters. However, despite the high rates of affective disorder in the general population, and the need for interventions expressed by a large number of clinicians from different disciplines, there are no preventive intervention programs available for families in which parents have an affective disorder. A consensus from a variety of sources, including clinicians who treat affective disorder in adults, supports the need for these programs (Anderson et al. 1986, Grunebaum 1984, Institute of Medicine 1989, Philips 1983).

This chapter discusses a prevention model based on a psychoeducational approach developed for use with families that have experienced recent parental affective disorder. The model is intended for clinical use among a wide range of practitioners, including psychologists, psychiatrists, internists, family practitioners, and pediatricians. The approach is based more on a public health model and less on a particular school of psychotherapy. It is not intended for families in the midst of an overwhelming life crisis because such families need treatment rather than preventive intervention. Furthermore, adolescents suffering acute depression need pharmacologic and/or psychotherapeutic intervention rather than preventive intervention. Therefore, this approach is best used by clinicians who are the first contact for families presenting with a parental affective illness.

As a psychoeducational prevention model, it involves educating parents and children in the biological/etiological aspects of depression, the psychosocial manifestations of the illness, and the risks to children. It aims to help children and adolescents develop plans for the future as well as understand the present course of the parental illness.

A central principle of the model is the belief that preventive intervention should incorporate information gained from the experience of resilient individuals. Studies of resiliency focus on the concept of self-understanding as the psychological process through which individuals make causal connections between experiences in the world at large and inner feelings. This process becomes an organizing principle that develops over time and eventually becomes a stable part of the individual's experience. Several theoretical and conceptual perspectives that contribute to the concept of self-understanding are briefly discussed. These perspectives include Hartmann's (1950, 1958) fundamental observation that there are a large number of internal psychological processes that are not defensive and do not rest on conflict. These processes are part of the conflict-free sphere of ego functioning, which includes adaptation, control, and integration. Self-understanding, seen as a cognitive function, is conceptualized as part of this conflict-free sphere. Self-understanding is partially rooted in a person's constitution and in life experience and is a part of the maturation process itself, independent of needs and life experience (Hartmann 1950, 1955).

Selman's (1980) theory of interpersonal negotiation contributes to an understanding of how resilient adolescents and adults utilize cognitive capacities in the development of mutuality in relationships. This emphasis on relationships outside the family is a major protective factor found in resilient individuals. Theoretical concepts from Beck (1963, 1967) and Seligman (1975, Seligman et al. 1979) on depressive cognitions and attributions provide a link to understanding the effect of depression on cognition and indicate some of the challenges faced by children whose parent has an affective disorder.

The four major components of the approach are (1) assessment of family members, (2) cognitive teaching about affective disorders and risks and resiliencies in children, (3) the child's experiences and development of plans for the future, and (4) family discussion. The goal is to link understanding of the illness to the development of concrete plans for helping the child cope in the future. Clinical methodology of the approach will be outlined and briefly discussed in another section of this chapter.

THE NEED FOR INTERVENTION

Empirical studies employing different conceptual frameworks and methods have demonstrated that children of parents with affective disorders fare much more poorly than controls. There is documentation of serious psychopathology in these children (Beardslee 1986; Beardslee et al. 1983, 1985, 1988b, Decina et al. 1983, Gershon et al. 1985, Keitner 1990, Keller et al. 1986, Merikangas et al. 1988, Orvaschel et al., 1988, Weissman et al. 1984a,b). Rates of affective disorder in the risk groups range from 11 percent to over 50 percent. A variety of reviews within the past 5 years have documented these figures (Lee and Gotlib 1989, Orvaschel et al. 1988, Rutter 1990, Waters 1987). In their summary of studies, Downey and Coyne (1990) report that children of affectively ill parents have a rate of depression that is several times that of control children. There is also increased awareness of the chronic nature of affective disorder in adults, particularly the combination of a chronic depression along with acute episodes (Keller et al. 1983).

Beardslee and colleagues (1983) and Keller and colleagues (1988) suggest that depression in such high-risk samples shows a strong resemblance to depression presenting for clinical treatment. Despite this clinical finding, only about one-fourth of the children receive treatment (Keller et al. 1991). In their longitudinal study of diagnoses in children of women with unipolar and bipolar affective disorder, Hammen and colleagues (1990) found that by age 18, approximately 80 percent of the children will receive a major psychiatric diagnosis.

Empirical findings suggest higher lifetime rates of diagnosable general psychopathology. Higher rates of episodes of major depression are reported in the offspring (ages 6–19) of parents who present for psychiatric treatment for affective disorder when compared with those in families without illness (Beardslee et al. 1985, Cytryn et al. 1982, Weissman et al. 1984a, Welner and Garrison 1985). The incidence of episodes of major depression in the children of parents with affective disorders increases significantly throughout adolescence. In the four above-cited studies, the occurrence of an episode of affective disorder ranged between 10 and 40 percent by the end of adolescence.

As part of a study of children of parents with affective disorder, Beardslee and colleagues (1985) examined the validity of the diagnosis of major depression in nine children and adolescents. They found that disruptions in multiple domains of functioning accompanied the depression. All the children reported persistent feelings of worthlessness, guilt, and self-reproach, and periods of social withdrawal. The social withdrawal ranged in severity from loss of interest in usual activities, to pervasive, withdrawn behavior and refusal to get out of bed. In all the children, symptoms lasted longer than the period of time during which the episode met full *DSM-III* criteria. These children had academic difficulties despite adequate intellectual competence and significant problems with compliance, attentiveness, concentration, and commitment to academic tasks (Beardslee et al. 1985).

As a complement to clinical samples used for research on the risks to children with parents who have affective disorders, Beardslee and colleagues (1988) undertook a study from an HMO population. This study of a nonreferred sample provides an important statement about growing up in families in which parents have an affective illness. The sample consisted of 153 youngsters from 81 families. The sample broke down into three groups: (1) families in which parents had never experienced any psychiatric disorder (twenty-one families with forty-five children), (2) families in which parents had experienced only nonaffective psychopathology (eleven families with nineteen children), and (3) families in which one or both parents had experienced affective disorder, sometimes in combination with other illnesses (forty-nine families with eighty-nine children).

There was considerable nonaffective psychopathology associated with the affective disorders. The most common diagnosis in the parents was major depressive disorder, followed by intermittent depressive disorder. The most common nonaffective diagnoses were alcoholism and different character pathology. Of the twenty-eight children in the sample diagnosed with either dysthymia or major depression, twenty-seven were in families in which parents had experienced serious affective disorder. Follow-up of this sample 4 years later with independent blind assessment of children further confirmed the powerful effect of parental affective illness on poor child outcome, because the rates of major depressive disorder were two and one-half times greater in children of parents with affective disorder, as opposed to children whose parents were not ill. It must be noted that parental affective disorder in this sample was strongly associated with nonaffective disorder and with divorce, as is often true clinically, hence, the youngsters were exposed to a constellation of risk factors (Beardslee et al. in press). This connection between affective disorder in parents and affective disorder in their children is striking, especially because it is obtained in a nonreferred sample. The findings draw added attention to the concern for children growing up in families in which parents do not present clinically for treatment.

RESILIENCY IN CHILDREN OF MENTALLY ILL PARENTS

Despite the many risk factors involved, there is evidence that children can and do successfully survive parental psychopathology through their own ability to adjust and cope. The terms *resilient* and *invulnerable* are commonly applied to these children. In his initial studies of invulnerability, Anthony (1976) noted that the children resisted becoming enmeshed in the parental psychopathology, showed intellectual curiosity in understanding what troubled the ill parent, maintained a compassionate but detached approach to the troubled parent, did not become overwhelmed by a series of interconnected troublesome life events, and were able to receive some emotional support from the well parent. Similar findings were reported in Garmezy's (1971, 1974, 1983) studies of resilient children of psychologically disturbed parents as well as in Rutter's (1979, 1981) studies of children of psychotic parents. These findings are more recently reported in the work of Garmezy. Rutter's (1986) work suggests that having a good relationship with the well parent is an important factor in resiliency. Beardslee and Podorefsky's (1988a) study of the use of other relationships in aiding resilience has added to the literature on coping with the stress and trauma of having an affectively disturbed parent. These studies provide background and structure for a preventive intervention approach with families because they indicate some of what is involved in surviving depression in the family.

Dimensions of Self-understanding from Studies of Resiliency

Findings from the studies of resiliency contribute to an understanding of how individuals adjust and cope with adverse conditions such as the presence of mental illness. Findings must always be interpreted in terms of the developmental period or life stage of the individuals involved because problem-solving skills and social cognitive skills undergo significant developmental changes. Variability in children's perception and response depends on their age and cognitive and emotional development.

A preschooler does not have the cognitive skills available to a child of school age and beyond. The younger child cannot strategize and many times is not even able to identify what the problem actually is. He or she responds out of sheer frustration because he or she has no sense of an inner world versus an outer world. The older child, if only through daily life experience, can absorb information and is more likely to think about situations, strategize, plan, and then act to solve a problem. The older child can likewise begin to understand motives and consequences (Maccoby 1987). He or she is able to assume the role of another and reflect back on an experience. The older child is aware of being able to put certain thoughts out of his or her mind as if to say he or she knows it but doesn't want to think or talk about it. This ego capacity helps the older child gain control of inner feelings and outer reactions to those feelings.

The studies of resiliency (Beardslee 1981, 1983, Beardslee and Podorefsky 1988) identify dimensions that might be amenable to preventive intervention. They reflect information based on adolescent and adult experiences of severe stress. The three studies underscore the presence of psychological qualities such as self-understanding and separateness in resilience. Together they provide information on the three main components of self-understanding. These include (1) a realistic appraisal of the stresses to be dealt with, (2) a realistic appraisal of the capacity to act and a sense of importance and effect of one's actions, and (3) actions that are congruent with one's view of one's parents' and one's own abilities.

Adequate Cognitive Appraisal

In these three studies of Beardslee (1981, 1983, 1988, Beardslee and Podorefsky 1988a), the individuals faced complex life situations: the turmoil of the civil rights movement, the struggle with childhood cancer, a life with parents who have an affective disorder. In each case, they had to appraise the stresses they faced and make the needed changes in response to these stresses. The children with parents who have an affective disorder also faced changing life situations, such as divorce, repeated parental hospitalization, and emotional loss of a parent to affective disorder. They were sensitive to factors in their family environment and recognized what their parents were experiencing. They changed their strategies for coping accordingly. In particular, these children had to distinguish between their own experience and that of their parents. They needed to form a separate identity and to not confuse their lives with those of their parents. They learned to talk about parental difficulties, be saddened by them, and remain empathic but not overwhelmed. They were aware that something was wrong with their parents but concluded that they themselves were not the cause of their parents' problems.

This appraisal and realization that it was not their fault were crucial and enhanced their ability to cope with the experience of having a mentally ill parent. Zahn-Waxler and colleagues (1990) point out that the symptoms of guilt that are expressed in the behaviors of depressed caregivers make them sensitive to issues of blame, suffering, and responsibility. In their attempt to handle tasks and responsibilities, these depressed caregivers are prone to share the burdens and blame with their children. The children inadvertently begin to feel responsible for negative events in the lives of their parents, simply by being there. This is especially difficult for the younger child, who quite readily assumes blame for a parent's unhappiness over something he or she has done.

Seligman's Learned Helplessness Model (1975) is relevant to

understanding this behavior in children. The Learned Helplessness Model asserts that the depressed person expects bad events to occur and that there is nothing he or she can do to prevent them. The depressed person, according to the model, expects failure to occur regardless of his or her behavior; therefore, he or she is not motivated to respond. Seligman's reformulated attribution theory, as discussed by Abramson and colleagues (1978), discusses the three attributional dimensions that govern when and where helplessness deficits appear. Depressed persons view the causes of negative events as internal; therefore, they see themselves as the cause. The causes of events are perceived by them as global and as, therefore, destroying everything they do. Lastly, depressed persons see the causes of events as stable and lasting forever. Children with parents who are depressed or have an affective disorder are exposed to these negative attributions as well as a whole range of depressive cognitions. They may inevitably begin to model their parents' way of viewing responsibility for the events around them and run the risk of feeling just as helpless. Furthermore, young children may not be able to distinguish between problems they have created and those that were started by or belong to another. They attempt to respond to this incomprehensible, depressed negative behavior by showing concern, internalizing responsibility, or attempting to change the situation by helping, sharing, or soothing the depressed parent (Radke-Yarrow and Zahn-Waxler 1984, Zahn-Waxler and Radke-Yarrow 1982, Zahn-Waxler et al. 1979). They may inadvertently become overly involved in or even identified with the depressed parent's problems. As a result of this overinvolvement, these children are deprived of the needed social and extrafamilial developmental experiences needed to protect or distance themselves from the parent's illness. This has serious implications for future adaptation in both family and social interaction. Children quickly acquire the idea that they are incapable of succeeding at tasks once they learned to be helpless, as the studies by Seligman and Maier (1967) have shown.

The Beardslee and Podorefsky (1988a) study of resilient adolescents discussed these adolescents' views of their lives as caretakers, peacemakers, and helpers in the family. However, these adolescents also described how they were able to differentiate themselves from their parents' experiences. In a sense, they developed empathy for the parents' experiences but did not lose their sense of identity or separateness from their parents. This cognitive competency is a key factor in helping children and adolescents adjust to their parent's illness. Resilient individuals display this ego strength, and it is therefore stressed in the intervention model with families.

Felsman and Vaillant (1987), in their report on resilient children as adults, note that one of the most intriguing qualities of the men with the best outcomes in the high-risk group was (and is) their apparent capacity to bear up to and endure multiple stresses. It has been shown in Rutter's (1979, Rutter et al. 1974) comparative studies of inner-city London and the Isle of Wight that what does lasting damage to a person's ability to cope is the experience of sustained emotional trauma. These studies seem to indicate that a multiplicity of stress factors actually determine a child's psychiatric risk. Anthony and Cohler (1987) suggest that two or three stress factors operating simultaneously increase the psychiatric risk factor fourfold (p. 307). The literature on risk for children with parents who have an affective disorder indicates multiple causality. Biological givens; parental personality and temperament factors; psychosocial stress factors including marital problems, diminished economic resources, and the loss of parental function and effectiveness — all contribute to the risks faced by children in these families.

Children form judgments about themselves based on their environment, and the environment of depression leads to negative evaluations of self and others. The idiosyncratic content and cognitive distortions that are present in the thinking of depressed individuals have an impact on a child's view of life. The depressed parent's experience of low self-regard, self-criticism, and self-blame, as well as the magnifications of duties and responsibilities, weighs heavily on his or her thinking and influences all his or her interactions. In his early work, Beck (1963, 1967) noted how the depressed individual's cognitions are filled with the "musts" and "shoulds" of responsibilities. These self-imposed commands get transferred to the children and form a large part of the tension in their interactions. Children whose parents have an affective disorder need help understanding that the injunctions are coming from the parent to the parent and are not really part of the child's responsibility. This helps them realistically appraise the situation, remain separate from it, and move on to problem-solve and plan a course of action.

Realistic appraisal of the capacity for and consequences of action

Resilient individuals had to assess their personal capacity for action and assess the effect of their personal actions. They learned to direct their energies to what they could do and not blame themselves for what was not accomplished. The children had to give up the dream of curing their parents and, at the same time, appraise how they could be of help, but in a limited way. This required a sense of identity and control over their situation. Perhaps a large part of this control was the knowledge gained through daily experience and the predictability of recurring events. There is a certain consistency and predictability to the course of depressive and affective disorder. Children can learn to expect certain behaviors and be prepared for consequences. This is not at all to minimize the adverse impact of parental affective disorder on a developing child's life; however, a child faced with a depressed parent can develop the capacity to overcome the trauma and, in time, adjust. Rather than viewing depression as a trauma that derails the child for life, it would appear that much can be done to help the child gain a sense of understanding and predictability in relation to the depression. Depression is an episodic, recurring illness. It has its expectable course of behaviors and extreme risks, and it can be treated with medication and therapy. In the course of family discussions, the family's experience of past events can be looked at and new strategies for coping can be developed. By gaining a better understanding of the parent's experience of the depression, the family can achieve some distance and express empathy. Identification with the depressed parent must be avoided at all costs.

Action

The three resiliency studies (Beardslee 1981, 1983, Beardslee and Podorefsky 1988a) show that resilient individuals are able to be engaged in actions in the world in addition to having an inner understanding of the complexities in their lives. These studies focused on adolescents and adults and, therefore, reflect competencies of those developmental periods. In view of this, the descriptive data collected in the follow-up assessment of the adolescents (Beardslee and Podorefsky 1988a), who were 14.6 to 22.8 years of age, provide a good example of these competencies. The researchers found that the adolescents and young adults were extensively and deeply involved in their academic pursuits, were deeply involved and committed to their jobs, and manifested the ability to persist in their work. The majority of them reported taking great pleasure in the varied activities they engaged in beyond work and school, and some even continued with athletics.

Another important aspect of resiliency and self-understanding is the ability to reach out to other relationships. This ability to form and maintain relationships outside the family indicates that individuals can function separately and independently of the family system. It also indicates that the adolescent (young adult) has reached a level of social-cognitive development in which he or she can understand and enter into the world of the other (i.e., through friendship and peer and family relationships) (Selman 1980). As Erikson (1963) points out, the mature sense of self includes a sense of mutuality or being able to give as well as receive. This is especially relevant for the adolescent's development because without this ability to form collaborative reciprocal relationships, the adolescent would have difficulty in personal, intimate relationships later in life. The existence of affective illness in the parent of an adolescent can impede the development of this capacity due to the impoverished interpersonal environment in the home. Beardslee and colleagues (1987) confirmed that there is a relationship between parental disorder and the adolescent's level of social-cognitive development. Adolescents do suffer in their capacity for interpersonal development in relation to the duration of the parental disorder. The parent's illness makes them neglect the essentials for mutual give-and-take. Modeling parental and family relationships is an especially important factor in the adolescent's development of social competence.

Adolescents should learn how to develop outside relationships because they offer the opportunity to make possible the developmental transition from focusing on the self to the understanding of and collaboration with others for the sake of mutual interest and intimacy (Broughton 1978, Damon and Hart, 1982, Selman 1980, Sullivan 1953, Youniss 1980). As shown in the Beardslee and Podorefsky (1988a) study of adolescents, these young people learned the importance of having relationships outside the family to turn to. Because their lives were full of disillusionment and confusion, and they suffered the loss of a role model or idealized loved one, they were left with considerable anger. Other relationships were crucial in allowing them to separate from their parents in an attempt to continue their own lives. Parentification of and identification with the ill parent are paramount obstacles to overcome when depression is in the family. The more resilient youngsters were able to understand the complexities in their situation and take appropriate action in order to avoid being enmeshed in the family illness. Very often, the child is inadvertently scapegoated into the situation or, even worse, pulled in as caretaker for the depressed parent. These resilient youngsters were helped by their cognitive competences, which made it possible to form healthier identifications and create new models for social relationships.

COMPONENTS OF THE PSYCHOEDUCATIONAL FAMILY INTERVENTION MODEL

The Psychoeducational Family Intervention Model was designed to be used by a number of different clinical disciplines. It is short-term and flexible in addressing the nature of explanations given to the family and in the kinds of intervention possible. Because it was conceived as an intervention based on the experience of resilient individuals, the knowledge gained from their experience was applied to the families.

In its present format, the intervention has been used in families in which parents have experienced a recent affective illness, often involving hospitalization. The children are in early to middle adolescence and have not yet become ill. This intervention can be flexibly applied to both single- and two-parent families. It can be performed by the primary clinician involved in treatment or by a separate clinician. The intervention covers four main areas: assessment, cognitive teaching, the child's present and future experience, and the family discussion of the parent's illness.

Format of the Model

The number of sessions is variable. Usually there are at least six but no more than ten. There is a combination of sessions involving parents alone, child (or children) alone, and parent and child (or children) together.

Assessment of Family Members

One or two parent-history sessions are held either with each spouse alone or with spouses together. The focus is on the parent's recent illness and past disorder and each spouse's experience and understanding of it.

Parents are asked to describe not only their histories but also how they think the children have experienced those histories. This helps the parent to take the child's perspective and elicits descriptive and useful information about everyday happenings, which is not always obtained from a traditional psychiatric history.

A vital element in the intervention is the family discussion. During the discussion, the child can gain a different perspective on the course of the illness and can understand that the behavior of depression is really discontinuous from normal behavior. The adolescents learn that their parents do not want to be the way they are, they are not the cause of the parent's behavior, and there is an alternative course in the future.

It is essential that the clinician demystify what has been a complex and confusing experience for the child. The children need to know that this event does not have to overwhelm them; they can understand it both cognitively and emotionally. This intervention model builds on known family and individual strengths, identifies risk factors, and helps the family plan for the future. It requires that the clinician be flexible in approach and able to be honest and open in discussing whatever the family feels is relevant. All need to work together to help the child or children adjust and cope with the family's situation.

In sessions with the children, the child's overall experience in school, with friends, in the family, and in outside activities, and major symptoms if any are explored. The clinician attempts to elicit the child's concerns about the parent's illness and his experience of the parent's recent illness. This is a form of family history construction through family sharing. Information about anniversary reactions to the parent's hospitalization is sensitively probed. It is important to ask what the children have actually seen and experienced, for example, suicide attempts, electroconvulsive therapy, and so forth.

Cognitive Teaching

In sessions with the parents alone, the clinician reviews what is known about the etiology of depression, its psychosocial manifestations, and the risks to children growing up in families with serious affective illness. The adaptive capacities of youngsters who function well in this and related risk situations are described.

The Child's Experience and Development of Plans for the Future

Sessions are conducted with both parents and specifically explore strategies that the family can use in discussing the parent's illness and planning for the future. The major areas covered include:

1. Need for clarity on the child's part as to what has happened to the parent and to the family
2. Provision to ensure that the child does not feel guilty or responsible
3. Encouragement of the child's understanding of the nature of the illness, and that the parent's unavailability and incapacity need not limit the child
4. Encouragement of explorations of networks of support for the child, particularly reestablishment of those that may have been disrupted by parental illness
5. Discussion of difficulties the child may face
6. Discussion of how to anticipate future development of illness in the child and seek prompt treatment
7. Discussion of how to continue the ongoing process of understanding in the family. At the end of these sessions, the parents define together what they hope to accomplish in the family sessions with the children.

Family Discussion

Two family sessions are held to present the above-listed material to the child. Special attention is given to explain that the child is not to blame. During these sessions, there is discussion of aspects of the depression that may have been confusing or frightening to the child. For example, a child may ask how someone becomes depressed and if he or she will also become depressed. A depressed mother may explain that when she was acting irritated, she was not angry at her family. She could not do anything about her irritability because it was part of her illness. Plans for the future are discussed in terms of continued exploration of the best course to take in helping the family adjust to the illness.

If clear diagnosable disorders are identified in the children or spouse, appropriate referral is made with the continued backup and support of the referring clinician. The family meets with the clinician at 6 and 12 months to review both the intervention and progress since then.

PREVENTION AND APPLICABILITY

As part of the preventive focus of the Psychoeducational Family Intervention Model, there is a strong emphasis on educating families about affective disorders and making them more aware of the signs of depression. Family misunderstanding about affective disorder undoubtedly contributes to the lack of recognition by the parents of distress in the children. The long-term goal of this model is the prevention of psychiatric disorder in the children. Prevention must include educating the family about the course of the illness, supporting their efforts to cope with the multiple stresses caused by the illness, and encouraging them to address their fears and concerns about the transmission of depression in the family. Beardslee and colleagues (in press) conducted a study comparing two preventive interventions with twenty families in which a parent experienced depression. The hypothesis was that a "clinician-based intervention would be more effective than lectures in changing behavior and attitudes towards affective illness, towards children and towards the future in families with severe affective disorder" (p. 3).

Efforts toward prevention in adults include cognitive behavioral approaches (Lewinsohn 1987, Munoz 1987, Vega et al. 1987). Cognitive approaches include those by Beck and colleagues (1979) and Rush and Giles (1982). Goldstein and colleagues, (1990) have developed approaches for depressed mothers and their infants. Workshops and family therapy have also been used effectively with hospitalized patients (Anderson et al. 1986, Clarkin et al. 1990). No program concentrated on primary prevention for children ages 8–14 with mood-disordered parents using a clinician-implemented family approach that focused on the family's illness experience.

The lecture intervention approach was chosen as a comparison because it was the most widely used form of intervention offered to parents and because lectures provided cognitive information about individual risks to and potential resiliency of children. The approach, however, omitted the vital feature of the clinician-based intervention, the consideration of the family's perspective-taking in enhancing competence in the children and increasing understanding of the illness.

Beardslee's (1990) study focuses on attitude change, behavioral change, and communication affected by the interventions. The two attitude changes of increased knowledge about depression and increased knowledge of both risk and resiliency in children were rated. The clinician-based group reported significantly more attitude changes. The category "increased understanding of factual information or of parent's illness experienced by the children" was highly significant. Eighty-three percent of the clinician-based subjects reported this change in contrast to none of the lecture-based subjects. Other changes included:

1. Better understanding of their spouse's experience or feelings,
2. Increased mutual understanding in the marital relationship and with their children,
3. Increased understanding of their child's experience of the illness,
4. Increased emotional closeness in the marriage.

Proactive behavior changes in response to the intervention included:

1. The adoption of new strategies for coping with depression,
2. Taking action when problems were identified in the children,
3. Becoming informed about depression and related issues by reading/seeking out information.

In communication among family members, there was:

1. Increased talking with the children and spouse and among the family as a whole,
2. Increased openness about the illness outside the immediate family as well as during the therapy sessions.

Because the sample size was small and follow-up interval too short, the authors indicated that their study could not establish the primary prevention effects of the intervention in terms of decreased incidence of affective disorder in children of parents with the disorder. Continued follow-up that extends the interval and allows preliminary assessment of preventive effectiveness is needed.

The comparison study, however, indicates that more changes in attitude and proactive behavior, increased familial communication, and, in general, integration of the cognitive material were reported with the clinician-based intervention approach. Although both approaches reported some changes in the severely disturbed individuals, it appears that some families may need the added component of clinician-based intervention, not simply lecture-based information.

CONCLUSION

In view of the challenge to provide a *primary prevention* model, which interferes with the future transmission of the disorder, an integrative perspective is needed. The Psychoeducational Family Intervention Model is an attempt to integrate the biological, social, and family objectives in order to address the multiple needs of families faced with affective illness. This clinician-based intervention addresses *secondary prevention* because it aims to identify early signs of depressive illness and initiate treatment before negative signs are clearly manifested. *Tertiary prevention* is also addressed because it aims to ensure that children who are diagnosed receive treatment.

The Psychoeducational Family Intervention Model is one approach to intervention in the lives of families dealing with an affective disorder. The model takes actual strength and personal resilience and nurtures it in an effort to make the family more capable of handling its own problems. As such, this approach places the family in better control of the illness, which in itself is overpowering and debilitating to all who are involved.

REFERENCES

Abramson, L., Seligman, M., and Teasdale, J. (1978). Learned helplessness in humans. Critique and reformulation. *Journal of Abnormal Psychology* 87:49–74.

Anderson, C., Griffin, S., Rossi, A., et al. (1986). A comparative study of the impact of education vs. process groups for families of patients with affective disorders. *Family Process* 25:185–206.

Anthony, E. J. (1976). How children cope in families with a psychotic parent. In *Infant Psychiatry: A New Synth*, ed. E. Rexford and T. Shapiro. New Haven, CT: Yale University Press.

Anthony, E. J., and Cohler, B. J. (1987). *The Invulnerable Child*. New York.

Beardslee, W. R. (1981). Self-understanding and coping with cancer. In *The Damocles Syndrome: Psychosocial Consequences of Surviving Childhood Cancer*, ed. G. Koocher and J. O'Malley, pp. 144–163. New York: McGraw Hill.

_____ (1983). *The Way Out Must Lead In: Life Histories in the Civil Rights Movement*. 2nd ed. Westport, CT: Lawrence Hill.

_____ (1986). The need for the study of adaptation in children of parents with affective disorders. In *Depression in Young People*, ed. M. Rutter, C. E. Izard, and P. B. Read, pp. 189–204. New York: Guilford.

_____ (1990). Development of a clinician-based preventive intervention for families with affective disorders. *Journal of Preventive Psychiatry and Allied Disciplines* 4:39–61.

Beardslee, W. R., Bemporad, J., Keller, M. B. et al. (1983). Children of parents with major affective disorder: a review. *American Journal of Psychiatry* 140:825–832.

Beardslee, W. R., Keller, M. B., and Klerman, G. L. (1985). Children of parents with affective disorder. *International Journal of Family Psychiatry* 6:283–299.

Beardslee, W. R., Keller, M. B., Lavori, P. W., et al. (1988b). Psychiatric disorder in adolescent offspring of parents with affective disorder in a non-referred sample. *Journal of Affective Disorders* 15:313–322.

Beardslee, W. R., and Podorefsky, D. (1988a). Resilient adolescents whose parents have serious affective and other psychiatric disorders: importance of self-understanding and relationships. *American Journal of Psychiatry* 145:63–69.

Beardslee, W., Salt, P., Porterfield, K., et al. (in press). Comparison of preventive interventions for families with parental affective disorder. *Journal of the American Academy of Child and Adolescent Psychiatry*.

Beardslee, W. R., Schultz, L. H., and Selman, R. L., (1987). Level of social-cognitive development, adaptive functioning, and *DSM-III* diagnosis in adolescent offspring of parents with affective disorders: implication of the development capacity for mutuality. *Developmental Psychology* 23:807–815.

Beck, A. T., (1963). Thinking and depression: I. Idiosyncratic content and cognitive distortions. *Archives of General Psychiatry* 9:324–333.

_____ *Depression: Clinical, Experimental and Theoretical Aspects*. (1967). New York: Harper & Row.

Beck, A., Rush, A., Shaw, B., and Emery, G. (1979). *Cognitive Therapy of Depression*. New York: Guilford.

Broughton, J. (1978). Development of concepts of self, mind, reality, and knowledge. *New Directions for Child Development* 1:75–100.

Clarkin, J. F., Glick, I. D., Haas, G. L., and Spencer, J. H. (1990). Inpatient family intervention for affective disorder. In *Depression and Families: Impact and Treatment*, ed. G. I. Keitner, pp. 121-136. Washington, DC: American Psychiatric Press.

Cytryn, L., McKnew, D. H., Bartho, J., et al. (1982). Offspring of patients with affective disorders II. *American Academy of Child Psychiatry* 21:389-391.

Damon, W., and Hart, D. (1982). The development of self-understanding from infancy through adolescence. *Child Development* 53:831-857.

Decina, P., Kestenbaum, C. J., Farber, S., et al. (1983). Clinical and psychological assessment of children of bipolar probands. *American Journal of Psychiatry* 140:548-553.

Downey, G., and Coyne, J. C. (1990). Children of depressed parents: an integrative review. *Psychological Bulletin* 108:50-76.

Erikson, E. H. (1963). *Childhood and Society*. 2nd ed. New York: W. W. Norton.

Felsman, J., and Vaillant, G. (1987). Resilient children as adults: a 40-year study. In *The Invulnerable Child*, ed. J. Anthony and B. Cohler. New York: Guilford.

Garmezy, N. (1971). Vulnerability research and the issue of primary prevention. A *Journal of Orthopsychiatry* 41:101-116.

_____ (1974). *The Study of Competence in Children at Risk for Severe Psychopathology*. Vol 2. Minneapolis, MN: University of Minnesota.

_____ (1983). Stressors of childhood. In *Stress Coping and Development in Children*, ed. N. Garmezy and M. Rutter, pp. 43-84. New York: McGraw-Hill.

Gershon, E. S., McKnew, D., Cytryn, L., et al. (1985). Diagnoses in school-age children of bipolar affective disorder patients and normal controls. *Journal of Affective Disorders* 8:283-291.

Goldstein, E. S., Yager, J., Heinicke, C., and Pynoos, R. S. (1990). *Preventing Mental Health Disturbances in Childhood*. Washington, DC: American Psychiatric Press.

Grunebaum, H. (1984). Parenting and children at risk. In *Psychiatry Update*, vol. 3, ed. L. Grinspoon. Washington, DC: American Psychiatric Press.

Hammen, C., Burge, D., and Stansbury, K. (1990). Relationship of mother and child variables to child outcomes in a high risk sample: a causal modeling analysis. *Developmental Psychology* 26:24-30.

Hartmann, H. (1950). Psychoanalysis and developmental psychology. *The Psychoanalytic Study of the Child*. 1:7-17. New York: International Universities Press.

_____ (1955). Notes on a theory of sublimation. *Psychoanalytic Study of the Child* 10:9-29. New York: International Universities Press.

_____ (1958). *Ego Psychology and the Problem of Adaptation*. NY: International Universities Press.

Institute of Medicine (1989). *Research on Children and Adolescents with Mental, Behavioral, and Developmental Disorders*. Washington, DC: National Academy Press.

Keitner, G. (1990). *Depression and Families: Impact and Treatment*. Washington, DC: American Psychological Association.

Keller, M. B., Beardslee, W. R., Dorer, D.J., et al. (1986). Impact of severity and chronicity of parental affective illness on adaptive functioning and psychopathology in their children. *Archives of General Psychiatry* 43:930–937.

Keller, M.B., Beardslee, W.R., Lavori, P.W., et al. (1988). Course of major depression in nonreferred adolescents: a retrospective study. *Journal of Affective Disorders* 15:235–243.

Keller, M. B., Lavori, P. W., Endicott, J., et al. (1983). Double depression: a two-year follow-up. *American Journal of Psychiatry* 6:689–694.

Lee, C. M., and Gotlib, I. H. (1989). Clinical status and emotional adjustment of children of depressed mothers. *American Journal of Psychiatry* 146:478–483.

Lewinsohn, P. (1987). The coping-with-depression course. In *Depression Prevention: Research Directions*, ed. R. F. Munoz, pp. 159–170. Washington, DC: Hemisphere.

Maccoby, E. (1987). Social-emotional development and response to stressors. In *Stress, Coping and Development in Children* ed. N. Garmezy and M. Rutter, pp. 217–234. New York: McGraw-Hill.

Merikangas, K. R., Prusoff, B. A., and Weisman, M. M. (1988). Parental concordance for affective disorders: psychopathology in offspring. *Journal of Affective Disorders* 15:279–290.

Munoz, R. (1987). Depression prevention research. Conceptual and practical considerations. In *Depression Prevention: Research Directions*, ed. R. F. Munoz, pp. 3–29. New York: Hemisphere.

Orvaschel, H., Walsh-Allis, G., and Ye, W. (1988). Psychopathology in children of parents with recurrent depression. *Journal Abnormal of Child Psychology* 16:17–28.

Philips, I. (1983). Opportunities for prevention in the practice of psychiatry. *American Journal of Psychiatry* 140:389–395.

Radke-Yarrow, M., and Zahn-Waxler, C. (1984). Roots, motives and patterning in children's presocial behavior. In *The Development and Maintenance of Prosocial Behavior*, ed. E. Staub, D. Bar-Tal, J. Karylowski and J. Reykowski, pp.155-176. New York: Plenum.

Rush, A. and Gyles, D. (1982). Diagnosing depression. In *Short-Term Psychotherapies for Depression*, ed. A. J. Rush. New York: Guilford.

Rutter, M. (1979). Protective factors in children's response to stress and disadvantage. In *Primary Prevention of Psychopathology. Vol 3: Social Competence in Children*, ed. R. Rolf and M. D. Kent. Hanover: NH: University Press of New England.

―――― (1981). Stress, coping and development: some issues and some questions. *Journal of Child Psychology and Psychiatry* 22:323–356.

―――― (1986). Meyerian psychobiology, personality, development, and the role of life experiences. *American Journal of Psychiatry* 143:1077–1087.

―――― (1990). Commentary: some focus and process considerations regarding effects of parental depression on children. *Developmental Psychology* 26:60–67.

Rutter, M., Yule, B., and Quinton, D. (1974). Attainment and adjustment in two geographical areas III: some factors accounting for area differences. *British Journal of Psychiatry* 125:520–533.

Seligman, M., Abramson, L., Semmel, A., and Baeyer, C. (1979). Depressive attributional style. *Journal of Abnormal Psychology* 88:242–247.

Seligman, M. (1975). *Helplessness: On Depression, Development, and Death*. San Francisco: Freeman.

Seligman, M., and Maier, S. (1967). Failure to escape traumatic shock. *Journal of Experimental Psychology* 74:1–9.

Selman, R. L. (1980). *The Growth of Interpersonal Understanding*. New York: Academic.

Shaffer, D., Garland A., and Gould, M. (1990). Preventing teenage suicide: a cultural review. In *Annual Progress in Child Psychiatry and Development*, ed. S. Chess and M. Hertzig. New York: Brunner/Mazel.

Sullivan, H. S. (1953). *The Interpersonal Theory of Psychiatry*. New York: W. W. Norton.

Vega, W. A., Valle, R., Kolody, B., and Hough, R. (1987). The Hispanic social network prevention intervention study: a community-based randomized trial. In *Depression Prevention: Research Directors*, ed. R. F. Munoz, pp. 217–221. New York: Hemisphere.

Waters, B. G. (1987). Psychiatric disorders in the offspring of parents with affective disorder: a review. *Journal of Preventive Psychiatry* 3:191–206.

Weissman, M. M., Leckman, J. F., Merikangas K. R., et al. (1984a). Depression and anxiety disorders in parents and children. *Archives of General Psychiatry* 41:845–852.

Weissman, M. M., Prusoff, B. A., Gammon, G. D., et al. (1984b). Psychopathology in the children (ages 6–18) of depressed and normal parents. *Journal of the American Academy of Child Psychiatry* 23:78–84.

Welner, Z., and Garrison, W. T. (1985). Blind high-risk study of depressives' offspring: preliminary data. *International Journal of Family Psychiatry* 6:301–314.

Youniss, J. (1980). *Parents and Peers in Social Development: A Sullivan-Piaget perspective.* Chicago: University of Chicago Press.

Zahn-Waxler, C., and Radke-Yarrow, M. (1982). The development of altruism: alternative research strategies. In *The Development of Prosocial Behavior*, ed. N. Eisenberg-Berg, pp. 109–137. New York: Academic.

Zahn-Waxler, C., Radke-Yarrow, M., and King, R. (1979). Child rearing and children's prosocial initiations toward victims of distress. *Child Development* 50:319–330.

Zahn-Waxler, C., Kochanska, G., Krupnick, J., and McKnew, D. (1990) Patterns of guilt in children of depressed and well mothers. *Developmental Psychology* 26(1):51–59.

14: FUTURE DIRECTIONS

G. Pirooz Sholevar, M.D.

The combined role of biological, interpersonal, and psychological factors in the genesis of depressive disorders is increasingly recognized. It is also clear that individuals vulnerable to depression due to any of the above factors are prone to multiple episodes of clinical depression during their lifetime. The transmission of depression from parents to children in the absence of protective mechanisms is another recognized fact.

The future investigations of depression should address a number of factors. The interrelatedness of depression with other symptomatic behaviors, particularly aggression and anxiety, is one promising area and may resemble a return to the concepts of depressive equivalent syndromes or masked depression. The inquiry into such interrelated behaviors can build on the investigations of Patterson and his colleagues in the interrelationship between intrafamilial aggression and depression. Family systems theory is helpful in recognizing that such constellations of behavior may be present in different family members rather than in one individual concomitantly or in a cyclical form. The investigation of the psychological, interpersonal, and behavioral correlates of genetic and biochemical vulnerability to depression may also prove productive. The mutual selection of depression-prone people through assortative mating plays a significant role in the perpetuation of a depressive interpersonal system. Spouses vulnerable to depression do not succeed to form an intimate marital relationship and become clinically depressed under stressful situations, particularly due to the lack of protective intimacy.

The combined use of antidepressants and interpersonal and individual psychotherapies has already proved to be the most effective method to comprehensive treatment of depression. The existing therapeutic guidelines have delineated the interpersonal difficulties most responsive to interpersonal psychotherapies and the symptom clusters treated most effectively by antidepressant medication. Further progress in this area can result in the recognition of multiple interacting biological and psychological mechanisms and feedback loops that maintain depression. A sensitive realignment of pharmacological, interpersonal, psychodynamic, cognitive, and behavior therapies may then pave the way to the most efficient and effective way of alleviating depression and reducing the likelihood of relapse.

The early detection of depression in vulnerable younger children, particularly the offspring of depressed parents, may be the most sensible and efficient way of combating depressive disorders. The institution of protective measures in terms of supportive interpersonal figures and psychoeducational measures may result in a dramatic reduction in the rate of future depression. The effectiveness of interventions has to be measured against further studies of the natural course of depression in young children and continued throughout their life span.

Dysthymic patients, with the usual onset of their disorder in preadolescence, constitute a vulnerable group that is already exhibiting a variant form of depressive disorder. The therapeutic and preventive measures to reduce the depressive symptomatology and enhance the quality of life and productivity in this population require focused attention.

Recognizing the multiple faces of depression, the full impact of its resistance to interventions is one significant challenge of our time. This book exhibits multiple lines of productive investigation toward the recognition, treatment, and prevention of depression.

INDEX